IMPROVEMENT OF MYOCARDIAL PERFUSION

DEVELOPMENTS IN
CARDIOVASCULAR MEDICINE

Lancée CT, ed: Echocardiology, 1979. ISBN 90-247-2209-8.

Baan J, Arntzenius AC, Yellin EL, eds: Cardiac dynamics. 1980. ISBN 90-247-2212-8.

Thalen HJT, Meere CC, eds: Fundamentals of cardiac pacing. 1970. ISBN 90-247-2245-4.

Kulbertus HE, Wellens HJJ, eds: Sudden death. 1980. ISBN 90-247-2290-X.

Dreifus LS, Brest AN, eds: Clinical applications of cardiovascular drugs. 1980. ISBN 90-247-2295-0.

Spencer MP, Reid JM, eds: Cerebrovascular evaluation with Doppler ultrasound. 1981. ISBN 90-247-2348-1.

Zipes DP, Bailey JC, Elharrar V, eds: The slow inward current and cardiac arrhythmias. 1980. ISBN 90-247-2380-9.

Kesteloot H, Joossens JV, eds: Epidemiology of arterial blood pressure. 1980. ISBN 90-247-2386-8.

Wackers FJT, ed: Thallium-201 and technetium-99m-pyrophosphate myocardial imaging in the coronary care unit. 1980. ISBN 90-247-2396-5.

Maseri A, Marchesi C, Chierchia S, Trivella MG, eds: Coronary care units. 1981. ISBN 90-247-2456-2.

Morganroth J, Moore EN, Dreifus LS, Michelson EL, eds: The evaluation of new antiarrhythmic drugs. 1981. ISBN 90-247-2474-0.

Alboni P: Intraventricular conduction disturbances. 1981. ISBN 90-247-2484-X.

Rijsterborgh H, ed: Echocardiology. 1981. ISBN 90-247-2491-0.

Wagner GS, ed: Myocardial infarction: Measurement and intervention. 1982. ISBN 90-247-2513-5.

Meltzer RS, Roelandt J, eds: Contrast echocardiography. 1982. ISBN 90-247-2531-3.

Amery A, Fagard R, Lijnen R, Staessen J, eds: Hypertensive cardiovascular disease; pathophysiology and treatment. 1982. ISBN 90-247-2534-8.

Bouman LN, Jongsma HJ, eds: Cardiac rate and rhythm. 1982. ISBN 90-247-2626-3.

Morganroth J, Moore EN, eds: The evaluation of beta blocker and calcium antagonist drugs. 1982. ISBN 90-247-2642-5.

Rosenbaum MB, ed: Frontiers of cardiac electrophysiology. 1982. ISBN 90-247-2663-8.

Roelandt J, Hugenholtz PG, eds: Long-term ambulatory electrocardiography. 1982. ISBN 90-247-2664-8.

Adgey AAJ, ed: Acute phase of ischemic heart disease and myocardial infarction. 1982. ISBN 90-247-2675-1.

Hanrath P, Bleifeld W, Souquet, J. eds: Cardiovascular diagnosis by ultrasound. Transesophageal, computerized, contrast, Doppler echocardiography. 1982. ISBN 90-247-2692-1.

Roelandt J, ed: The practice of M-mode and two-dimensional echocardiography. 1983. ISBN 90-247-2745-6.

Meyer J, Schweizer P, Erbel R, eds: Advances in noninvasive cardiology. 1983. ISBN 0-89838-576-8.

Morganroth J, Moore EN, eds: Sudden cardiac death and congestive heart failure: Diagnosis and treatment. 1983. ISBN 0-89838-580-6.

Perry HM, ed: Lifelong management of hypertension. 1983. ISBN 0-89838-582-2.

Jaffe EA, ed: Biology of endothelial cells. 1984. ISBN 0-89838-587-3.

Surawicz B, Reddy CP, Prystowsky EN, eds: Tachycardias. ISBN 0-89838-588-1.

Spencer MP, ed: Cardiac Doppler diagnosis. 1983. ISBN 0-89838-591-1.

Villarreal H, Sambhi MP, eds: Topics in pathophysiology of hypertension. 1984. ISBN 0-89838-595-4.

Messerli FH, ed: Cardiovascular disease in the elderly. 1984. ISBN 0-89838-596-2.

Simoons ML, Reiber JHC, eds: Nuclear imaging in clinical cardiology. 1984. ISBN 0-89838-599-7.

Ter Keurs HEDJ, Schipperheyn JJ, eds: Cardiac left ventricular hypertrophy. 1983. ISBN 0-89838-612-8.

Sperelakis N, ed: Physiology and pathophysiology of the heart. ISBN 0-89838-615-2.

Messerli FH, ed: Kidney in essential hypertension. ISBN 0-89838-616-0.

Sambhi MP, ed: Fundamental fault in hypertension. ISBN 0-89838-638-1.

Marchesi C, ed: Ambulatory monitoring: Cardiovascular system and allied applications. ISBN 0-89838-642-X.

Kupper W, MacAlpin RN, Bleifeld W, eds: Coronary tone in ischemic heart disease. ISBN 0-89838-646-2.

Sperelakis N, Caulfield JB, eds: Calcium antagonists: Mechanisms of action on cardiac muscle and vascular smooth muscle. ISBN 0-89838-655-1.

Godfraind T, Herman AS, Wellens D, eds: Calcium entry blockers in cardiovascular and cerebral dysfunctions. ISBN 0-89838-658-6.

Morganroth J, Moore EN, eds: Interventions in the acute phase of myocardial infarction. ISBN 0-89838-659-4.

Abel FL, Newman WH, eds: Functional aspects of the normal, hypertrophied, and failing heart. ISBN 0-89838-665-9.

Sideman S, Beyar R, eds: Simulation and imaging of the cardiac system. ISBN 0-89838-687-X.

Van der Wall E, Lie KI, eds: Recent views on hypertrophic cardiomyopathy. ISBN 0-89838-694-2.

Mathes E, ed: Secondary prevention in coronary artery disease and myocardial infarction. 1985. ISBN 0-89838-736-1.

Meyer J, Erbel R, Rupprecht HJ, eds: Improvement of myocardial perfusion. ISBN 0-89838-748-5.

IMPROVEMENT OF MYOCARDIAL PERFUSION

Thrombolysis, angioplasty, bypass surgery

edited by

JÜRGEN MEYER MD, RAIMUND ERBEL MD,
HANS JÜRGEN RUPPRECHT MD

Department of Internal Medicine II
Johannes Gutenberg University
Mainz, Federal Republic of Germany

1985 SPRINGER-SCIENCE+BUSINESS MEDIA, B.V.

Library of Congress Cataloging in Publication Data

Main entry under title:

Improvement of myocardial perfusion.

(Developments in cardiovascular medicine)
Includes index.
1. Coronary heart disease--Treatment. 2. Heart--
Infarction--Treatment. 3. Fibrinolysis. 4. Transluminal
angioplasty. 5. Aortocoronary bypass. I. Meyer,
Jürgen. II. Erbel, Raimund. III. Rupprecht, Hans
Jürgen. IV. Series. [DNLM: 1. Heart--pathophysiology.
2. Myocardium. 3. Perfusion. W1 DE997VME / WG 280 I34]
RC685.C6I45 1985   617'.412   85-13834

ISBN 978-94-010-8729-2   ISBN 978-94-009-5032-0 (eBook)
DOI 10.1007/978-94-009-5032-0

Copyright

Preface

This book contains the manuscripts of the majority of the papers given during the symposium 'Improvement of Myocardial Perfusion' which was held from September 27–29, 1984 in Mainz/Germany. It has been the purpose of this meeting to focus the interest of scientifically and clinically interested cardiologists on the new developments in this field. We therefore chose the subtitle 'Medical - Mechanical - Surgical Approach'.

The medical improvements in myocardial perfusion have been brought about by the application of streptokinase, urokinase and tissue-type plasminogen activator in the first hours after the onset of an acute myocardial infarction. The different modes of application and the possibilities to evaluate and eventually to quantify the results of these treatments were addressed during the first part of the meeting.

The mechanical way to improve perfusion nowadays mainly consists of the application of intracoronary balloon angioplasty. Although since 1977 the treatment has become a routine method, several questions are still open such as the exact mode of action, the reaction of the vessel wall, the optimal pressure and balloon size as well as the long term results and the prevention of restenosis.

The third mode of action is bypass-surgery. The operative technique has meanwhile gained a high and reliable level. Because of this, the borderlines to very old patients, to those with severely reduced myocardial function, to multivessel disease and to interventions in the acute phase of a myocardial infarction have been put forward more and more. New technical developments like endarteriectomy and laser technique are under way or even in clinical use.

This book does not give a definite answer to the question how myocardial perfusion in the acute and chronic ischemic status can be improved. It rather gives an overview of the state of the art at this moment. It shows what has been reached, what is still unclear, and what the unsolved problems are.

Jürgen Meyer, M.D.

Table of contents

X

List of contributors

Arnim, Th. von
  Medical Department I, University of Munich, Grosshadern Clinic, Marchioni-
  strasse 15, 8000 Munich, F.R.G.
  co-authors: B. Kemkes, B. Höfling

Bahawar, H.
  Kerckhoff-Clinic, Max-Planck-Gesellschaft, 6350 Bad Nauheim, F.R.G.
  co-authors: J. Lang, M. Kindler, G. Staemmler, M. Schlepper

Berclaz, S.
  Cardiology Center, University Hospital, 1211 Geneva 4, Switzerland

Block, P.C.
  Cardiac Catheterization Laboratory, Massachusetts General Hospital, Boston
  MA 02114, U.S.A.

Brückner, U.B.
  Department of Experimental Surgery, Surgical Center, University of Heidelberg, Im Neuenheimer Feld 347, 6900 Heidelberg 1, F.R.G.
  co-authors: U. Mittmann, W.W. Saggau

Busch, U.W.
  Medical Clinic I, Clinic 'Rechts der Isar', Ismaniger Strasse 22, 8000 Munich,
  F.R.G.
  co-authors: R. Erbel, U. Pfeiffer, J. Meyer, G. Blümel, H. Blömer, R.
  Heinze, H. Sebening, U. Kusawe

Castaneda-Zuniga, W.
  Department of Radiology, Mayo Medical Building, University of Minnesota,
  Box 292, 420 Delaware Street S.E., Minneapolis MN 55455, U.S.A.

Collen, D.

Department of Medical Research, Center for Thrombosis and Vascular Research, University of Leuven, 3000 Leuven, Belgium

Cosgrove, D.M.

Department of Thoracic and Cardiovascular Surgery, The Cleveland Clinic Foundation, 9500 Euclid Avenue, Cleveland OH 44106, U.S.A.
co-author: F.D. Loop

Dörr, R.

Department of Internal Medicine I, RWTH Aachen, Pauwelstrasse 1, 5100 Aachen, F.R.G.
co-authors: R. von Essen, S. Effert, F. Ahnert, T. Tolxdorff

Düber, C.

Institute of Pathology and Anatomy, Johannes Gutenberg University, Langenbeckstrasse 1, 6500 Mainz, F.R.G.
co-authors: H.-J. Rumpelt, R. Erbel

Elayda, M.A.

Division of Cardiology, Texas Heart Institute of St. Luke's Episcopal, P.O. Box 20345, Houston TX 77225, U.S.A.
co-authors: R.J. Hall, V.S. Mathur, G.L. Hallman, A.G. Gray, D.A. Cooley

El Gamal, M.I.

Department of Cardiology, Catharina Hospital, Michelangelolaan 2, 5623 EJ Eindhoven, The Netherlands
co-authors: H.R. Bonnier, H.R. Michels, J.M. Heyman, E.G. Stassen

Erbel, R.

Medical Clinic II, Johannes Gutenberg University, Langenbeckstrasse 1, 6500 Mainz, F.R.G.
co-authors: T. Pop, B. Henkel, G. Schreiner, C. Steuernagel, F. Beck, L. Henrichs, J. Meyer

Essen, R. von

Department of Internal Medicine I, RWTH Aachen, Pauwelstrasse 1, 5100 Aachen, F.R.G.
co-authors: W. Schmidt, R. Uebis, B. Edelmann, S. Effert, J. Silny, G. Rau

Frilling, A.

Department of Surgery B, University of Düsseldorf, Moorenstrasse 5, 4000 Düsseldorf, F.R.G.
co-authors: W. Bircks, R. Körfer, K. Minami, H.D. Schulte

Fuchs, M.
Internal Medicine III, University of Cologne, Joseph-Stelzmannstrasse 9, 5000 Cologne 41, F.R.G.
co-authors: F.M. McDonald, H.W. Höpp, A. Heinen, J. Kreuzer, G. Arnold, L. Heymans, V. Hombach, Hj. Hirche, V. Hossmann, H.H. Hilger

Glogar, D.
Cardiology Clinic, University of Vienna, Garnisongasse 13, 1097 Vienna, Austria
co-authors: W. Mohl, H. Mayr, P. Schindler, F. Kaindl, E. Wolner

Gould, K.L.
Division of Cardiology, Positron Diagnostic and Research Center, University of Texas Health Science Center, P.O. Box 20708, Houston, TX 77025, U.S.A.
co-authors: R.W. Smalling, N. Mullani, R.A. Goldstein, F. Fuentes, G. Wong, M. Matthews

Hartzler, G.O.
St. Luke's Hospital, Mid-American Heart Institute, Kansas City MO, U.S.A.
co-authors: B.D. Rutherford, D.R. McConahay, W.L. Johnson

Henkel, B.
Medical Clinic II, Johannes Gutenberg University, Langenbeckstrasse 1, 6500 Mainz, F.R.G.
co-authors: R. Erbel, W. Clas, G. Schreiner, H. Kopp, T. Pop, J. Meyer

Henrichs, K.J.
Medical Clinic II, Johannes Gutenberg University, Langenbeckstrasse 1, 6500 Mainz, F.R.G.
co-authors: R. Erbel, C. Steuernagel, J. Meyer

Jones, E.L.
Emory University School of Medicine, 1364 Clifton Road N.E., Atlanta GA 30322, U.S.A.

Kober, G.
Department of Cardiology, Center of Internal Medicine, Johann Wolfgang Goethe University School of Medicine, Theodor-Stern-Kai 7, 6000 Frankfurt a.M. 70, F.R.G.
co-authors: C. Vallbracht, M. Kaltenbach

Krause, E.
Department of Thoracic and Cardiovascular Surgery, University Medical Center, Theodor-Stern-Kai 7, 6000 Frankfurt a.M. 70, F.R.G.
co-author: D. Scherer

Leimgruber, P.P.
Department of Medicine, Emory University School of Medicine, 1364 Clifton Road N.E., Atlanta GA 30322, U.S.A.
co-author: A.R. Grüntzig

Lew, A.S.
Division of Cardiology room 5314, Cedars-Sinai Medical Center, 8700 Beverly Boulevard, Los Angeles CA 90048, U.S.A.
co-author: W. Ganz

Livesay, J.J.
Division of Cardiovascular Surgery, Texas Heart Institute of St. Luke's Episcopal, P.O. Box 20345, Houston TX 77225, U.S.A.
co-authors: O.H. Frazier, D.A. Cooley

Marra, S.
Division of Cardiology, Maggiore Hospital, Via Cavour 31, I-10123 Torino, Italy
co-authors: V. Paolillo, P.F. Angelino, T. Varetto, G. Piccioto, P.G. Defilippi, B. Doronzo, R. Schmitt, M. Sabatier, V. Dor

McDonald, F.M.
Institute of Physiology, University of Cologne, Robert-Koch-Strasse 39, 5000 Köln 41, F.R.G.
co-authors: M. Fuchs, J. Kreuzer, A. Heinen, H.W. Höpp, Hj. Hirche, V. Hombach, V. Hossmann, H.H. Hilger

Meerbaum, S.
Cedars-Sinai Medical Center, Halper Building 325, 8700 Beverly Boulevard, Los Angeles CA 90048, U.S.A.

Messmer, B.J.
Department of Thoracic and Cardiovascular Surgery, RWTH Aachen, Pauwelstrasse 1, 5100 Aachen, F.R.G.
co-authors: R. von Essen, R. Dörr, W. Merx, J. Meyer, P. Bardos, C. Minale, S. Effert

Meyer, J.
Medical Clinic II, Johannes Gutenberg University, Langenbeckstrasse 1, 6500 Mainz, F.R.G.
co-authors: R. Erbel, H.J. Schmitz, T. Pop, K. von Olshausen, B. Henkel, H.J. Rupprecht, H. Kopp, S. Effert

Minale, C.
Department of Thoracic and Cardiovascular Surgery, RWTH Aachen, Pauwelstrasse 1, 5100 Aachen, F.R.G.
co-author: B.J. Messmer

Oelert, H.
Clinic for Thoracic and Cardiovascular Surgery, Hannover Medical School, Konstanty-Gutschow-Strasse 8, 3000 Hannover 61, F.R.G.
co-authors: A. Haverich, S. Iversen, J. Schulze, R. Hetzer

Poole-Wilson, P.A.
Cardiothoracic Institute, 2 Beaumount Street, London W1N 2DX, U.K.
co-author: S.C. Webb

Probst, P.
Cardiology Clinic, University of Vienna, Garnisongasse 13, 1097 Vienna, Austria
co-authors: W. Zangl, O. Pachinger

Rafflenbeul, W.
Department of Cardiology, Hannover Medical School, Karl-Wiechert-Allee 9, 3000 Hannover 61, F.R.G.

Rey, F.J. van
Department of Cardiology, Catharina Hospital, Michelangelolaan 2, 5623 EJ Eindhoven, The Netherlands
co-authors: H.J. Bonnier, H.R. Michels, M.I. El Gamal, H.J. Hoffmann

Rupprecht, H.J.
Medical Clinic II, Johannes Gutenberg University, Langenbeckstrasse 1, 6500 Mainz, F.R.G.
co-authors: R. Erbel, K.-H. Schöter, B. Schreiner, K.-L. Henrichs, J. Meyer

Samama, M.
Central Laboratory of Hematology, Hôtel-Dieu, 1 Place du Parvis Notre-Dame, 75181 Paris Cédex 04, France
co-author: E. Szwarcer

Sandring, K.-H.
Humboldt University, Hospital Charité, Schumannstrasse 20/21, 1040 Berlin, G.D.R.
co-authors: V. Gliech, W. Dänschel, C. Müller, K.H. Günther

Schanzenbächer, P.
Medical Clinic, Joseph-Schneider-Strasse 2, 8700 Würzburg, F.R.G.

Scheld, H.H.
Clinic for Cardiovascular Surgery, Justus Liebig Universität, Klinikstrasse 29, 6300 Giessen, F.R.G.
co-authors: M. Gottwik, G. Görlach, U. Bauer, J. Mulch, R. Höge, D. Kling, F.W. Hehrlein

Scherer, H.-E.
Medical and Cardiac Surgery Clinic Hospital Links der Weser, Senator-Wessling-Strasse 1, 2800 Bremen, F.R.G.
co-authors: H.-J. Engel, E. Hörmann, H. Oster, K. Leitz

Schmitz, H.J.
Department of Internal Medicine I, RWTH Aachen, Pauwelstrasse 1, 5100 Aachen, F.R.G.
co-authors: J. Meyer, R. von Essen, S. Effert

Schofer, J.
Department of Cardiology, University Hospital Eppendorf, Martinistrasse 52, 3000 Hamburg 20, F.R.G.
co-authors: R. Montz, D.G. Mathey, W. Bleifeld

Schröder, R.
Department of Cardiology, Steglitz Clinic, Free University Berlin, Hindenburgdamm 30, 1000 Berlin 45, F.R.G.

Serruys, P.W.
Catheterization Laboratory, Thorax Center, Erasmus University, P.O. Box 1738, 3000 DR Rotterdam, The Netherlands
co-authors: W. Wijns, M. van den Brand, C. Slager, J. Grimm, B.E. Jaski, R.W. Brower, O.M. Hess, P.G. Hugenholtz, V. Ulmans, G.P. Heyndrickx, P.J. de Feyter

Spiller, P.
Medical Clinic B, University of Düsseldorf, Moorenstrasse 5, 4000 Düsseldorf, F.R.G.
co-authors: E. Schwammentahl, J. Jehle, A. Lauber, B. Lösse, F. Loogen

Systemic streptolysis of acute myocardial infarction

ROLF SCHRÖDER

There was considerable scepticism and even criticism a few years ago, when I reported about successful early recanalization of an thrombotically occluded coronary artery by high-dose brief duration intravenous streptokinase infusion [1].

Nowadays, the effectiveness of intravenous streptokinase is generally accepted (Table 1). However, the angiographically proven recanalization success rate of about 60% with the intravenous approach is less than that reported for intracoronary streptokinase application [2, 3, 4, 5, 6]. Yet, the figure 'about 60%' is probably not correct because lysis of an intracoronary clot lasts somewhat longer with the intravenous approach as compared to intracoronary streptokinase. Naturally, during the acute phase of infarction, the angiographic observation time was limited, mostly to about 1 hour. Recanalizations occurring somewhat delayed were, therefore, not detected.

Table 2 shows data from four authors, who compared recanalization rates achieved by intracoronary streptokinase application with restoration of coronary blood flow by high-dose brief duration intravenous streptokinase infusion [7, 8, 9,

Table 1. Angiographically confirmed recanalization rates of completely occluded coronary arteries in patients with acute myocardial infarction treated with brief duration high-dose intravenous streptokinase within 6 hours after symptom onset. Comparison with intracoronary streptokinase application by three authors.

	IV STK recanalization no of pts	Time to recanal. minutes	IC STK recanalization no of pts	Time to recanal. minutes
Schröder et al. [2]	11/21 (52%)	44 ± 19	–	–
Neuhaus et al. [3]	24/38 (63%)	48	28/37 (76%)	28
Spann et al. [4]	21/43 (49%)	30 – 60	–	–
Blunda et al. [5]	7/10 (70%)	54 ± 28	10/12 (80%)	27 ± 14
Alderman et al. [6]	8/13 (62%)	39	11/15 (73%)	28
	71/125(57%)		49/64(77%)	

Table 2. Comparison of restoration of coronary blood flow in patients with evolving myocardial infarction treated with intravenous or intracoronary streptokinase. Abbreviation: IRA = infarct-related artery.

		Patent IRA	Symptom onset to STK (min.)	Angiography performed
Geft et al. [7]	IC–STK	65/78 (84%)	207 ± 61	2–7 days later
	IV–STK	55/57 (96%)	144 ± 57	
Taylor et al. [8]	IC–STK	48/63 (76%)	214 ± 83	1 h to 3 days
	IV–STK	53/63 (84%)	170 ± 79	later (59/63 ≤24 hrs)
Rogers et al. [9]	IC–STK	9/14 (64%)	IV 66 min	10 days post
	IV–STK	12/14 (86%)	earlier	MI
Anderson et al. [10]	IC–STK	13/18 (72%)	246 ± 90	predischarge
	IV–STK	15/20 (75%)	162 ± 66	

10]. In the intravenously treated groups no coronary angiography was performed before initiation of streptokinase infusion, but treatment was started as soon as possible. Although there was no direct angiographic confirmation of a recanalization, clinical signs of reperfusion and early elevation and peaking of serial serum CK–MB activity highly suggested an early restoration of coronary blood flow. Patency of the infarctrelated coronary artery was angiographically confirmed between 1 hour and 10 days later.

The first two studies used historical controls, the two studies at the bottom were performed in an at-random fashion.

Restoration of coronary blood flow tended to be higher with intracoronary streptokinase application. This may be explained by the fact that some of the intravenously treated patients may have had only incomplete or intermittent thrombotic obstructions.

Without need for prior catheterization, intravenous thrombolysis could be initiated 44–84 minutes earlier than intracoronary streptokinase application. It has been shown that the differences in clot lysis time between the intravenous and the intracoronary approach are small if treatment is initiated early (Table 1). Thus, the somewhat longer lasting clot lysis time with the intravenous approach probably can be more than balanced by the earlier begin of treatment and should lead to an earlier restoration of coronary blood flow in many patients. Since most groups who attempt early recanalization by intracoronary streptokinase infusion today begin as soon as possible with an intravenous pretreatment with streptokinase or urokinase, it also seems generally accepted that expeditious initiation of intravenous thrombolysis may potentially salvage more myocardium.

Do we have data which could support this hypothesis? In Table 3, data from

Table 3. Data from three authors from Table 2 with some measures of functional improvement following intravenous streptokinase infusion as compared to intracoronary application.

Functional improvement		
Geft: Peak CK–MB	IC 161 ± 122	
	IV 100 ± 168	$p<0.001$
Rogers: EF improved 7 days post MI	IC 3/13 (23%)	
	IV 8/13 (62%)	$p<0.05$
Anderson: Change EF day 1–10	IC + 1.4%	
	IV + 6.4%	$p<0.02$

Abbreviation: EF = radionuclide ejection fraction.

three authors from Table 2 are listed with some measures of functional improvement following intravenous streptokinase infusion as compared to intracoronary application.

Thrombolysis, either by the intracoronary or by the intravenous route has a potential of myocardial salvage during the first hours of myocardial infarction. However, an improvement in short- and long-term mortality has not yet been clearly demonstrated. Most studies of either intracoronary or intravenous streptokinase reported to date are non-randomized and use historical controls, and thus are likely to overestimate any true benefit on mortality and even morbidity.

Some smaller randomized controlled trials have shown promising but inconclusive results.

In May 1981, Muller et al. published an editorial on the problem related to coronary artery recanalization in the acute phase of myocardial infarction with the thought-provoking title 'Let's not let the genie escape from the bottle – again.' [11]. Inspite of this warning we are presently confronted with the dissemination of this new technique for treatment of ischemic heart disease before scientific proof of its beneficial effects has been unequivocally demonstrated by conclusive data from large controlled randomized trials. The concept of limiting infarct size by early restoration of coronary blood flow obviously is so fascinating – and in the individual patient clinically impressing improvement has been observed with early thrombolysis by everybody who used this mode of therapy – the widespread dissemination of this new technique does not surprise us. However, the optimal management course after successful thrombolytic therapy has not been defined.

Successful thrombolysis, even with satisfactory myocardial salvage, does not modify the underlying coronary artery disease. A high incidence up to more than 20% of reinfarctions and late reocclusions has been reported after successful intracoronary streptokinase treatment. Probably it was Meyer et al. who introduced the combined procedure of intracoronary streptokinase infusion and PTCA directly at the same time when recanalization had been achieved by thrombolysis [12]. However, an additional mechanical recanalization probably is not mandatory for all patients. Furthermore, the rate of early reocclusion after angioplasty might be as high as 20% [13]. Although angioplasty may improve the coronary artery patency after administration of intracoronary streptokinase, the long-term stability of this combined therapy is yet still unknown.

Quantitative angiographic analysis at the end of intracoronary streptokinase infusion has been applied by Serruys et al. [14]. Reocclusion in the short term and reinfaction in the long term was frequent only in patients with a residual mean diameter stenosis of 58% or more of the infarct-related coronary artery. Harrison et al. measured the percent area stenosis in 24 patients with successful intracoronary thrombolysis [15]. Reangiography was performed 2 weeks later. Seven of 14 patients with residual lesions causing a more than 90% area stenosis in the acute phase had rethrombosis, while none of the 10 patients with a less than 90% area stenosis had rethrombosis. A 90% area stenosis is about a 68% diameter stenosis. In both studies, patients had been on continuous intravenous heparin, followed by oral coumarin in the study of Serruys et al.

From these data it appears that reocclusion and recurrent myocardial infarction is frequent in patients with highergraded residual stenosis despite anticoagulants. The marginal line lying somewhere between a diameter stenosis of 58–68%. In patients with a lesser degree of post lysis stenosis, and this was the majority of patients in the study of Serruys et al., there was no reocclusion and thus, PTCA during the acute stage of myocardial infarction does not seem to be mandatory in these patients or may not even be justified.

The complexity of this issue is further compounded by the fact that the appearance of lesions immediately after streptokinase reperfusion may not reflect the eventual geometry of the lesions several days or weeks later. An improvement in the luminal diameter, after one or more weeks in comparison to immediate post intracoronary streptokinase, has been shown by Gandadharan et al. [16], Karsch et al. [17], and Serruys et al. [14]. Figure 1 shows changes in the area stenosis post successful lysis and two weeks later in 17 patients of Harrison et al. [15] and, in comparison, changes in area stenosis 24 hours after intravenous successful thrombolysis to reangiography in the 4th week after the acute event in 15 of our patients. Because probably most of the readers are more familiar with the diameter stenosis rather than the area stenosis, the changes in diameter stenosis in the same 15 patients are shown on the right side. The stenotic lesions are measured with a computer-added method, not eye-balled. Harrison found a significant decrease in the area stenosis from a mean value of about 85–76%, the bars represent standard error of the mean. We found a significant decrease from a mean value of 84% after 24 hours to 79% in the 4th week, the bars represent the standard deviation. Expressed as diameter stenosis, there was a decrease from 62% to 55%. In one patient, the diameter stenosis increased to more than 65% in

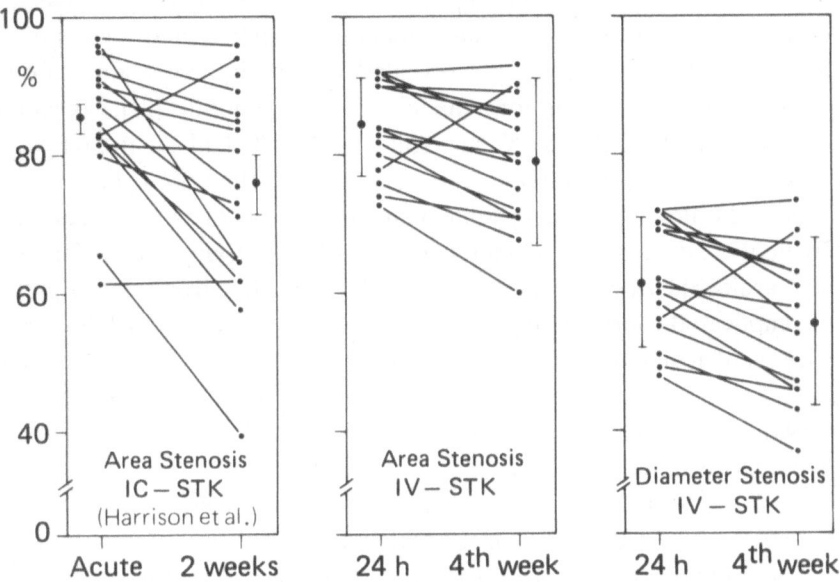

Figure 1. Changes in area stenosis immediately post successful intracoronary lysis and 2 weeks later in 17 patients of Harrison et al. [15] – left side – and changes of the area stenosis and the corresponding diameter stenosis – right side – 24 hours after successful intravenous thrombolysis to reangiography in the 4th week in 15 of our patients (mean value ± SD; Harrison: mean value ± SEM).

the 4th week, and in two it remained above 65%. In one of these three patients subsequent successful PTCA had been performed. In the two others, at re-angiography several months later the infarct-related artery was found occluded.

There are two conflicting attitudes about patients who have undergone success-ful thrombolytic reperfusion: 1) definitive treatment requires additional mechan-ical therapy, 2) proper anticoagulant therapy provided, patients are no different from other patients with myocardial infarction secondary to coronary artery disease. In patients with intracoronary streptokinase, the option exists for im-mediate PTCA. In patients with intravenous streptokinase, the anatomical con-ditions of the coronary artery before and after treatment are not known. Desi-cions, therefore, must be made on clinical grounds. It is of interest that the early re-occlusion and re-infarction rate after intravenous streptokinase treatment seems to be considerably lower than after intracoronary streptokinase [2, 3, 18]. Actually, it is in the same order as in patients after intracoronary streptokinase and additional PTCA [12, 13, 14, 19, 20]. If, after intravenous thrombolysis unstable angina remains, immediate coronary angiography should be performed with appropriate subsequent surgical or mechanical interventions. If patients suffer an early re-infarction, a second successful intravenous thrombolysis, per-haps with additional PTCA, can be performed. With this regimen, results proba-bly can be obtained that are comparable with those obtained with intracoronary streptokinase and perhaps additional PTCA.

6

Generally, in all patients angiography should be performed 1–3 weeks after intravenous streptolysis. Until February 1982, we have performed angiography in the 4th week [2]. Sixty-three patients revealed a patent infarct-related coronary artery. They were followed-up for a mean of 33.6 ± 10 months [21]. Six patients were followed-up until death, 57 are still alive. 59% had an infarct-related residual stenosis of less than 65%, and 41% of more than 65%. Patients with uncomplicated follow-up had a residual diameter stenosis of $57 \pm 13\%$; eleven of the 36 patients had a residual diameter stenosis of more than 65%. In 5 patients with late cardiac death the residual stenosis did not differ from that in patients with uncomplicated course. However, all 5 patients had multi-vessel disease and severe left ventricular impairment. Thus, cardiac death is related to poor left ventricular function rather than to the residual size of the infarct-related coronary artery lesion. In patients who suffered a re-infarction during follow-up, the diameter stenosis in 4 out of 5 was greater than 65%.

Figure 2 shows the changes in diameter stenosis from the 4th week to re-study, on the average 26 months later, in 18 patients who had no bypass surgery or PTCA. The broken lines represent patients with reinfarctions. All patients with a

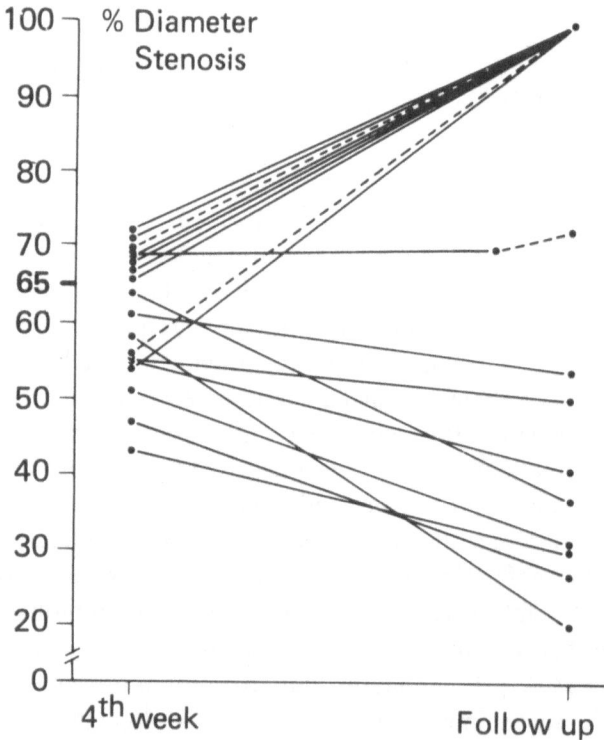

Figure 2. Changes in diameter stenosis from the 4th week to restudy 26 ± 9 months later in patients without bypass surgery or PTCA. The broken lines represent patients with late post intervention reinfarctions.

residual diameter stenosis greater than 65% had either reocclusion or reinfarction. Six exhibited a clinically silent reocclusion, and in one the artery was found occluded after reinfarction. The eighth patient had a high-graded stenosis of a diagonal branch in the 4th week. After an uneventful course of 27 months, he was restudied and the coronary artery lesion was almost the same. The patient was completely free of symptoms and had a negative exercise-ECG up to 200 Watts. Ten months later, that means 37 months after the first successfully treated infarction, he suffered a sudden re-ischemia which could be successfully treated with intravenous streptokinase. Because he remained unstable, angiography and successful PTCA were performed the next day.

Ten patients revealed a residual diameter stenosis of 64% or less in the 4th week after the acute event. In 8, the residual diameter stenosis decreased significantly from a mean value of 54 to 36%. In 2 patients the infarct-related coronary artery was occluded. In one of them after a reinfarction, which was not treated with thrombolysis. Both patients had multi-vessel disease and more than one stenosis of the infarct-related coronary artery. In both patients aortocoronary bypass surgery had been recommended previously, but both had refused. From these data it appears that reocclusion and recurrent myocardial infarction during long-term follow-up frequently occur in patients with a residual diameter stenosis of the infarctrelated coronary artery of 65% or more in the 4th week after successful intravenous thrombolysis. Therefore, if there is no firm indication for bypass surgery, it seems to be advisable to perform PTCA in these patients. On the other hand, in keeping with the findings of Serruys et al. with intracoronary streptokinase, there seems to be no need for an additional PTCA in patients with less severe residual stenosis in the 4th week after successful intravenous streptokinase. This suggestion is supported by the fact that in the 8 patients with residual diameter stenosis of less than 65%, which further decreased during follow-up, there was also a substantial and significant improvement in the left ventricular function. Figure 3 shows the changes in the infarctrelated dyssynergic area of the left ventricle.

However, late reocclusion of an infarct-related coronary artery does not necessarily imply worsening of the left ventricular function. On the contrary, some patients showed considerable improvement, probably because they had developed sufficient collateral flow. Figure 4 shows the changes in the regional wall motion disorders during follow-up of the 10 patients, who suffered a reocclusion or reinfarction. If should be kept in mind that 8 of these 10 patients had a residual diameter stenosis in the 4th week of more than 65%. Even afterwards we were not able to predict, in which particular patient the left ventricular function would improve during long-term follow-up, even if a subsequent occlusion of the infarct-related coronary artery would occur. Therefore it may be advisable to perform PTCA in all patients with a residual infarct-related coronary artery stenosis greater than 65%, if there is evidence that at-risk myocardium has been salvaged. Thallium-scintigraphy may help to identify patients with silent isch-

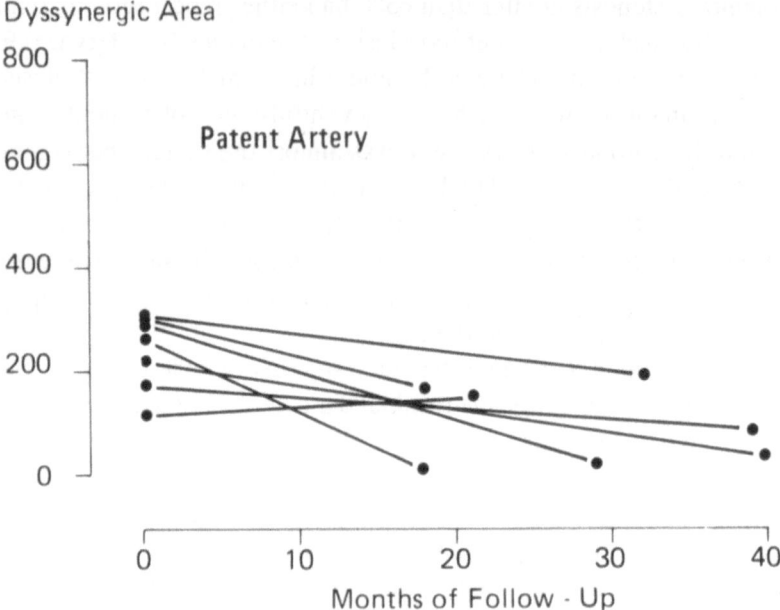

Figure 3. Changes in the infarct-related regional wall motion abnormalities (dyssynergic area, for method see ref. no. 2) during follow-up in patients with a diameter stenosis of less than 65% in the 4th week and remaining patency.

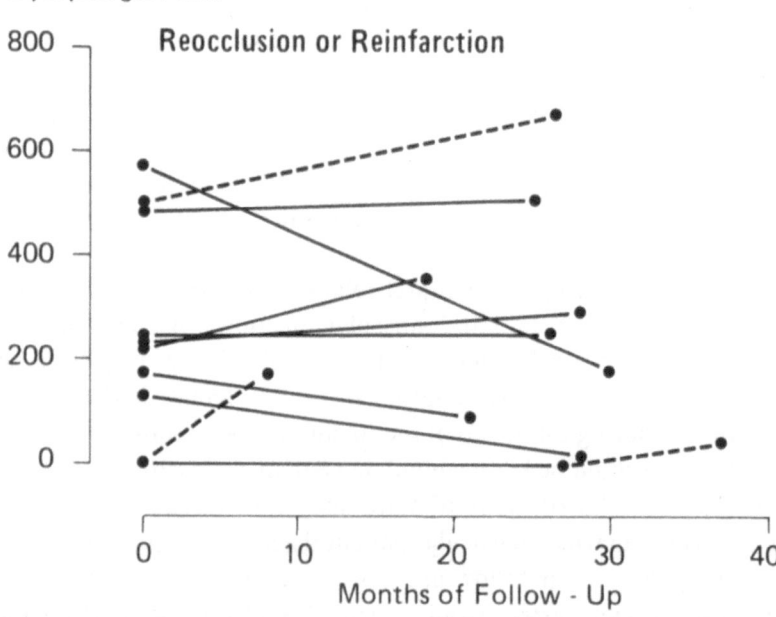

Figure 4. Changes in the infarct-related regional wall motion abnormalities during follow-up in patients with a late reinfaction (broken lines) or reocclusion. 8 out of 10 have had a diameter stenosis of more than 65% in the 4th week.

emia. Re-angiography should be performed in patients with recurrent angina with repeated PTCA in case of re-stenosis. PTCA may also be considered a preliminary step in patients intended for elective bypass surgery in order to minimize the risk of reinfarction before surgery.

It must be underlined, however, that these suggestions are based on limited clinical experience. Further results must be obtained and critically evaluated. It is necessary to assess efficacy and safety of additional PTCA or aortocoronary bypass surgery in controlled randomized trials of sufficient scope with longterm follow-up.

Summary

A brief review is given about the results obtained with high-dose brief duration intravenous streptokinase infusion in patients with evolving myocardial infarction. Actual successful lysis of a coronary clot probably occurs as frequently with the intravenous approach as with intracoronary streptokinase application. A longer clot lysis time often will be more than compensated by the earlier initiation of intravenous therapy. Expeditious initiation of intravenous thrombolysis may potentially salvage more myocardium.

From limited data in patients with angiographic long-term follow-up it appears that following successful intravenous restoration of coronary blood flow in patients with a residual diameter stenosis of less than 65% in the 4th week late reocclusions or reinfarctions are a rare event, while it is frequent in patients with a more severe residual stenosis. Although late reocclusion does not necessarily lead to a worsening of the left ventricular function, PTCA might be advisable in patients with higher-graded residual infarctrelated stenosis 1–3 weeks after infarction.

References

1. Schröder R, Biamino G, v. Leitner ER, Linderer T, Prokein E, Schäfer J–H, Sörensen R, Grassot A (1981) Comparison of the effects of intracoronary and systemic streptokinase infusion in acute myocardial infarction: Preliminary results. In: Myocardial revascularization, medical and surgical advances in coronary disease. Eds. Mason DT, Collins JJ. Publisher: Yorke Medical Books, U.S.A. pp. 464–479
2. Schröder R, Biamino G, v. Leitner ER, Linderer T, Brüggemann T, Heitz J, Vöhringer HF, Wegscheider K (1983) Intravenous short-term infusion of streptokinase in acute myocardial infarction. Circulation 67: 536–548
3. Neuhaus KL, Kreuzer H, Sauer G, Thiemann U, Köstering H (1983) Intravenöse Streptokinase-Kurzinfusion beim akuten Myokardinfarkt. Hämostaseologie 2: 38–43
4. Spann JF, Sherry S, Carabello BA, Denenberg BS, Mann RH, McCann WD, Gault JH, Gentzler RD, Belber AD, Maurer AH, Cooper EM. (1984) Coronary thrombolysis by intravenous streptokinase in acute myocardial infarction: Acute and follow-up studies. Am J Cardiol 53: 655–661

5. Blunda M, Wolf NM, Singh S, Mandelkorn J, Kersh R, Pickering N, Shechter J, Rodgers D, Workman M, Meister SG (1982) Intravenous vs intracoronary streptokinase to reopen occluded coronary arteries: Preliminary results. Circulation 66: 11–184

6. Alderman EL, Jutzy KR, Berte LE, Miller RG, Friedman JP, Creger WP, Eliastam M (1984) Randomized comparison of intravenous versus intracoronary streptokinase for myocardial infarction. Am J Cardiol 54: 14–19

7. Geft I, Rodriguez PK, Shah Y, Charuzi Y, Sasaki H, Weiss A, Maddahi J, Berman DS, Swan HJC, Ganz W (1983) Comparison of intravenous and intracoronary streptokinase in evolving myocardial infarction. Circulation 68: III–326

8. Taylor GJ, Mikell FL, Moses HW, Dove JI, Batchelder JE, Thull A, Schneider JA, Wellons HA (1983) Intravenous and intracoronary streptokinase for MI. Circulation 68: III–314

9. Rodgers WJ, Hood WP, Reeves RC, Whitlow PL (1984) Randomized trial of intracoronary versus intravenous streptokinase in acute myocardial infarction. JACC 3(2): 525

10. Anderson JL, Marshall HW, Lutz JR, Sorensen SG, Askins JC, Hagan AD (1984) A randomized trial of intracoronary versus intravenous streptokinase in myocardial infarction. JACC 3(2): 526

11. Muller JE, Stone PH, Markis JE, Braunwald E (1981) 'Let's not let the genie escape from the bottle – again.' N Engl J Med 304: 1294–1296

12. Meyer J, Merx W, Schmitz H, Erbel R, Kiesslich T, Dörr R, Lambertz H, Bethge C, Krebs W, Bardos P, Minale C, Messmer BJ, Effert S (1982) Percutaneous transluminal coronary angioplasty immediately after intracoronary streptolysis of transmural myocardial infarction. Circulation 66: 905–913

13. Papapietro SE, McLean WAH, Stanley AWN Jr. (1983) Percutaneous transluminal coronary angioplasty in acute myocardial infarction. J Am Coll Cardiol 1: 580

14. Serruys PW, Wijns W, van den Brand M, Ribeiro V, Fioretti P, Simoons ML, Kooijman CJ, Reiber JHC, Hugenholtz PG (1983) Is transluminal coronary angioplasty mandatory after successful thrombolysis? Br Heart J 50: 257–265

15. Harrison DG, Ferguson DW, Collins SM, Skorton DJ, Ericksen E, Kioschos M, Marcus ML, White CW (1984) Rethrombosis after reperfusion with streptokinase: importance of geometry of residual lesions. Circulation 69: 991–999

16. Gangadharan V, Ramos RG, Hauser AM, Westveer DC, Timmis GC, Gordon S (1982) Intracoronary streptokinase: evidence for continued iatrogenic or spontaneous thrombolysis after termination of infusion. Am J Cardiol 49: 973

17. Karsch K, Blanke H, Pichard A, Driesman M, Gorlin R, Teichholz LE, Rentrop KP (1981) Changes in the degree of stenosis of the infarct vessel following intracoronary streptokinase. Circulation 64: IV–107

18. Ganz W, Geft I, Shah PK, Lew AS, Rodriguez L, Weiss T, Maddahi J, Berman DS, Charuzi Y, Swan HJC (1984) Am J Cardiol 53: 1209–1216

19. Gold HK, Cowley MJ, Palacios IF, Vetrovec GW, Akins CW, Block PC, Leinbach RC (1984) Combined intracoronary streptokinase infusion and coronary angioplasty during acute myocardial infarction. Am J Cardiol 53: 122–125

20. Hartzler GO, Rutherford BD, McConohay RD (1982) Percutaneous coronary angioplasty with and without prior streptokinase infusion for treatment of acute myocardial infarction. Am J Cardiol 49: 1033

21. Schröder R, Vöhringer HF, Linderer T, Biamino G, Brüggemann T, v. Leitner ER (in press) Follow-up after reperfusion with intravenous streptokinase: quantitative angiographic study. Am J Cardiol

Efficacy of BRL 26921, a new fibrinolytic agent for intravenous infusion, in acute myocardial infarction

FRANK J. VAN REY, HANS J. BONNIER, HERMAN R. MICHELS, MAMDOUH I. EL GAMAL and HANS J. HOFFMANN

The main goal of therapeutic thrombolysis in acute myocardial infarction is early reperfusion of acutely obstructed coronary arteries, thus reducing the size of myocardial infarction. Intracoronary thrombolysis has shown to be more successful than intravenous fibrinolysis [1, 2]. The major disadvantage of the technique is the delay in starting the treatment, caused by the need for selective coronary angiography.

BRL 26921 is an acylated streptokinase-human plasminogen complex that does not interact with plasminogen in the systemic circulation. After binding to fibrin the active thrombolytic complex is released by deacylation [3].

We studied the efficacy of 30 mg BRL 26921 given intravenously, and the degree of systemic fibrinolytic activation in thirteen patients (10 male, 3 female, aged 51 to 71 years), who were admitted with acute myocardial infarction of less then 3 hours duration. After an occluded coronary artery was identified by selective coronary angiography, 30 mg of BRL 26921 was given in a short iv infusion. Coronary angiography was repeated every 15 min. Levels of fibrinogen, fibrin degradation products (FDP), α_2-antiplasmin and plasminogen were determined before, and 1, 4, 12, 24 and 48 hours after infusion. The time delay from onset of symptoms till treatment was 70–230 min (mean 155 min). Reperfusion was seen in 11 patients (85%) within 5–60 min (mean 33 min). In 9 patients control angiography was performed 1–75 days (mean 22 days) after treatment. In 3 of

Table 1. Plasma levels of fibrinogen, FDP, plasminogen and α_2-antiplasmin in 12 patients before and at several moments after 30 mg BRL 26921 iv. Figures indicate mean values ± SEM.

	Fibrinogen (g/l)	FDP (mg/l)	Plasminogen (U/ml)	α_2-antiplasmin (U/ml)
before	2.70 ± 0.65	3.8 (1.5–9.8)	88 ± 12	91 ± 14
after 1 hr	0.24 ± 0.30	512 (105–2487)	12 ± 6	50 ± 11
4 hrs	0.27 ± 0.27	375 (135–917)	8 ± 6	49 ± 12
12 hrs	0.46 ± 0.34	128 (39–416)	24 ± 19	38 ± 13
24 hrs	0.77 ± 0.29	79 (28–221)	33 ± 9	38 ± 10
48 hrs	1.93 ± 0.38	16 (3.9–66)	53 ± 16	54 ± 9

12

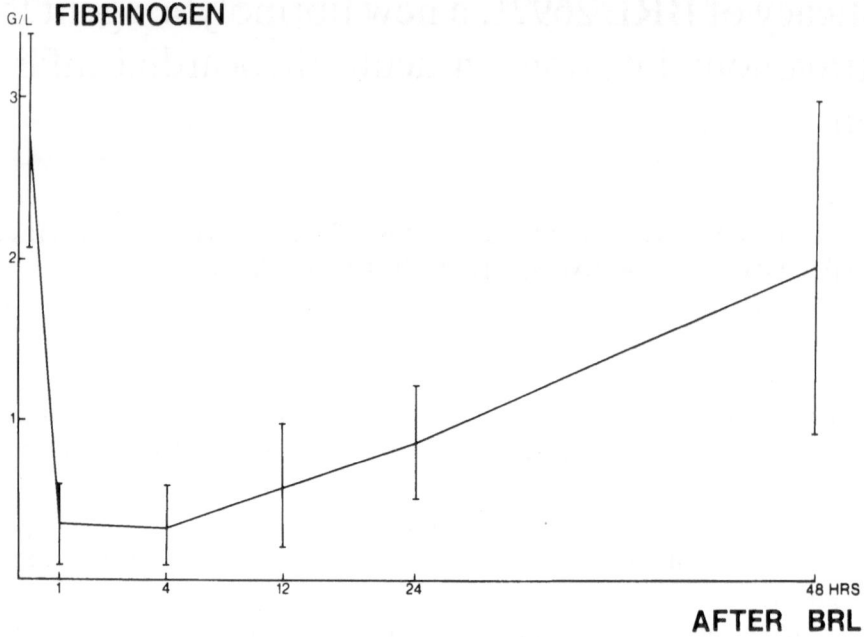

Figure 1. Fibrinogen levels before and after 30 mg BRL 26921 iv in g/l. Mean values ± SEM. (Clauss method).

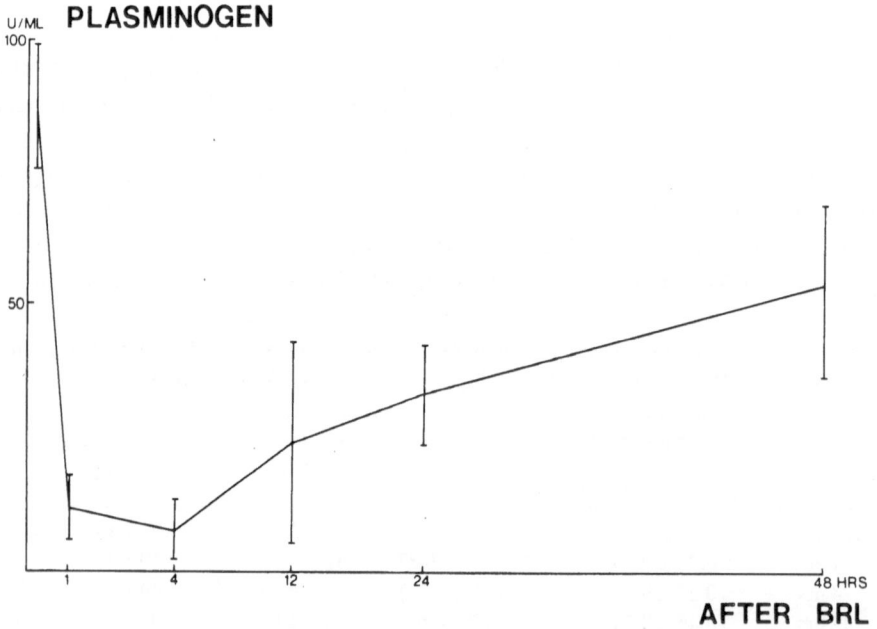

Figure 2. Plasminogen levels before and after 30 mg BRL 26921 iv in U/ml. Mean values ± SEM (Chromogen-substrate S-2251, Kabi).

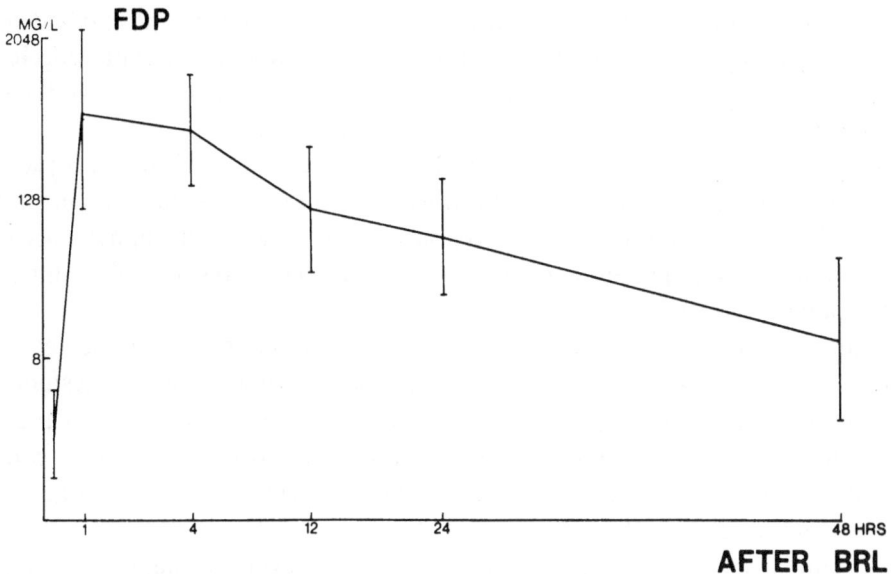

Figure 3. Fibrinogen degradation products before and after 30 mg BRL 26921 iv in mg/l. Mean values and range. (Thrombo-Wellcotest, Wellcome).

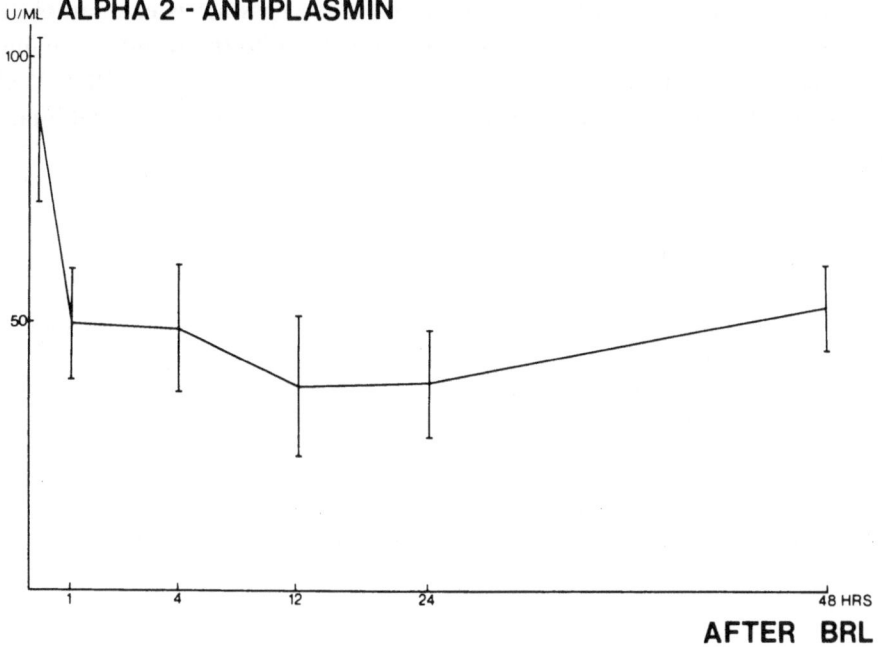

Figure 4. α_2-antiplasmin levels before and after 30 mg BRL 26921 iv in U/ml. Mean values $\pm$ SEM. (Laurell method).

them the infarct related coronary artery was reoccluded. One patient who had no control angiography had clinical signs of reocclusion. Two patients with reocclusion were treated conservatively, one patient had coronary angioplasty, and one patient underwent emergency coronary bypass operation.

In 6 patients hypotension (i.e. 25% reduction in systolic aortic pressure) was seen, which responded in all cases to infusion of inotropics. One patient had gastric bleeding, treated conservatively, one patient developed staphylococcus septiceamia, and one patient had fatal aortic bleeding due to complicated intra-aortic balloon insertion.

Systemic fibrinolytic activation was seen in 12 of 13 patients, as indicated in table 1. Only one patient had successful reperfusion without signs of systemic fibrinolysis. There was a reduction in plasma levels of fibrinogen and plasminogen to about 10% of initial value one hour after BRL 26921 and a concomitant rise in FDP, indicating binding of the active enzyme to plasminogen in the systemic circulation (Figures 1, 2 and 3).

We found a significant reduction in α_2-antiplasmin levels, lasting for 48 hours after treatment, which is in keeping with marked systemic fibrinolysis (Figure 4).

Conclusions

30 mg of BRL 26921 given intravenously is an effective thrombolytic agent in patients with acute myocardial infarction and its successrate is comparable to equivalent doses of intracoronary streptokinase. Despite the results of animal experiments and results obtained in healthy volunteers [4] this dosis of BRL 26921 produces marked systemic fibrinolysis in patients with acute myocardial infarction.

References

1. Spann JF et al. (1984) Coronary thrombolysis by intravenous streptokinase in acute myocardial infarction: acute and follow-up studies. Am J Cardiol 53: 655–661.
2. Rentrop P et al. (1979) Acute myocardial infarction: intracoronary application of nitroglycerin and streptokinase in combination with transluminal recanalization. Clin Cardiol 2: 354–363.
3. Matsuo O, Collen D, Verstraete M (1981) On the fibrinolytic and thrombolytic properties of active-site-p-anisoylated streptokinase – plasminogen complex (BRL 26921). Thromb Res 24: 347–358.
4. Prowse CV, Hornsey V, Ruckley CV, Boulton FE (1982) A comparison of acylated streptokinase – plasminogen complex and streptokinase in healthy volunteers. Thromb Haemostas 47: 132–135.

Coronary venous retroperfusion support of reperfusion following acute coronary occlusion

SAMUEL MEERBAUM

Abstract

Synchronized coronary venous retroperfusion with arterial blood and supplemental retroinfusions are described and discussed in relation to treatment of acute myocardial ischemia following coronary occlusions. Experimental studies indicate safety of the technique, and demonstrated 1) significant preferential retrograde supply to and enhanced washout from the acutely ischemic zone, 2) prompt improvement of regional ischemic and global cardiac function, and 3) extended viability of the jeopardized myocardium. Since retroperfusion provides a partial return in ischemic zone perfusion, and in view of experimental evidence that a staged reperfusion minimizes the derangements associated with sudden reflow, the retrograde method was explored as a pretreatment of full reperfusion. Comprehensive investigation in closed chest dogs corroborated the benefits of such an approach during intracoronary balloon occlusion and reperfusion. Supplementation of retroperfusion with streptokinase retroinfusion via the great cardiac vein was found to provide retrograde lysis of an occlusive trombus instituted in the LAD coronary artery of dogs. Retroperfusion and retroinfusion are believed to offer substantial potential as an alternate treatment of acute myocardial ischemia.

Many investigators have pursued the concept of coronary venous retroperfusion treatment of ischemic myocardium, jeopardized by extremely poor access via severely obstructed coronary arteries and insufficient collaterals. One of the best known series of investigations was performed some forty years ago under the leadership of Claude Beck, and pertained to surgical retroperfusion procedures [1–3]. These were exhaustively studied in the laboratory and then applied in about 200 patients. The initial enthusiasm of these investigators eventually waned, and the method was abandoned at about the time coronary artery bypass revascularization appeared to be the most promising procedure. A recognized problem with the retroperfusion technique was the inherently high and persisting coronary venous blood pressure. This obviously interferes with coronary venous drainage, and can cause major damage as a result of vascular trauma and engorgement, edema, and myocardial hemorrhages.

Synchronized coronary venous retroperfusion

A synchronized retroperfusion (SRP) approach was developed in the early 70's [4–5]. It addressed the evident need to allow coronary venous drainage during retroperfusion, and was designed as a temporary catheter-based circulatory support technique. The primary object was to promptly supply oxygen and substrates to critically jeopardized myocardium, and at least partly reestablish circulation in the acutely ischemic region distal to a coronary obstruction. We have been studying various aspects of an ECG-synchronized diastolic retroperfusion system [6–8]. We designed a special single lumen autoinflatable balloon catheter which can be readily placed in the regional coronary veins. Balloon deflation in systole facilitates coronary venous drainage, while diastolic balloon inflation allows unidirectional retroinfusate propulsion toward the jeopardized zone (Figure 1).

Numerous experimental studies performed by us and others during acute myocardial ischemia have extablished that this method provides significant improvement of regional and global cardiac function, and that it significantly extends myocardial viability as demonstrated through measurements of infarct salvage after a 6 hour SRP-treated coronary occlusion [6–8]. Additional recent studies investigated SRP with regional moderate hypothermia [9–10], cardioactive drug or thrombolytic agent retroinfusion [11–13], and retrograde administration of antiarrhythmic agents [14]. Both catheters and pumping systems are now being professionally manufactured for future clinical applications [15]. We have performed safety studies [8] and, pending US Federal Drug Administration review and approval, we expect the SRP system to be clinically applied in the near future.

Several potential SRP applications have been identified. As a derivative of the extensive and promising SRP studies during experimental coronary artery occlusions, SRP should be considered in the setting of evolving acute myocardial infarction, e.g. in the presence of thrombotic occlusion of the left anterior descending and/or left circumflex coronary arteries. SRP might be applied in conjunction with other currently investigated nonsurgical thrombolytic reperfusion techniques. An attractive use of SRP is to protect myocardium during complex PTCA procedures involving significant periods of coronary occlusion, with a similar rationale applying to potential future intracoronary laser techniques. Coronary venous retroinfusion of cardioplegic solutions is already being evaluated by cardiovascular surgeons, when severe obstruction of major coronary arteries leads to undesirable myocardial nonuniformities with current procedures [16–17]. Retroperfusion prior to or during surgical coronary artery revascularization can also be considered as a temporary support and to avoid complications.

We have recently reported on promising results with cardioactive agent delivery via the coronary veins. While such coronary venous retroinfusion appears to

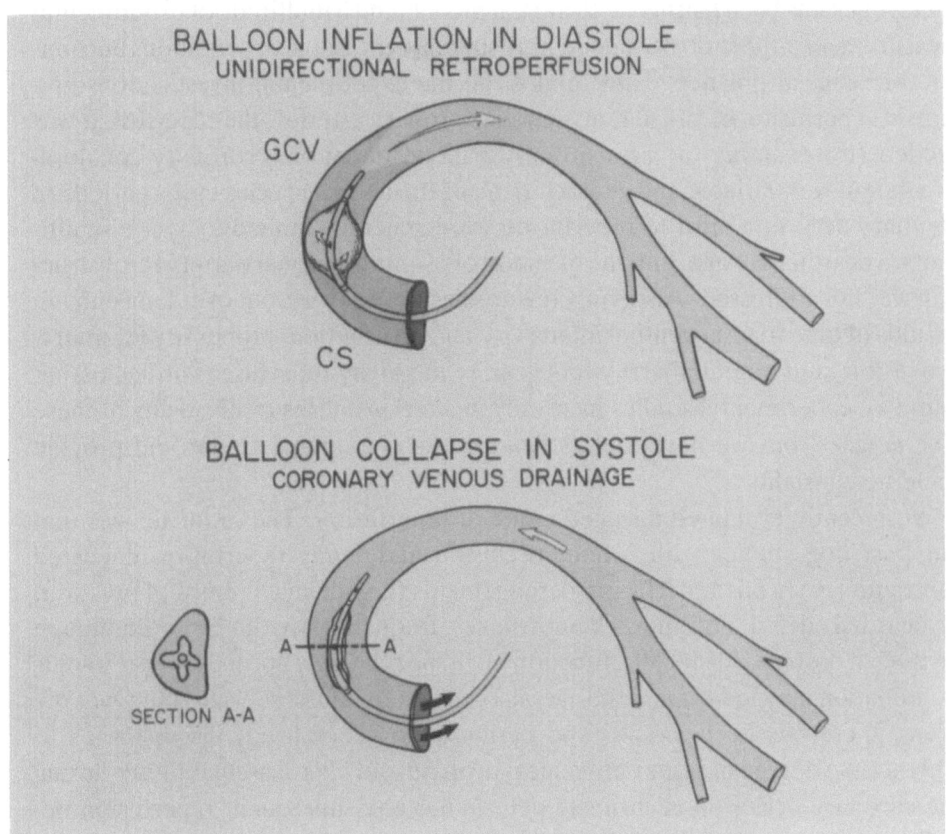

Figure 1. Phasic operation of synchronized retroperfusion. During cardiac diastole, arterial blood is pumped through the catheter placed within a regional coronary vein such as the great cardiac vein (GCV). This also inflates the catheter balloon, ensuring unidirectionality of the retrograde flow. During systole, the electrocardiographic synchronized pump stops forward flow, causing a sharp decrease in pressure within the catheter. This leads to rapid balloon collapse, which facilitates coronary venous drainage. Note the characteristic mode of balloon folding in the form of a star around the body of the catheter (SECTION A–A). CS = coronary sinus. [6]

be an interesting alternate technique for delivering pharmaceutics to the ischemic myocardium, the primary goal of treating acute ischemia remains the reestablishment of coronary perfusion. Thus, we have been interested in the general relationship of retroperfusion to reperfusion, and this paper attempts to address this particular question.

Reperfusion in evolving acute myocardial infarction

It is necessary to put in perspective the many experimental studies of reperfusion, including recent clinical studies of thrombolytic methods [18–20]. Certainly, while much has been learned with animal models and a multitude of experimental measurements, these do not adequately simulate the range of conditions encountered in clinical practice. Thus, almost all the experimental investigations employed reperfusion of single non-stenotic coronary arteries, the reperfusion was sudden (for example by intracoronary balloon deflation), coronary collateral circulation was variable and characteristic of the animal species used, periods of coronary occlusion prior to reperfusion were generally limited to assure significant myocardial salvage, and the question of eventual coronary artery re-obstruction was not addressed. Also, only few studies were carried out over long enough periods of time to test eventual infarct size and distribution, propensity for infarct expansion, and potential arrhythmogeneity in patchy reperfused cardiac tissue. Our own experimental studies have only in a few instances resolved any of these divergencies, but we nevertheless believe that the animal studies did provide some new insights.

We recently evaluated a staged mode of reperfusion. The rationale was that our past dog studies with 3 hour occlusion and 7 day reperfusion indicated substantial early postreperfusion derangements (e.g. delayed return of function, myocardial edema, intramural hemorrhages, frequent arrhythmias) even though on the 7th postreperfusion day function might be relatively normal and pathologic examination may indicate on the average significant infarct salvage [18]. Over the years, there has been ample (and perhaps too generalized) discussion as to whether the degree of prior ischemic myocardial and microvascular injury during the coronary occlusion exclusively determines any subsequent reperfusion derangements and damage, or whether reperfusion per se might also contribute derangements because of the stunned myocardium, arrhythmias, etc, even when the ischemic damage prior to reperfusion was still largely reversible. The latter cannot be excluded, although there can be little question that the ischemic injury is primarily implicated in the extent to which reperfusion can be effective. We did not address this question and merely compared staged vs sudden modes of reperfusion following acute coronary occlusion. We accepted results of prior research indicating that sudden reperfusion is associated with major calcium reflow, myocardial cell swelling and potential microvascular damage, and we reasoned that damage could be minimized by interposing a partial reperfusion stage with lower reflow at lesser blood pressure.

An initial study with relatively short coronary occlusion periods followed by reperfusion appeared encouraging in terms of the course of postreperfusion function [21]. In our more recent closed chest experimental preparation, a partial reflow was instituted in dogs 3 hours after coronary artery occlusion by interim stage pumping of arterial blood through the center lumen of the occlusive intracoronary balloon catheter. This was followed by full reperfusion through intracoronary balloon deflation. Early experiments with a 10 cc/min stage maintained for 2 hours proved inconclusive, presumably because any advantage derived through the gradual reperfusion was cancelled out by an extended period of ischemia, particularly in dogs with limited pre-existing coronary collaterals. Recent study with a 2 hour period of an interposed 20–30 cc/min coronary reflow stage (normal LAD flow in the dogs averaged about 60 cc/min) provided clear evidence of significant benefits (Table 1). Thus, we were able to show that the staged reperfusion resulted in a significantly smaller increase in early postreperfusion end diastolic wall thickness of the ischemic myocardium, implying less edema, and we also demonstrated a more rapid return of regional segmental function (by sequential 2D echo studies). We noted a sharp and highly significant reduction in early postreperfusion arrhythmias (minimal premature ventricular contractions), when compared to sudden reperfusion 3 hours postocclusion. Both the sudden and staged reperfusion groups of dogs were followed for 3 weeks, and at that time no significant differences were seen in function. With only a few in each of the groups, variations of infarct size were such as to preclude inferences as to statistical differences in measured infarction.

Table 1. Sudden (Su) vs Staged (St) reperfusion in closed chest dogs 2DE measurements of LV ischemic zone function.

		LAD Occlusion 3 hrs	LAD Reperfusion 2 hrs	7 days
Systolic fractional area change (%)	Su	1.0 ± 4.3	6.0 ± 5.2	19.3 ± 9.3
	St	-2.2 ± 8.9	12.2 ± 7.8	$29.4 \pm 4.8^*$
End diastolic wall thickness (mm)	Su	$6.8 \pm .1$	10.4 ± 2.7	$8.3 \pm .3$
	St	$7.0 \pm .6$	$8.0 \pm .4^*$	$7.6 \pm .9$

* $p < .05$

Retroperfusion treatment of reperfusion derangements

Several investigations demonstrated that synchronized retroperfusion provided an increase in acutely ischemic myocardial perfusion, to a level which was significantly higher than in an untreated control group with coronary artery occlusion, although perfusion remained still far below normal [22]. Thus, when acute LAD occlusion reduced regional myocardial perfusion from $1.14 \pm .09$ to $.32 \pm .05$ cc/min/g tissue, retroperfusion increased the level to $.51 \pm .04$ cc/min/g tissue ($p < .05$). We might consider this a first stage of myocardial reperfusion, perhaps capable of significantly extending viability and improving cardiac function during a stepwise or gradual transition to a complete reperfusion.

In a specific study performed in our laboratory in 12 closed chest dogs, moderately hypothermic SRP was begun 30 minutes after proximal LAD occlusion, when the acutely ischemic regional myocardium was presumed to be still fully viable [23]. SRP was continued for $2^1/_2$ hours with maintained coronary occlusion, and full and sudden reperfusion was instituted at 3 hours postocclusion by intracoronary balloon deflation. Reperfusion was then carried out for 7 days. An equivalent reperfusion control series of 13 dogs had no SRP pretreatment, and sudden reperfusion was instituted 3 hours after LAD occlusion. In addition to hemodynamic and ECG measurements, we studied in detail changes in global and regional cardiac function, at several levels of the left ventricle, and in both ischemic as well as nonischemic segments of each level. Results of this study are illustrated in Tables 2 and 3.

We found that pretreatment with SRP significantly enhanced the course and consequences of reperfusion. Thus, left ventricular volumes were reduced and ejection fraction increased by SRP. Ischemic zone function was significantly improved. The SRP treated group of dogs had about half the mortality exhibited by the untreated series over 7 days, and infarct size after 7 days reperfusion was significantly reduced by the pretreatment (4.2 ± 5.9 vs 12.0 ± 6.5 of the LV). The most dramatic difference seen was the rapid improvement of ischemic zone function after reperfusion to a near normal level at 24 hours postreperfusion, whereas without treatment ischemic zone akinesis and thinning persisted for 7 days. Equally significant was the absence of serious arrhythmias and minor

Table 2. Hypothermic retroperfusion (RTP) pretreatment of LAD reperfusion global cardiac effects in closed chest dogs.

| | | LAD Occlusion | | LAD Reperfusion | |
		30 min	3 hrs	1 hr	7 days
LV Ejection fraction (%)	Controls	36 ± 7	35 ± 5	31 ± 5	43 ± 7
	RTP	35 ± 7	$49 \pm 6^*$	$43 \pm 9^*$	$55 \pm 5^*$
LV dp/dt (mmHg/sec)	Controls	1487 ± 234	1524 ± 332	1307 ± 272	1569 ± 338
	RTP	1737 ± 314	1856 ± 524	1513 ± 497	$2183 \pm 416^*$

* p<.05

Table 3. Hypothermic retroperfusion (RTP) pretreatment of LAD reperfusion ischemic zone function in closed chest dogs.

| | | LAD Occlusion | | LAD Reperfusion | |
		30 min	3 hrs	1 hr	7 days
Systolic fractional area change (%)	Controls	1 ± 8	-1 ± 12	-8 ± 7	11 ± 20
	RTP	3 ± 11	$25 \pm 22^*$	$24 \pm 22^*$	$40 \pm 17^*$
Systolic wall thickening (%)	Controls	-2 ± 11	$-.4 \pm 6$	-8 ± 8	-2 ± 17
	RTP	2 ± 7	$17 \pm 16^*$	$11 \pm 17^*$	$25 \pm 24^*$
End diastolic wall thickness (mm)	Controls	7.3 ± 7	8.2 ± 1	12.6 ± 2	11.2 ± 2
	RTP	8.1 ± 9	9.3 ± 1	$10.3 \pm 1^*$	8.8 ± 1

* p<.05

postreperfusion increase in end diastolic ischemic zone wall thickness in the pretreated dogs, whereas a major increase was noted in the untreated group, reflecting frequent myocardial edema caused by sudden reperfusion.

Lysis of a coronary artery thrombus by regional coronary vein streptokinase retroinfusion

Indirect, and more recently direct, measurements during great cardiac vein retroinfusion of arterial blood indicate that a fraction (possibly 20%) of the retroinfusate may transverse the myocardial microcirculation and appear in the LAD coronary artery distal to its occlusion, particularly when the antegrade flow and pressure are severely diminished by the coronary occlusion. We theorized that by adding streptokinase to SRP we could not only provide improved function and extend viability with retroperfusion, as previously demonstrated, but that we might also enhance the process of coronary artery thrombolysis. Therefore, in a small series of closed chest dogs [24], we placed a thrombogenic copper coil in the LAD, which led to full thrombotic coronary artery occlusion within 10–60 minutes. After a further interval to extend the coronary occlusion to 90 min from coil insertion, we began SRP with streptokinase. Alternately, we intermittently

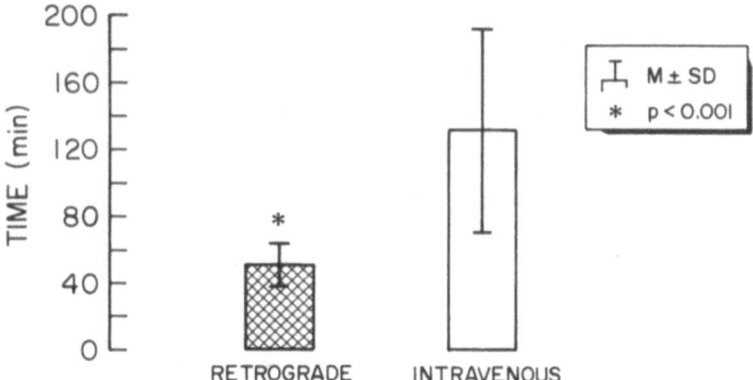

Figure 2. Time from start of streptokinase administration to full lysis of coronary artery thrombus. Individual data, as well as mean ± standard deviation, are shown for the three approaches of streptokinase administration: intermittent coronary venous retroinfusion, synchronized venous retroperfusion and intravenous method. The dog preparation and dosage were equivalent. Note the apparent repeatability and promptness of the retroperfusion modality, followed by equally short but somewhat more variable results with intermittent retroinfusion, and substantial scatter and significant longer time to lysis when streptokinase was administered intravenously. [24]

(10 min on–10 min off) retroinjected arterial blood along with streptokinase. Drug dosage in the dogs was 1–2000 IU/min, and we also studied such streptokinase administration intravenously to test whether effects noted with SRP were truly retrograde or else largely produced via systemic shunting.

Results of this initial study are shown in Figure 2. We found that thrombolysis took place in all 15 dogs studied (5 dogs per group). Lysis was significantly delayed when streptokinase was administered intravenously (131.6 ± 60.0 min, range 65–200 min), whereas it was similarly and significantly more rapid with the two retrograde infusion methods (combining date, full and stable reperfusion in 50.5 ± 13.2, range 27 to 75 min). Initial thrombolysis was often seen much earlier, in 26.7 ± 9.2 minutes after retrograde streptokinase administration. Figure 3 illustrates the sequence in one dog with SRP plus streptokinase; early lysis was noted within 18 minutes from the time of streptokinase administration, and reperfusion was fully established after 50 minutes. Although statistical evaluation

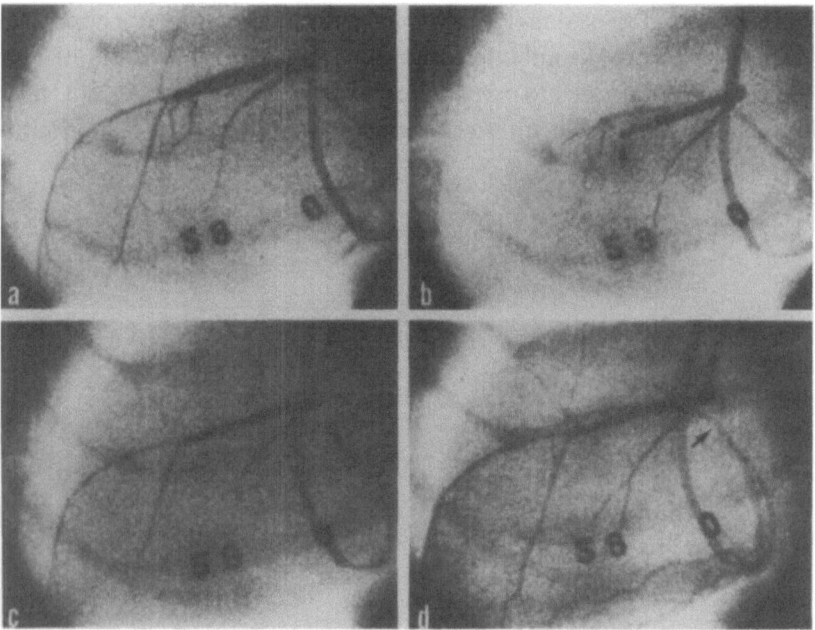

Figure 3. Angiographic documentation of an experimental sequence of coronary artery events before and after streptokinase retroperfusion-induced thrombolysis in one closed chest dog: a) selective coronary angiography in the control state, showing the left anterior descending coronary artery and its branches; b) total thrombotic obstruction of the left anterior descending artery (see arrow) beyond the small copper coil placed at a relatively proximal site; c) initial left anterior descending coronary reflow after streptokinase treatment by way of coronary venous retroperfusion; and d) fully reestablished coronary flow noted 50 minutes after start of the streptokinase retroperfusion via great cardiac vein (see arrow). Similar coronary artery thrombolysis was achieved in all dogs treated with retrograde coronary venous streptokinase infusion. [24]

of all the reperfusion effects cannot be derived from this study because of the small groups and varying periods of occlusion and lysis, the observed results were very much in consonance with those previously noted in controlled studies of untreated vs. SRP treated reperfusion. We found no reperfusion arrhythmias after the retrograde thrombolysis, and we were impressed with a rapid return of ischemic zone function shortly after the retrograde thrombolytic reperfusion, something we seldom see with untreated sudden reperfusion following similar periods of coronary occlusion. A more extended series will provide further evaluation of this interesting retrograde application, and we also hope to shortly examine different thrombolytic agents. It would be premature at this time to draw conclusions relative to a potential use of this method, alone or in conjunction with other techniques, but it does seem worthwhile to reemphasize the two aspects of our coronary venous streptokinase retroinfusion along with SRP: 1) it provided protection of jeopardized myocardium pending effective reperfusion, and 2) it caused rapid retrograde lysis of an intracoronary artery clot.

Current directions

Synchronized and other modes of coronary venous retroperfusion appear ready for selected clinical applications. At the same time, substantial research is still seeking clarification of the mechanisms underlying the reported effectiveness of this treatment during acute myocardial ischemia. New concepts of retroperfusion and retroinfusion are currently broadening the potentials of this methodology, and will necessitate further development along with critical review.

References

1. Gross L, Blun L, Silberman G (1937) Experimental attempts to increase the blood supply to the dog's heart by means of coronary sinus occlusion. J Exper Med 65: 91
2. Beck CS, Hahn RS, Leighninger DS, McAllister FF (1951) Operation for coronary artery disease. JAMA 147: 1726
3. Bakst AA, Costas-Durieux J, Goldberg H, Bailey CP (1954) Protection of the heart by arterialization of the coronary sinus. I. Coronary collateral flow in normal dogs and in dogs having had previous nondescript cardiac surgery. J Thoracic Surg 27: 433
4. Meerbaum S, Uchiyama T, Lang TW (1980) Extension of myocardial viability by closed-chest regional hypothermic retroperfusion early after coronary occlusion (abstr). Circulation 62 (suppl III): III–316
5. Meerbaum S, Lang TW, Osher JV (1976) Diastolic retroperfusion of acutely ischemic myocardim. Am J Cardiol 37: 558–98
6. Farcot JC, Meerbaum S, Lang T, Kaplan L, Corday E (1978) Synchronized retroperfusion of coronary veins for circulatory support of jeopardized ischemic myocardium. Am J Cardiol 21: 1191–202
7. Smith GT, Geary GG, Blanchard W, McNamara JJ (1981) Reduction in infarct size by synchronized selective coronary venous retroperfusion of arterialized blood. Am J Cardiol 48: 1064–70

8. Yamazaki S, Drury JK, Meerbaum S, Corday E (1984) Effects of synchronized retroperfusion on left ventricular function measured by two dimensional echocardiography. In: The coronary sinus. Proceedings of the 1st International Symposium on Myocardial Protection via the Coronary Sinus, 375–9, (Mohl W, Wolner E, Glogar D eds), Steinkopff Verlag, Darmstadt

9. Haendchen RV, Aosaki N, Uchiyama T (1981): Hypothermic retroperfusion treatment of acute myocardial ischemia: effects on cardiac function and infarct size (abstr). Am J Cardiol 47: 436

10. Meerbaum S, Haendchen RV, Corday E (1982): Hypothermic coronary venous phased retroperfusion: a closed chest treatment of acute regional ischemic myocardium. Circulation 65: 1435–45

11. Povzhitkov M, Haendchen RV, Meerbaum S, Fishbein M, Rit J, Corday E (1982) Mannitol coronary venous retroperfusion: improvement in ischemic left ventricular function in acute occlusion (abstr). Clin Res 30: 17A

12. Povzhitkov M, Haendchen RV, Meerbaum S, Fishbein M, Rit J, Corday E (1982) Protective effect of coronary venous prostaglandin E_1 retroperfusion during acute myocardial ischemia (abstr). Am J Cardiol 49: 1017

13. Meerbaum S, Povzhitkov M, Haendchen RV, Broffman J, Lang TW, Corday E (1982) Coronary artery thrombolysis by streptokinase coronary venous retroinfusion or systemic administration (abstr). Am J Cardiol 49: 1046

14. Karagueuzian HS, Ohta M, Drury JK, Fishbein MC, Corday E, Meerbaum S, Mandel WJ, Peter T (1984) Coronary venous retroinfusion of procainamide in the management of inducible ventricular tachyarrhythmias in conscious dogs, during chronic myocardial infarction. In: The coronary sinus. Proceedings of the 1st International Symposium on Myocardial Protection via the Coronary Sinus, 385–91 (Mohl W, Wolner E, Glogar D eds), Steinkopff Verlag, Darmstadt

15. Drury JK, Yamazaki S, Meerbaum S, Fishbein M, Corday E (1984) Synchronized coronary venous retroperfusion: A safe and effective treatment of acute myocardial ischemia. In: The coronary sinus. Proceedings of the 1st International Symposium on Myocardial Protection via the Coronary Sinus, 347–53, (Mohl W, Wolner E, Glogar D eds), Steinkopff Verlag, Darmstadt

16. Gundry SR, Kirsh MM (1984): Myocardial compliance following retrograde versus antegrade cardioplegia in the presence of coronary artery obstruction. In: The coronary sinus. Proceedings of the 1st International Symposium on Myocardial Protection via the Coronary Sinus, 270–4, (Mohl W, Wolner E, Glogar D eds), Steinkopff Verlag, Darmstadt

17. Fuentes M. Batanero J, Robles D, Martinez JA, Garcia J, Casinello N (1984) Cardioplegia via the coronary sinus, our experience in 331 cases. In: The coronary sinus. Proceedings of the 1st International Symposium on Myocardial Protection via the Coronary Sinus, 316–9, (Mohl W, Wolner E, Glogar D eds), Steinkopff Verlag, Darmstadt

18. Costantini C, Corday E, Lang TW (1975) Revascularization after 3 hours of coronary arterial occlusion: effects on regional cardiac metabolic function and infarct size. Am J Cardiol 36: 368–84

19. Theroux P, Ross J Jr, Franklin D, Kemper WS, Sasayama S (1976) Coronary arterial reperfusion. III. Early and late effects on regional myocardial function and dimensions in conscious dogs. Am J Cardiol 38: 599–606

20. Ganz W, Buchbinder N, Marcus H (1981) Coronary thrombolysis in evolving myocardial infarction. Am Heart J 101: 4–13

21. Aosaki N, Haendchen RV, Wyatt HL (1981) Accelerated return of cardiac function with gradual reperfusion after brief coronary occlusion abstr). Clin Res 29: 175A

22. Berdeaux A, Farcot JC, Bourdarias JP, Barry M, Bardet J, Giudicelli JD (1981) Effects of diastolic synchronized retroperfusion on regional coronary blood flow in experimental myocardial ischemia. Am J Cardiol 47: 1033–40

23. Haendchen RV, Corday E, Meerbaum S, Povzhitkov M, Rit J, Fishbein MC (1983) Prevention of ischemic injury an early reperfusion derangements by hypothermic retroperfusion. JACC 1(4): 1067–80

24. Meerbaum S, Lang T, Povzhitkov M, Haendchen RV, Uchiyama T, Broffman J, Corday E (1983) Retrograde lysis of coronary artery thrombus by coronary venous streptokinase administration. JACC 1(5): 1262–7

Elevation of coronary sinus pressure improves myocardial protection

U.B. BRÜCKNER, U. MITTMANN and W.W. SAGGAU

Introduction

Despite the use of cardioplegic solutions tissue areas remain unprotected in the presence of a severe coronary stenosis [1], particularly in the subendocardial layer [2]. Retrograde coronary sinus perfusion [3] may protect such ischemic areas during cardiopulmonary bypass. However, this method available requires additional facilities [4].

Therefore, the aim of our study was to investigate whether transient elevation of coronary sinus pressure (CSP) improves the cooling efficacy and tissue preservation of orthograde cardioplegic perfusion.

Methods

In 12 mongrel dogs ($23 \pm 2\,\text{kg}$) the left anterior descending coronary artery (LAD) was ligated followed by clamping of the aorta and orthograde myocardial

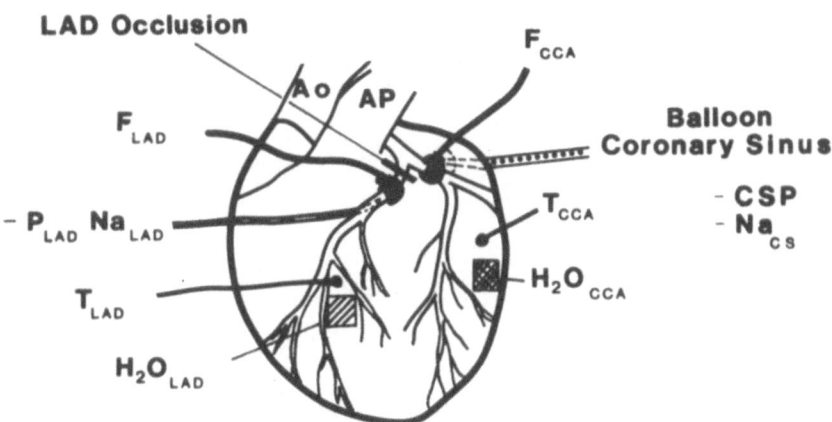

Figure 1. Scheme of the experimental procedure. F_{LAD} = retrograde flow LAD; P_{LAD} = distal pressure LAD; Na_{LAD} = distal sodium concentration LAD; T_{LAD} = tissue temperature LAD area; H_2O_{LAD} = tissue water content LAD area; CSP = coronary sinus pressure; Na_{cs} = sodium concentration coronary sinus; F_{CCA} = flow CCA; T_{CCA} = tissue temperature CCA area; H_2O_{CCA} = tissue water content CCA area.

protection with cold (4° C) Bretschneider's low sodium HP-solution. Coronary artery pressure, coronary flow, and arterial sodium concentration were measured distal to the occlusion (Figure 1). Myocardial tissue temperature and tissue water content were determined both in the LAD-dependent area and in a control region supplied by the left circumflex coronary artery (CCA). In 8 dogs CSP was elevated by a balloon placed into the coronary sinus, whereas 4 animals without CSP elevation served as controls.

Results

Myocardial tissue temperature fell in the CCA region below 15° C within 2 min but the decrease in the LAD area was delayed. Elevation of CSP from initially 11.2 to 25.8 mmHg doubled the slope of temperature decrease from initially 0.9 to 2.0° C/ min ($p<0.05$) in the LAD area (Figure 2).

CSP elevation also caused an increase in retrograde coronary flow by 123% to 2.6 ml/min ($p<0.05$) and augmented distal LAD pressure by 58% to 19.3 mmHg ($p<0.05$). Plasma Na-concentration distal to the LAD occlusion was 52 mmol/l

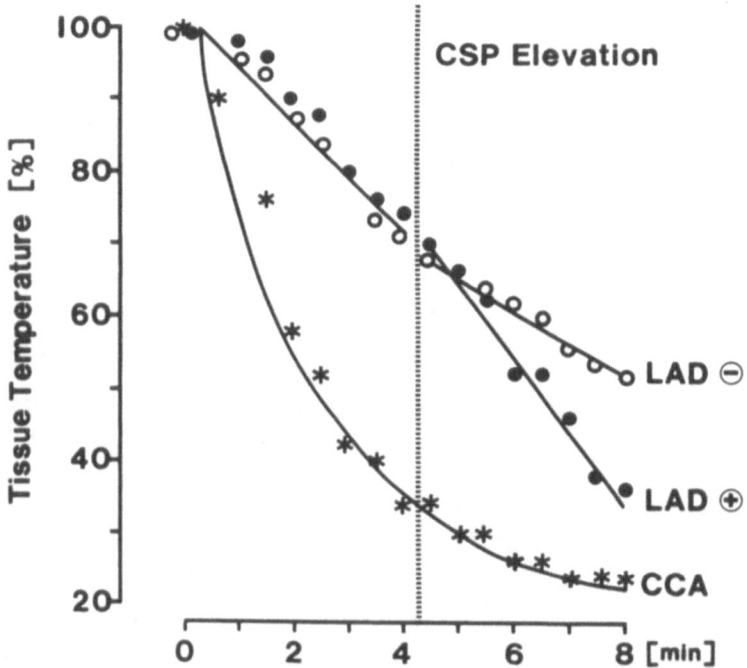

Figure 2. Decrease in myocardial tissue temperature before and after CSP elevation during 8-min cardioplegic perfusion. CCA = control area supplied by the unaffected CCA; LAD ⊖ = ischemic LAD region without CSP elevation; LAD ⊕ = after CSP elevation.

Table 1. Regional changes in the LAD-dependent ischemic area and in the unaffected control region supplied by the CCA prior and 4 min after elevation of the coronary sinus pressure (CSP).

	CSP elevation Prior		After	
	LAD	CCA	LAD	CCA
Pressure (mmHg)	12 ± 5 distal	100 ± 14	19 ± 6 distal	99 ± 14
Flow (ml/min)	1.2 ± 0.6 retrograde	55 ± 29	2.6 ± 1.2 retrograde	50 ± 25
Plasma Na-Concentration (mmol/l)	52 ± 22 distal	29 ± 20	33 ± 26 distal	27 ± 22
Tissue Temperature (°C)	23.8 ± 3.5	11.4 ± 2.5	10.9 ± 2.9	8.2 ± 3.6
Tissue Water Content (%)	81 ± 2	79 ± 1	79 ± 1	78 ± 1

and dropped by 40% to 33 mmol/l after CSP elevation. Myocardial tissue water content was identical in both areas measured either at normal or at elevated CSP.

Discussion

The delayed temperature decrease in the ischemic LAD area was abolished after CSP elevation which might be due to a better venous filling. However, the increased distal coronary pressure and flow together with an intracoronary sodium concentration identical to that of the CCA clearly indicate that the cardioplegic solution had passed the exchange vessels. Therefore, the efficacy of cooling was accelerated.

This beneficial CSP elevation, which may be obtained rapidly by supporting the sinus on the finger-tip during cardiosurgery, did not augment myocardial water content, neither in the ischemic nor in the control area.

References

1. Mittmann U et al. (1980) Thorac Cardiovasc Surgeon 28: 184
2. Flameng W et al. (1974) Basic Res Cardiol 69: 435
3. Solorzano J et al. (1978) Ann Thorac Surg 25: 201
4. Bates RJ et al. (1977) Ann Thorac Surg 23: 83

Improvement of myocardial perfusion and enhancement of washout during coronary artery occlusion by intermittent pressure controlled coronary sinus occlusions

D. GLOGAR, W. MOHL, H. MAYR, P. SCHINDLER, F. KAINDL
and E. WOLNER

Introduction

Pressure controlled intermittent coronary sinus occlusion (PICSO) is performed using a catheter pump device that allows for cyclic inflation of a balloon catheter, placed into the orifice of the coronary sinus [1, 2, 3], until the coronary sinus pressure (CSP) reaches a plateau. Following the phase of inflation, balloon deflation allows coronary sinus drainage until the CSP has reached the baseline values. Previous studies have shown that this method leads to an improvement of regional myocardial function in ischemic myocardial segments [4] and to an improvement of washout measured by continuous coronary sinus blood outflow density measurements [5]. The present study was devised to evaluate the effects of PICSO on

1) myocardial perfusion during acute experimental coronary artery occlusion (LAD), and
2) on myocardial washout of metabolites.

Methods

Two series of experiments are included in this paper. Group A consisted of anaesthetised dogs that were submitted to 6 hours of CAO. The myocardium at risk (MR I) was determined at 15 minutes CAO by injecting 99 mCi Technetium labelled albumine microspheres and prior to sacrifice after 6 hours CAO (MR II) by injecting Monastral blue dye into the left atrium [6]. Infarct size was determined postmortem with the TTC technique. Regional myocardial blood flow was measured using radioactive plastic microspheres. PICSO was begun after 15 minutes CAO (n = 13), 12 experiments served as controls.

Group B consisted of 6 further animal experiments in which PICSO was begun 2 hours post CAO and was maintained for 4 hours. In these experiments we sampled at time of sacrifice numerous tissue biopsies from ischemic and non-ischemic myocardium to determine the tissue electrolyte content (Na^+, K^+, Cl^-, Mg^{++}) using Neutron Activation Analysis.

Results

In group A PICSO reduced infarct size to $55.9 \pm 6.5\%$ of the pretreatment myocardium at risk (MR I) compared to $99.0 \pm 3.3\%$ in controls (p<0.001). While the myocardium at risk remained unchanged in controls during the evolution of the infarct, PICSO led to a reduction of the myocardium at risk (MR I vs MR II) by 20% (p<0.05) indicating and improvement of perfusion of border zone by PICSO. RMBF measuring antegrade perfusion using radioactive microspheres showed no significant changes in the center and the margin of the infarction, the noninfarcted border zone and the normal myocardium showed an improvement of myocardial perfusion between 20–60% (Figure 1).

In group A PICSO was begun 2 hours after CAO and continued for 4 hours. Infarct size was also reduced significantly in this model with $17 \pm 1.9\%$ of the respective myocardium at risk protected from necrosis by the intervention. Tissue electrolytes that were measured by Neutron Activation Analysis were determined from the center of the infarction and the nonischemic region (Figure 2). Tissue concentrations measured reflect total tissue concentrations including both extracellular and intracellular spaces. We found significant differences in the pattern of tissue electrolytes between infarcted and noninfarcted regions. Particularly the reduction of total tissue potassium and magnesium lost from the intracellular space during ischemia may indicate a washout of these elements from the infarcted region that may reflect the therapeutic effects of PICSO.

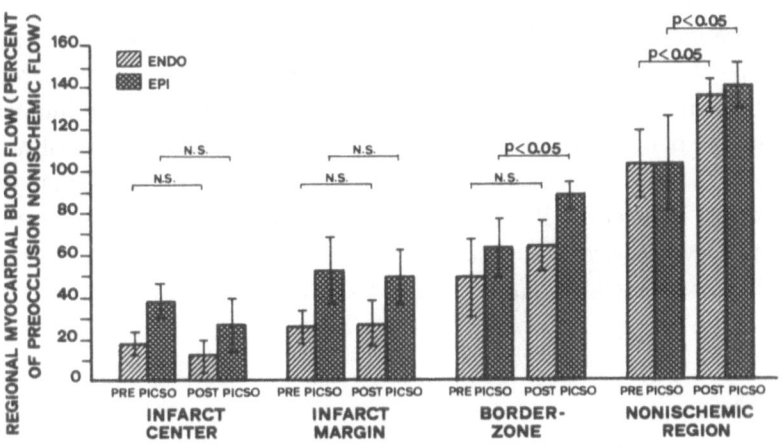

Figure 1. Effect of 6 hours PICSO on regional myocardial blood flow. RMBF expressed as the percentage of RMBF measured prior to CAO. PRE PICSO represents RMBF measured after 15 Min CAO prior to intervention and POST PICSO represents RMBF measured during PICSO treatment after 6 hours CAO.

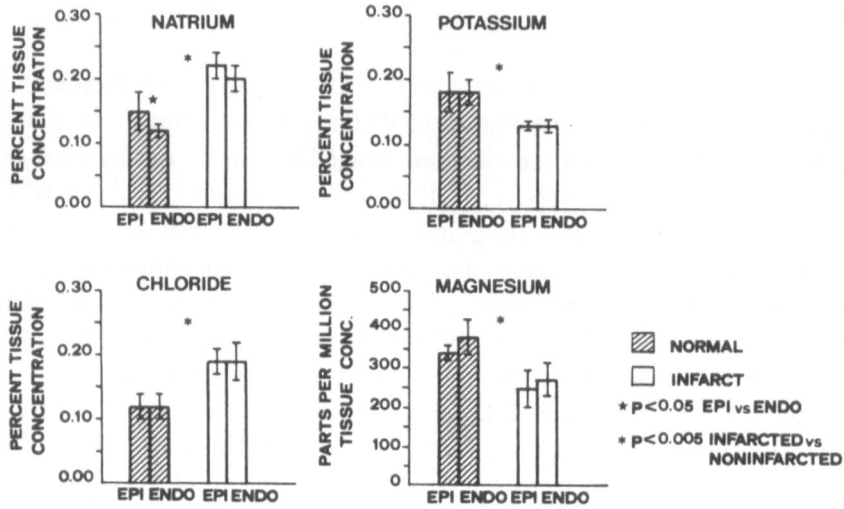

Figure 2. Tissue concentration of sodium, potassium, chloride and magnesium measured by neutron activation analysis.

Discussion

Pressure controlled intermittent coronary sinus occlusion has been shown to significantly reduce myocardial ischemia and improve ischemic myocardial function. The present paper demonstrates that at least one of the mechanisms involved by which PICSO effectively decreases infarct size may be due to an improvement of regional myocardial blood flow (experimental group A). The microsphere method, however, only allows the measurement of antegrad blood flow; during PICSO retrograde perfusion via the coronary venous circulation may be operative additionally. Another mechanism that could be important in explaining the beneficial effects of PICSO may be the improvement of washout. Particularly the reduction of total tissue potassium and magnesium may point to such on effect induced by PICSO treatment. If this loss of electrolytes may also lead to negative consequences such as aggravation of arrhythmias was not addressed in this investigation and remains to be clarified.

References

1. Mohl W, Güggi M, Haberzeth K, Losert H, Pachinger O, Schabert A, Borek H, Wolner E, Kessler M (1980) Effects of intermittent coronary sinus occlusion (PICSO) on tissue parameters after ligation of LAD. Bibliotheca Anatomica 20: 517–521
2. Mohl W, Glogar D, Mayr H, Losert U, Sochor H, Pachinger O, Kaindl F, Wolner E (1984)

Reduction of infarct size induced by pressure-controlled intermittent coronary sinus occlusion. Am J Cardiol 53: 923–928

3. Glogar D, Mohl W, Mayr H, Losert U, Sochor H, Wolner E, Kaindl F (1982) Pressure controlled intermittent coronary sinus occlusion reduces myocardial necrosis (abstr) Am J Cardiol 49: 1017

4. Heimisch W, Mohl W, Mendler N, Hagl S (1984) Intermittent coronary sinus occlusion (ICSO): Effects on regional normal and ischemic myocardium. In: The coronary sinus, D. Steinkopff-Verlag, Darmstadt, pp 465–472

5. Mohl W, Moser M, Schuster J, Kenner T, Klepetko W, Moritz A, Müller M, Glogar D, Aigner A, Wolner E (1984) Enhancement of washout induced by intermittent coronary sinus occlusion (PICSO) in the canine and human heart. In: Mohl W, Wolner E, Glogar D; The Coronary Sinus, D. Steinkopff-Verlag, Darmstadt, pp 537–548

6. Glogar D, Ertl G, DeBoer LWV, Darsee SR, Kloner RA (1980) Characterisation of the myocardium protected by collateral flow in experimental coronary occlusion. A comparison of in vivo and vitro methods for the determination of the myocardium at risk. Clin Research (abstr) 28: 174

7. Farcot JC, Meerbaum S, Lang TW, Kaplan L, Corday E (1978) Synchronized retroperfusion of coronary veins for circulatory support of jeopardized ischemic myocardium. Am J Cardiol 41: 1191–1201

Medical-mechanical treatment of myocardial infarction

R. ERBEL, T. POP, B. HENKEL, G. SCHREINER, C. STEUERNAGEL, F. BECK, K.L. HENRICHS and J. MEYER

Introduction

The aim of therapy in acute myocardial infarction is the restoration of coronary blood flow. By streptolysis therapy a reperfusion rate for intracoronary administration between 60% [1] and 86% [2] for intravenous administration between 50% [3] and 67% [4] using acute coronary angiography and 96% using indirect clinical criteria were reached [5]. From start of therapy until reperfusion 23 ± 12 min [6] to 36 ± 8 min [7] were reported.

In order to increase reperfusion rate and to reduce infarct times streptolysis therapy was combined with mechanical approach by 3 F and 4 F balloon catheters providing the possibility of angioplasty immediately after reperfusion.

Methods

Patients

In the study 127 patients were included who reached hospital within 6 h after onset of symptoms of acute myocardial infarction. Diagnosis was based on (1) acute chest pain lasting for more than 30 minutes, (2) persistent ST segment elevation of more than 0.3 mV in leads V1–V6/or 0.2 mV in leads I–III, aVL or AVF. All patients received premedication with 5.000 U heparin, 250 mg prednisolon, 3 mg/h nitroglycerine, 1 g acetyl salicylate acid. 250.000 U streptokinase were infused intravenously prior to heart catheterization within 20 min.

Heart catheterization started with the introduction of a pacing catheter. In a random fashion coronary angiography was performed via a 7 F catheter (group I) or 9 F guide catheter (group II). After opacification of the occluded vessel, streptokinase infusion started immediately at a dose of 4.000 U/min. In case of an open coronary artery infusion rate was increased to 12.000 U/min. The total dose was 250.000 U. During the streptolysis therapy, 3 F recanalization catheters (Schneider, Zürich) or 4 F Gruentzig balloon catheters (Schneider, Zürich) were prepared. As soon as possible the catheters were introduced into the occluded coronary artery for mechanical recanalization. Immediately after the recanalization streptokinase was administered superselectively via the 3 F or the 4 F catheters. After administration of the total dose of streptokinase, coronary angioplasty was attempted in all cases in group II. Cineangiography was performed with 30 to 40 ml meglumine ioxaglate acid (Hexabrix°) at 12–15 ml/s and a frame rate of 50/s. The patients were managed in the coronary care unit, serial ECG, systemic and pulmonary artery pressures monitored and cardiac index calculated.

Heparin therapy started within 5–6 h after lysis. Full dose was given for 4–5 days. Overlapping phenprocoumon therapy started and was held between 15–25%.

Before discharge right and left heart catheterization with coronary angiography was repeated [9]. Cineangiography of the left ventricle was filmed during atrial pacing corresponding to initial angiography in the acute stage to exclude possible heart rate – related effects on left ventricular volumes and ejection fraction [8].

Calculation

Left ventricular volumes were determined using a disc method, as previously described [9]. End-diastole was taken at the peak of the R-wave, end-systole defined as the smallest silhouette of the ventricle. Stroke volume and ejection fraction were calculated.

For regional wall motion analysis a floating system was used with diastolic long axis as a center point, creating 28 radii. Percentage shortening of the 28 segments was calculated, normal values established in 30 controls.

Statistics

All results are given as mean ± standard deviation. Students t-test for unpaired and the Wilcoxon test for paired data were used, as well as the Chi-square test: a p-value <0.05 was regarded as significant.

Results

Analysis of clinical data demonstrated no significant difference between group I and II related to mean age (56 ± 11 and 57 + 10 years), sex (54 M/1 OF and 56 M/7 F) – 17% of patients were older than 70 years – infarct location (anterior myocardial infarction 30 and 30 patients, inferior infarcts 34 and 93 patients), 2 patients demonstrated infarcts of anterior and posterior location. Time between onset of symptoms and admission to hospital measured 156 ± 11 min and 153 ± 58 min, time until iv streptokinase therapy 18 ± 23 min and 14 ± 15 min, time until i c streptolysis was 39 ± 15 min and 39 ± 20 min, further 13 ± 27 min and 14 ± 16 min were found until reperfusion (Figure 1).

First coronary angiography demonstrated an open vessel in 23/64 patients (36%) in group I and in 12/63 (19%) in group II. Mechanical recanalization with 3 F catheters was succesful in 27/41 patients (66%) in group I and 26/51 patients

Medical-Mechanical Recanalisation		
	Group I	Group II
onset of symptoms		
	156 ±71	153 ± 58 min
admission		
	18±23	14±16 min
IV lysis		
	39±15	39±20 min
IC lysis		
	13±27	14±16 min
recanalisation		

Figure 1. Time delay from onset of symptoms until admission to hospital (X ± SD), until intravenous (iv), until intracoronary (ic) streptokinase administration and until reperfusion.

(51%) of group II. In 9/41 patients in group I (22%) and 18/51 patients (35%) in group II reperfusion took place before mechanical recanalization could be performed or occurred during superselective streptolysis therapy when mechanical recanalization failed. Thus, reperfusion rate in group I measured 59/64 patients (52%) and 56/63 patients (89%) in group II (Figure 2).

	Group I	Group II
open vessel	23/64 (36%)	12/63 (19%)
mech. RE	27/41 (66%)	26/51 (51%)
med. RE	9/41 (22%)	18/51 (35%)
reperfusion rate	59/64 (92%)	56/63 (89%)

Figure 2. Percentage of open coronary vessels at the first coronary angiography, of successful mechanical recanalization (RE), of occluded vessels, of thrombolysis (medial RE), of occluded vessels in which mechanical RE failed or lysis took place before mechanical RE could be performed.

Coronary angioplasty

In group II immediately after the end of the streptokinase infusion, angioplasty was performed in 55/56 patients with reopening of coronary vessels. Angioplasty was successful in 36/55 patients (65%) and unsuccessful in 19/55 patients (35%) taking into account an improvement of 20% of coronary luminal narrowing as significant. In 2/55 patients (4%) coronary vessel reocclusion occurred during angioplasty.

Coronary anatomy

In group I coronary luminal narrowing measured 94,2 ± 8,6% before and 78 ± 11.9% after recanalization. In 47/64 patients control before discharge revealed a narrowing of 77.2 ± 14.8%. In group II coronary luminal narrowing measured 96.9 ± 6,6% before and 82.8 ± 6% after medical mechanical recanalization. After angioplasty coronary stenosis measured 46.9 ± 30.5%. Dividing in the subgroup with successful angioplasty revealed a coronary narrowing of 28.0 ± 16.3% and with unsuccessful PTCA of 84.7 ± 7.6%. The control before discharge performed in 43/63 patients (79%) with reperfusion of occluded coro-

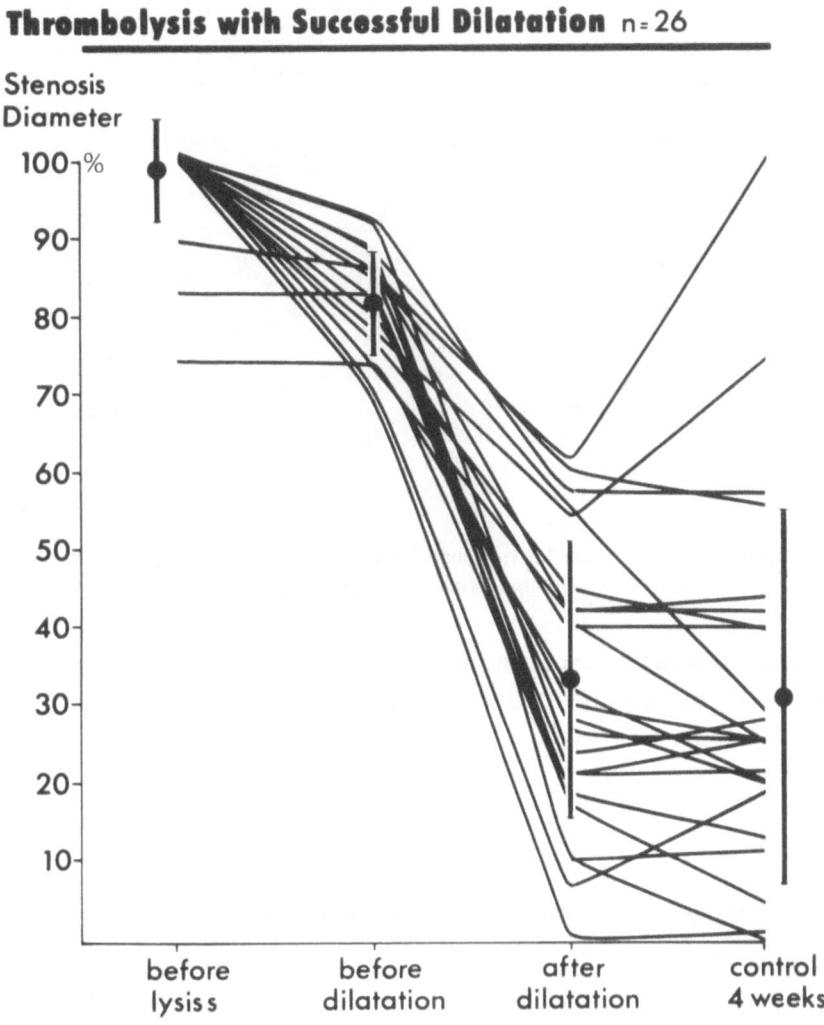

Figure 3. Degree of coronary luminal diameter narrowing before and after medical-mechanical recanalization and at the control 4 weeks later in group I.

36

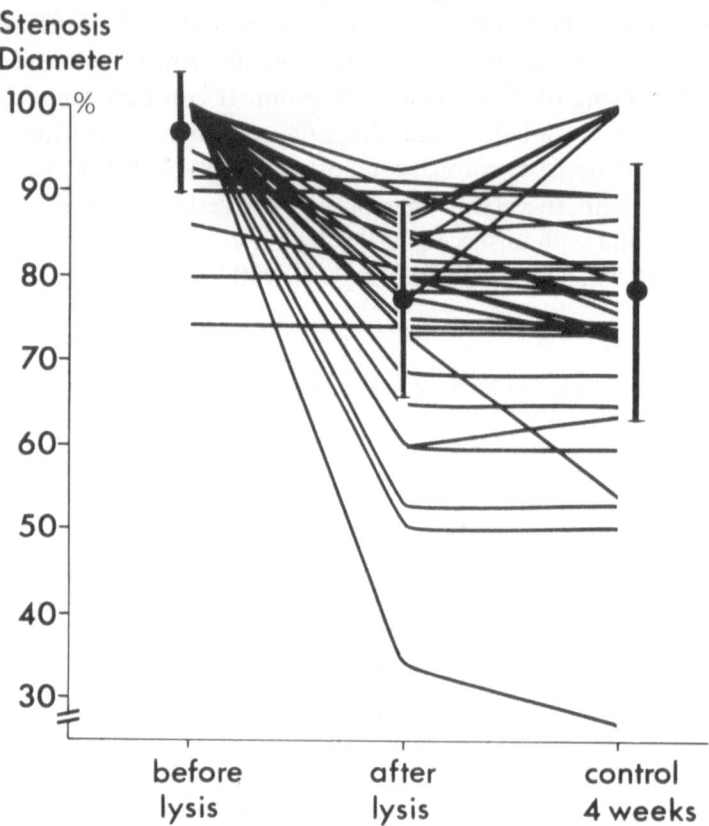

Thrombolysis without Dilatation n=47

Stenosis
Diameter
100%

Figure 4. Degree of coronary luminal narrowing before and after medical-mechanical recanalization and at the control 4 weeks later in group II with additional percutaneous transluminal angioplasty.

nary arteries showed that in patients with successful and unsuccessful angioplasty mean value of coronary luminal narrowing remained constant with 29.8 ± 22.4% and 87.2 ± 12% (Figures 3, 4).

Coronary thrombus

Incidence of filling defects, suggesting coronary thrombus, are listed in Figure 5, indicating percentage of dissolvement and coronary embolism.

Coronary Thrombus _____

35/127 patients (**28**%)

20/35 persistent thrombus (**57**%)
  6/20 reocclusion (**30**%)
15/35 dissolvement (**43**%)
  4/35 peripheral coronary
             embolization (**11**%)

Figure 5. Coronary thrombus opacification, indicated by filling defects, after successful medical-mechanical recanalization.

Early reocclusion and reinfarction

Acute stage: In 6/62 patients (10%) in whom coronary vessels were open at the first coronary angiogram or reopened during medical therapy without mechanical intervention reocclusion occurred in the cath lab. Mechanical recanalization was successful in all patients. In 4 patients with a G 20–30 balloon catheter and in 2 with 3 F Steerable catheters. In 10/52 patients (19%) reocclusion occurred after mechanical recanalization. The difference to those demonstrating reocclusion after medical reperfusion was not significant. Mechanical reopening was possible in all patients twice with J 20–30, twice with G 20–30 and six times with 3 F recanalization catheters.

Late reocclusion

During hospital stay reocclusion occurred in group I in 10/59 patients (17%) and in group II in 9/55 patients (16%). Dividing patients in a group II with successful and unsuccessful angioplasty reocclusion was found in 3/36 patients (8%) and in 6/17 patients (38%) respectively (p<0.001) (Figures 6–8).

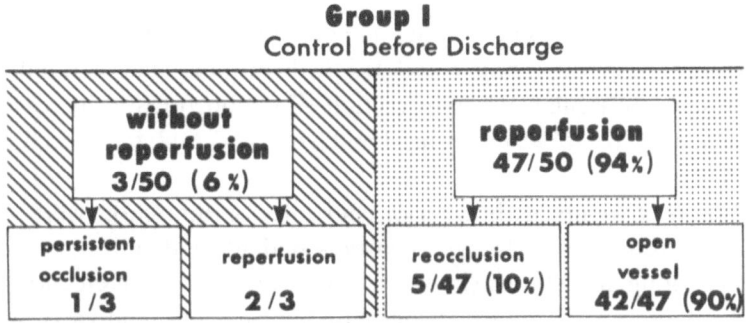

Figure 6. Follow-up of group I during hospital stay. Included are only patients in whom control coronary angiography before discharge could be performed.

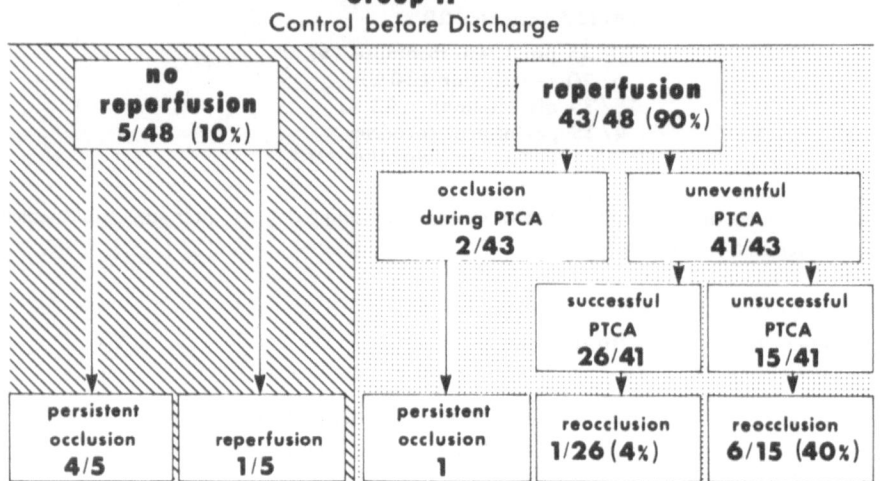

Figure 7. Follow-up of group II during hospital stay. Included are only patients in whom control coronary angiography before discharge could be performed.

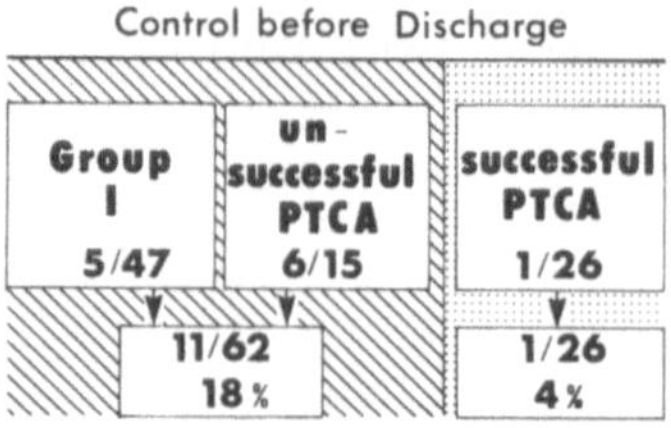

Figure 8. Reocclusion rate in patients of group I and patients of group II with unsuccessful angioplasty compared to patients of group II with successful angioplasty.

Left ventricular function

Comparison of left ventricular volumes and ejection fraction revealed no significant difference between group I and II. Both groups demonstrated a slight increase of left ventricular ejection fraction. Ejection fraction increased from $55.9 \pm 10.6\%$ to $56.6 \pm 12.8\%$ in group I and from $52.8 \pm 12.4\%$ to $55.3 \pm 13.8\%$ in group II.

Subgroups of patients with anterior and inferior infarction were also not significant different. Successful angioplasty in patients with anterior myocardial infarction and long infarct time showed a significant increase of ejection fraction from $45.3 \pm 9.8\%$ to $59.1 \pm 14\%$, while patients without angioplasty showed a constant ejection fraction of $49.6 \pm 6.6\%$ and $49.4 \pm 16.2\%$ ($p < 0.05$).

Hospital mortality

During hospital stay 7/64 (11%) in group I had a cardiac death and 4/63 (6%) in group II. In group II in addition 3 cases of acute respiratory distress syndrome and one subarachnoidal bleeding was observed. In group I 1 case demonstrated an anaphylactic reaction during acute catheterization and 1 rupture during resuscitation occurring with hemorrhagic shock. In group I 1 ventricular septum defekt and 1 free wall rupture and in group II 1 free wall rupture was observed. The latter could be acute operated. Patient died later on septic shock.

Discussion

Mechanical recanalization was attempted with coronary angiography catheters [4] and guide wires [2, 3, 7, 10, 11, 12], complicated by perforation of coronary arteries in 4% [11]. Previous studies demonstrated that mechanical recanalization can safely be performed by angioplasty catheters in acute myocardial infarction and the chronic stage [13]. Even main stem occlusions could be recanalized [14]. Combining medical streptolysis therapy with mechanical approach reperfusion rate could be increased up to 90% [15]. Recanalization was possible with 4 F balloon angioplasty catheters but also with 3 F specially designed recanalzation catheters which were available with G and J as well as Steerable wires. The advantage of 3 F catheters is that they can be guided by 7 F catheters whereas for 4 F balloon catheters 8 F or 9 F guide catheters are necessary. In addition time of preparation of a 3 F recanalization catheter is much shorter than of a balloon catheter. Recanalization with balloon catheters possess however the possibility of consecutive angioplasty without an additional change of guide catheters. With both types of catheters no side effects, no perforation was observed.

For both groups only in the mean a time of 13 and 14 minutes was found between start of ic streptolysis therapy and reperfusion of the vessel. This time is lower than the time reported for streptolysis therapy alone with time intervals of 23 ± 12 min [2] and 36 ± 8 min [7].

In more than 50% of the patients, in group I up to 66%, were mechanically recanalized. Only in few cases mechanical approach failed. In 2 patients in group I and 7 patients in group II reperfusion took place before recanalization could be performed. During superselective streptolysis therapy after failing of mechanical recanalization reperfusion was found in 2 patients in group I and 7 patients in group II, as suggested by others [5].

Combining medical mechanical recanalization reperfusion rate could be increased to 92% in group I and 89% in group II. By conventional streptolysis therapy reperfusion rate ranged from 60% [3] to 86% [2], in the mean about 70%.

Combination of intravenous and intracoronary streptolysis therapy was performed according to reports of others [15]. Also in our study values of open vessels at the first coronary angiogram was higher than previously reported [2, 16, 17, 18].

After opening of the vessel coronary thrombus was observed in 28% of our patients clearly underlining the concept of combining mechanical recanalization with streptolysis therapy. These results are in agreement with other reports [16, 18]. Coronary embolization was observed in 11% with consecutive lysis of the embolism. Dissolution of the coronary thrombus was found in 43%.

In patients with mechanical recanalization reocclusionrate was performed higher than in patients with open coronary arteries and those in whom reperfusion took place during ic streptolysis therapy (10 and 19% respectively). But in all patients mechanical recanalization was again successful leading to permanent perfusion. Also in patients with reocclusion during continuous streptolysis therapy recanalization was mechanically successful.

Reocclusion during hospital stay occurred in group I in 17%, in group II in 16% of patients with successful reperfusion. The difference was not significant different. In group II a significant difference was found between reocclusion and reinfarction rate in those with successful angioplasty (8%) and those with unsuccessful reocclusion (38%). Angioplasty was complicated by 3.6% occlusion during the procedure.

Regarding left ventricular function no significant difference between group I and II were found. Both groups showed a slight improvement of left ventricular ejection fraction during hospital stay [16, 18].

In the subgroup of patients with long infarct times and anterior myocardial infarction, left ventricular ejection fraction increased significantly higher in the group with angioplasty than in those without this additional procedure. This is of course related to the left ventricular function in these patients with salvage of myocardium by using angioplasty in addition to recanalization.

Conclusion

This randomized study demonstrates that by combination of intravenous and intracoronary streptolysis therapy with mechanical approach for recanalization, reperfusion rate could be increased and infarct times shortened. Reocclusion and infarct rate could be significantly reduced by angioplasty with low side effects. In patients with critical left ventricular function salvage of myocardium could be increased by additional angioplasty.

References

1. Kjaha F, Walton J, Brymer JF, Lo E, Osterberger L, O'Neill W, Colfer T, Weiss R, Lee Te, Kurian Th, Goldberg D, Pitt B, Goldstein S (1983) Intracoronary fibrinolytic therapy in acute

myocardial infarction. Report of a prospective randomized trial. New Engl J of Med 308: 1305

2. Timmis GC, Gangadharan V, Hauser A, Ramos RG, Westveer DC, Gordon S (1982) Intracoronary streptokinase in clinical practise. Am Heart J 104: 925

3. Spann JF, Sherry S, Blase A, Mann RH, McCann WD, Gault JH, Gentzler RD, Rosenberg KM, Maurer AH, Denenberg BS, Warner WF, Rubin RN, Malmud LS, Comerota A (1982) High-Dose, brief intravenous streptokinase early in acute myocardial infarction. Am Heart J 104: 939

4. Neuhaus KL, Köstering H, Tebbe U, Sauer G, Kreuzer H (1981) Intravenöse urzzeitstreptokinase-Therapy beim frischen Myocardinfarkt. Z. Kardiol. 70: 791

5. Ganz W, Buchbinder N, Marcus, Mondkar A, Moddohi J, Charuzi Y, O'Connor L, Shell W, Fischbein MC, Kass R, Miyamoto A, Swan HJC (1981) Intracoronary thrombolysis in evolving myocardial infarction. Am Heart J 101: 4

6. Tennant ST, Dixon J, Venable TH C, Page HL, Roach A, Kaiser A, Frederiksen R, Tacogue L, Kaplan P, Babu S, Anderson E, Wooten E, Hennings S, Breinig J, Campbell WB (1983) Intracoronary thromboylsis in patients with acute myocardial infarction: comparison of the efficacy of urokinase with streptokinase. Circulation 69: 756

7. Reduto L, Smalling R, Freund GC, Gould Kl: Intracoronary infusion of streptokinase in patients with acute myocardial infarction (1981) Effects of reperfusion on left ventricular performance. Am J Cardiol 48: 403

8. Erbel R, Schweizer P, Krebs S, Langen HJ, Meyer, Effert S (1984) Effects of heart rate changes on left ventricular volume and ejection fraction. Am J Cardiol 53: 590

9. Erbel R, Rebs W, Schweizer, Richter HA, Meyer, Effert S (1982) Comparison of single plane and biplane volume determination by two-dimensional echocardiography: A study in asymmetric model hearts. Eur Heart J 3: 469

10. Mathey DG, Schofer J, Kuck KH, Beil UL, Klöppel G (1982) Transmural haemorrhagic myocardial infarction after intracoronary streptokinase. Clinical, angiographic and necropsy findings. Br Heart J 48: 546

11. Rutsch W, Schartl M, Mathey D, Kuck K, Merx W, Dörr R, Rentrop P, Blanke H, Karsch K (1982) Perkutane transluminale koronare Rekanalisation: Methodik, Ergebnisse und Komplikationen. Z Kardiol 71: 7

12. Kasper W, Erbel R, Meinertz T, Drexler M, Rückel A, Pop T, Prellwitz W, Meyer J: Intracoronary thrombolysis with a new acylated streptokinase-plasminogen complex (BRL 26921) in patients with acute myocardial infarction. J Am Coll Cardiol (in press).

13. Schreiner G, Erbel R, Meyer J (1984) Bedeutung von Koronarspasmen bei der percutanen transluminalen coronaren Angioplastie (PTCA). Z Kardiol 73, Suppl. 1, 32 (abstr)

14. Erbel R, Meinertz T, Wessler J, Meyer J, Seybold-Epting W (1984) Recanalization of occluded left main coronary artery in unstable angina pectoris. Am Cardiol J 53: 1725–1727

15. Schwarz F, Hofmann M, Schuler G, v. Olshausen K, Zimmermann K, Kübler W (1984) Thrombolysis in acute myocardial infarction: Effect of intravenous followed by intracoronary streptokinase application on estimates of infarct size. Am J Cardiol 53: 1505

16. Rentrop P, Blanke H, Karsch R, Kaiser H, Köstering H, Leitz K (1982) Selective intracoronary thrombolysis in acute myocardial infarction and unstable angina pectoris. Circulation 63: 307

17. Mathey DG, Kuck KH, Tilsner V, Krebber HJ, Bleifeld W (1981) Nonsurgical coronary artery recanalization in acute transluminal myocardial infarction. Circulation 63: 489

18. Mathey DG, Kuck KH, Remmecke J, Tilsner V, Bleifeld W (1980) Transluminal recanalization of coronary artery thrombosis: a preliminary report of its application in cardiogenic shock. Eur Heart J 1: 207

Autopsy findings in 14 patients with myocardial infarction treated with thrombolysis or combined thrombolysis and PTCA

CHRISTOPH DÜBER, HANS-JOACHIM RUMPELT and
RAIMUND ERBEL

Patients

From March 1 (1983) to June 15 (1984) 127 patients with evolving myocardial infarction (MI) entered a randomized clinical trial at the II. Medizinische Klinik, Johannes Gutenberg-Universität, Mainz.

Medical-mechanical recanalization (group A) of the infarct-related artery (including systemic and intracoronary thrombolysis and catheter probing) was compared with medical-mechanical recanalization and subsequent PTCA (group B).

In-hospital death (within 4 weeks) occured in 19 cases (15%).

Fourteen patients (12 men, 2 women; age 45–75 years, mean: 63 years; interval from infarct to recanalization 85–510 min, mean: 4 h; interval from infarction to death 0–22 days, mean: 8 days), who underwent complete necropsy examination within 48 hours after death at the Pathologisch-Anatomisches Institut, Johannes Gutenberg-Universität, Mainz form the basis of this study.

Methods

The heart was removed by transsection of the large arteries and veins. The epicardial coronary arteries were carefully excised, fixed in formalin decalcified, cut into 2–3 mm long segments, and then processed for microscopy. Interesting segments (site of thrombosis or angioplasty) were step-sectioned. The sections were stained with hematoxylin and eosin and Elastica van Gieson/Goldner.

The heart was packed with cellulose, fixed in formalin, and then sectioned according to the apical four chamber-view of echocardiography. For complete assessment of the myocardium the heart was sliced transversely from apex to base at 1 cm intervals. Sections from normal appearing myocardium, the junction of normal and infarcted tissue, and the central portion of the infarct were stained with hematoxylin and eosin, van Gieson, and Goldner.

Results

Clinical data, and autopsy findings of the coronary arteries and the myocardial infarcts are listed in Table 1.

A large tear of the interventricular septum with hemorrhagic pericardial effusion and tamponade in one patient (group A) and rupture of the ventricular wall and anterior papillary muscle in another case (group B) were noted as complications of myocardial infarction.

A massive bleeding at the puncture site of the femoral artery extending to the retroperitoneum was referred to thrombolytic therapy in one patient (group A).

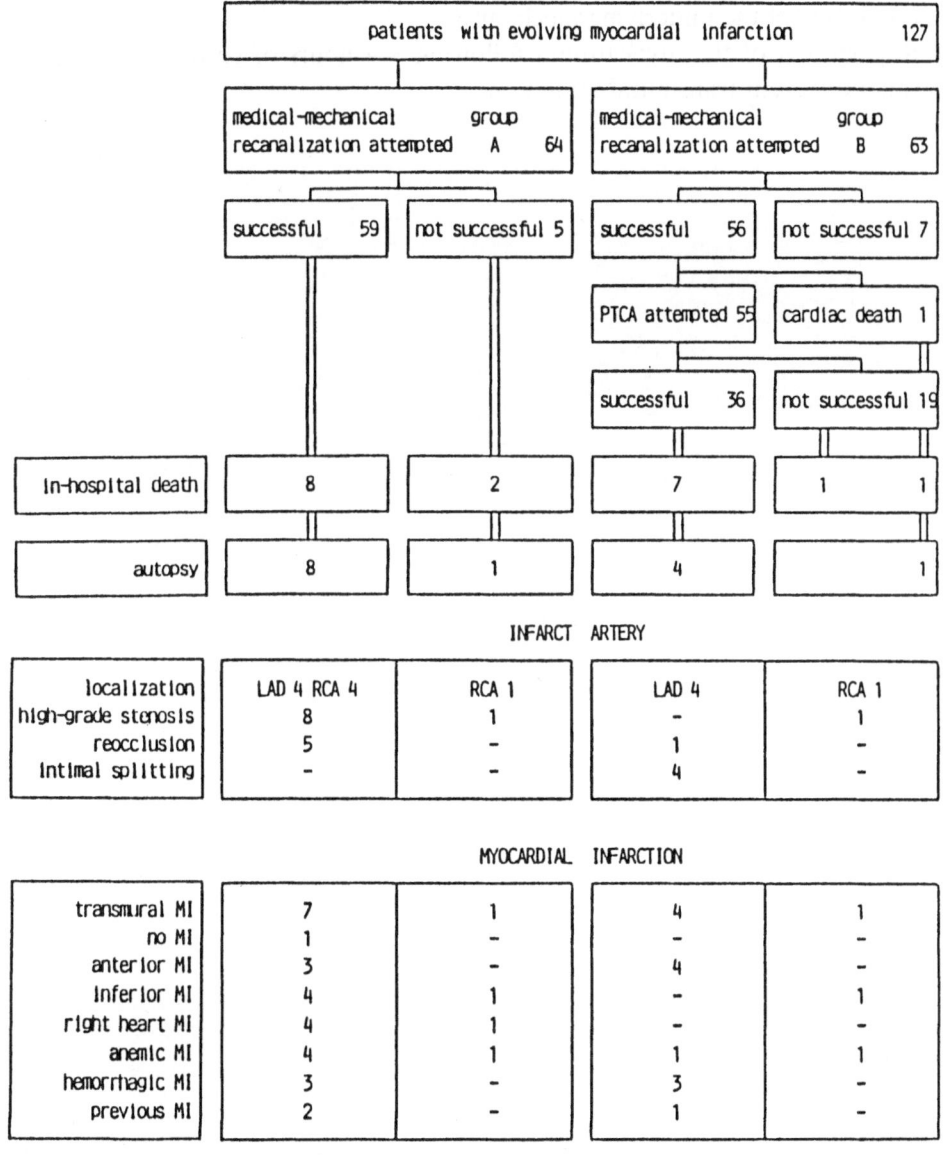

patients with evolving myocardial infarction			127
medical-mechanical group recanalization attempted A 64		medical-mechanical group recanalization attempted B 63	
successful 59	not successful 5	successful 56	not successful 7
		PTCA attempted 55	cardiac death 1
		successful 36	not successful 19

in-hospital death	8	2	7	1 1
autopsy	8	1	4	1

INFARCT ARTERY

localization	LAD 4 RCA 4	RCA 1	LAD 4	RCA 1
high-grade stenosis	8	1	–	1
reocclusion	5	–	1	–
intimal splitting	–	–	4	–

MYOCARDIAL INFARCTION

transmural MI	7	1	4	1
no MI	1	–	–	–
anterior MI	3	–	4	–
inferior MI	4	1	–	1
right heart MI	4	1	–	–
anemic MI	4	1	1	1
hemorrhagic MI	3	–	3	–
previous MI	2	–	1	–

There was cardiac death in all patients from group A while there were noncardiac causes (ARDS: 3 patients; postoperative multiple organ failure: 1 patient) in group B.

Conclusions

– High grade atheromatous stenosis of the infarct-related artery is a common finding after successful thrombolysis with a considerable risk of early reocclusion.
– PTCA can effectively reduce coronary obstruction. Intimal (and medial) splitting is one of the underlying mechanisms.
– Reperfusion of the myocardium following 3–4 hours of coronary occlusion cannot prevent transmural infarction.

Thrombolytic therapy in myocardial infarction: Are fibrinolytic drugs comparable, and similarly effective?

M. SAMAMA and E. SZWARCER

Introduction

Many authors consider that SK and UK are both useful thrombolytic agents [1]. They also consider that the choice between SK and UK is influenced by economic considerations [2].

A recent excellent review in the New England Journal of Medicine states that its (UK) major advantages over streptokinase is that it is not antigenic or pyrogenic, but its cost is more than five times as high [2].

The aim of this presentation is to demonstrate that each of these drugs has several different characteristics which should be taken into consideration by cardiologists.

Moreover, three more promising thrombolytic agents have become available. Streptokinase-plasminogen acylated complex and tissue plasminogen activator are now available for clinical trials. Also, pro-Urokinase is ready for experimental usage. We will come back to these later.

The four important differences between SK and UK are the following:

– Doses although expressed in I.U. for SK and UK are really not truly comparable.

– Laboratory control is sharply different because of vast differences in fibrinogen lowering effect.

– The frequency of side effects mainly bleeding accidents seems also quite different.

– Finally, combination with heparin has to be much more careful with SK compared to UK.

Doses in I.U. are not comparable

The mechanisms of action of UK and SK are very different where UK has a direct action on plasminogen with a possible plasma inhibitor while SK has an indirect action on plasminogen with no plasma inhibitor [1, 3].

In vitro, it has been shown in our lab and in the laboratory of Robbins that 1 I.U. of SK generates 10 times as much plasmin as 1 I.U. of UK [4].

In vivo, in acute myocardial infarction, the comparative dosages of UK and SK are not well documented at present.

We have produced some data showing that the active dosage of UK necessary to achieve reopening of the coronary arteries by intracoronary infusion may be at least two and half times higher than the dose per minute of SK [5]. However, in this trial, Lys-plasminogen was added to the UK dosage to increase its activity.

More recently, Tennant et al. in a similar comparison demonstrates that 3 times as much of UK produces similar results on coronary reopening compared to SK. However, as expected, fibrinogen depletion under 1 g/l was much more common with SK than with UK [6].

Laboratory control and fibrinogen lowering

SK causes a rapid and dramatic decrease in plasma fibrinogen and plasminogen which is almost independent of dosage.

In contrast, while using UK, there is a less rapid and less dramatic drop in fibrinogen and plasminogen which is dose-dependent and therefore titratable. This was clearly demonstrated by our group and others [5, 7, 8, 9].

Therefore, the proper laboratory procedures will include: Plasma fibrinogen (however, different methods can give different results due to interference of FDP), thrombin clotting time (and/or reptilase clotting time), FDP measurement in serum, as well as prothrombin time (PT) and activated partial thromboplastin time (APTT).

Side effects are mostly bleeding problems

The hemorrhagic risk seems theoretically higher when fibrinogen is depleted (under 1 g/l) and thus should be more probable with SK than with UK.

This is strongly suggested by our personal experience [10] as well as that seen in the literature [11]. Table 1 illustrates bleeding problems occurring at various dosages of intracoronary and intravenous streptokinase with or without heparin.

Combination with heparin

It is generally accepted that the risk is increased when heparin is used especially with SK.

However, heparin does have a value even though we have to consider the hazards.

For example, there is a rate of recurrence of myocardial infarction after successful thrombolysis (15 to 35%) and this rate might be reducible by heparin

Table 1. Bleeding complications during intracoronary (I.C.) and intravenous (I.V.) SK therapy with and without heparin.

Authors	Patients n	SK dose × 10^3 I.U.	Bleeding
Breddin et al. 1973	102	250/h × 3 I.V.	4% 2 epixtaxis, 1 intestinal, 1 hematuria
Kennedy et al. 1983	134 SK 116 C	250 to 350 Intracoronary + Heparin	5,2% Puncture site
Merx et al.	204	25 to 400 Intraconorary + Heparin about 800/h.	7.4% (complications → transfusions)
Rentrop et al. 1981	29	I.C. 15 to 200	oozing (rare), bleedings at puncture site (2)
Meyer et al. 1982	21	I.C. 130	no accident
Cowley et al. 1983	23	I.C. 200 ± 74	Hemopericardium (1) cerebral hemorrhages (2) with heparin Hemorrhage (2) and one death.
Khaja et al. 1983	20	I.C. 250	No accident
Rogers et al. 1983	51	I.C. 240 I.V. 500 to 1.000	Hematoma Blood transfusion 10%
Alderman et al. 1984	28	I.C. 340 I.V.725	Episodes with heparin (4) Hematuria, retroperitoneal hematoma, intestinal bleeding, hematoma.

C = control

administration [12, 13]. However, we must be careful since full doses of heparin immediatly after SK are known to produce bleeding accidents within the first 24 to 72 hours.

UK and heparin are often used together in Europe and seems to be safer when compared to SK usage [14].

In order to reduce the risk of bleeding manifestations, heparin should be given in continuous infusion but the dosage reduced during any severe hypofibrinogenemia (under 1 g/l). The dose later may be progressively increased as the fibrinogen elevates.

For example, as the graph illustrates, immediately after SK administration, heparin dosage should be low but gradually increased as the fibrinogen level climbs as time elapses (Figure 1).

Of course, the laboratory control will include fibrinogen, Partial Thromboplastin Time (APTT) or recalcification clotting time in order to monitor properly this early critical stage.

48

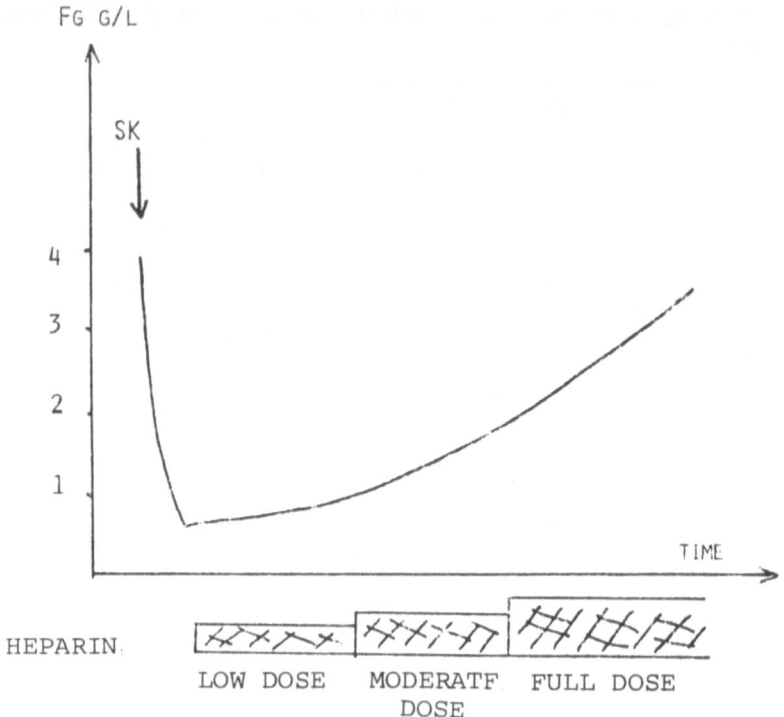

Figure 1. Plasma fibrinogen level evolution during and after SK therapy. Adjustment of heparin dosage according to fibrinogen level.

The actual dosage of heparin in these situations is not totally worked out and will require laboratory and clinical judgement. Using this theorical scheme, this appears to us to be the most reasonable approach at this time.

Let us now return to the most recent thrombolytic developments which may well become of greater significance than all that we have mentioned previously.

If we consider the fibrinolytic system, two important plasminogen activators are tissue plasminogen activator (t-PA) and pro-Urokinase, both have been obtained by genetic engineering [15, 16].

The modality which has recently come in to considerable prominence is t-PA.

This physiological endogenous compound is available for pharmacological studies and clinical trials [17, 18]. It converts directly plasminogen bound to fibrin into plasmin. However, a plasma inhibitor does exist.

Its activity can be demonstrated in vitro through the usage of a standard hanging clot suspended in a plasma environment containing one of these thrombolytic agents.

This clot should be prepared with a known amount of labelled fibrinogen. The rate of lysis can be followed by the measurements of radioactivity released during thrombolysis. Moreover fibrinogen and plasminogen in the surrounding plasma can also be measured to confirm the fibrinogen degradation.

t-PA was found by Collen's group [19] and by ourselves to be more active than UK in thrombolysis (unpublished results).

It is noted that plasma fibrinogen level does not decrease markedly during this process using t-PA unlike comparable use of UK or SK.

Therefore since fibrinogen is not lowered, laboratory monitoring of fibrinogen or plasminogen may not be necessary.

Side effects so far are not evaluated sufficiently since very few patients have received this modality.

Doctor Collen will undoubtelly discuss this problem further in the same issue. Finally, combination with heparin does seems logical and, we hope, will prove safe.

Two other compounds, acylated streptokinase plasminogen and pro-urokinase, exhibit similar potential as t-PA, i.d., being able to lyse clots without producing a severe systemic lytic state [20, 21].

Very few clinical data are, at present, available [22] and only well conducted randomized trials will be able to determine the therapeutic value of these new thrombolytic agents.

In conclusion, a proper choice of drug, SK or UK, is often difficult and not fully documented.

Differences between SK and UK cannot be ignored and t-PA therapy may bring a solution to this whole problem and may be the future in thrombolytic therapy.

With SK and UK, lab monitoring is important for heparin dosage and a fine balance must be achieved to reduce clotting but maintain safety.

The three new compounds on the horizon must be watched with close attention since at least one of them will probably replace these older agents and be only the next in a series of progressions.

Summary

Acute myocardial infarction is actually treated by intracoronary or intravenous routes with SK, UK (alone or associated with lys-plasminogen), or t-PA (tissue plasminogen activator).

Activity of these fibrinolytic agents is expressed in apparently equivalent international units, but they are clearly different. For instance, 1 I.U. of SK generates 10 times more plasmin than 1 I.U. of UK; SK has an indirect mechanism of action on plasminogen, while UK acts directly, and T-PA has the particularity of requiring fibrin for its activity; and the in vivo effect on circulating plasminogen and fibrinogen is different: they decrease more importantly when using SK than UK, nearly no modifications occuring when using t-PA.

Also, hemorrhagic complications seem more frequent with SK than with UK, experience with t-PA being still needed.

The fibrinolytic activity of these activators can be measured using different methods: fibrin plates (using bovine or human fibrinogen); fibrinogen-plasminogen clot lysis assays in the presence of one lytic agent (recorded visually, with thromboelastography or otherwise), and, doing so, t-PA was found more active than HMW UK or LMW UK.

Comparison of results using intracoronary SK or UK in personal work and in the literature, suggest that higher amounts of UK are needed for coronary reopenings. Moreover, combination of heparin with moderate doses of UK seems possible while contraindicated with SK. Finally, the dosage of heparin to be used after completion of SK or UK treatment should be adjusted taking into account the evolution of plasma fibrinogen level.

References

1. Sharma GVRK, Cella G, Parisi AF, Sasahara AA (1982) Thrombolytic therapy. N. Engl. J. Med. 306: 1268–1276
2. Laffel GL, Braunwald E (1984) Thrombolytic therapy: a new strategy for the treatment of acute myocardial infarction (first of two parts). N. Engl. J. Med. 311: 710–717
3. Samama M, Szwarcer E, Conard J, Horellou MH (1984) Thrombolysis. In: Recent advances in blood coagulation; n° 4, L. Poller (ed) Churchill Livingstone, pp 267–299
4. Robbins KC (1982) Fibrinolysis. In: Kwaan HC, Bowie EJW (ed) Thrombosis. W.B. Sanders Company, Philadelphia pp 23–28
5. de Prost D, Guerot C, Laffay N, Horellou MH, Samama M (1983) Intra coronary thrombolysis with streptokinase or lys-plasminogen/urokinase in acute myocardial infarction: effects on recanalization and blood fibrinolysis. Thromb. haemostas. 50: 792–796
6. Tennant SN, Dixon J, Venable JC, Page HL, Roach A, Kaiser AB et al. (1984) Intra coronary thrombolysis in patients with acute myocardial infarction: comparison of the efficacy of urokinase with streptokinase. Circulation 69: 756–760
7. Conard J, Samama M (1972) Laboratory control of SK therapy in Losito R. Ed. Present status of thrombosis its pathophysiology, diagnosis and treatment. Proceedings of International Symposium on intravascular coagulation and fibrinolysis. Sherbrooke Schattauer – Verlag, Stuttgart pp 191–198
8. Marder VJ (1979) Use of thrombolytic agents choice of patient, drug, administration, laboratory monitoring. Annals Intern Med 90: 802–808
9. Samama M, Conard J (1977) Biological results during UK therapy at different doses. In Paoletti R., Sherry S. (eds) Thrombosis and Urokinase. Academic Press, New York, 1977, 243–244
10. Conard J, Samama M, Milochevitch R, Horellou MH, Chabrun B, Prestat J (1979) Complicactions hémorragiques au cours de 98 traitements par la SK. Place de la surveillance biologique. Nouv Presse Méd 8: 1319–1325
11. Timmis GP, Bandagharan V, Ramos RG (1984) Hemorrhage and the products of fibrinogen digestion after intra-coronary administration of streptokinase. Circulation 69: 1146–1152
12. Gold HK, Leinbac RC, Palacios IF (1983) Coronary reocclusion after selective administration of streptokinase. Circulation 68: 150–154
13. Lee G, Low RI, Takeda P (1982) Importance of follow-up medical and surgical approaches to prevent reinfaction, reocclusion, and recurrent angina following intracoronary thrombolysis with streptokinase in acute myocardial infarction. Am Heart J 104: 921–924

14. Serradimigni A, Romani A, Chiche B, Aubry J, Philip F (1981) Les indications des thrombolytiques dans les thromboses veineuses et l'embolie pulmonaire. Rev. Prat. 31: 3793–3804

15. Pennica D, Holmes WE, Kohr WJ, Harkins RN, Vehar GA, Ward CA, Bennett WF, Yelverton E, Seeburg PH, Heyneker HL, Goeddel DV, Collen D (1983) Cloning and expression of human tissue-type plasminogen activator cDNA in E. Coli. Nature 301: 214–220

16. Zamarron C, Lijnen HR, Van Hoef B, Collen D (1984) Biological and thrombolytic properties of proenzyme and active forms of human urokinase. I. Fibrinolytic and fibrinogenolytic properties in human plasma in vitro of urokinases obtained from human urine or by recombinant DNA technology. Thromb. Haemostas. 52: 19–23

17. Sobel BE, Gross RW, Robison AK (1984) Thrombolysis, clot selectivity and kinetics. Circulation 70: 160–164

18. Sobel BE, Geltman EM, Tiefenbrunn AJ (1984) Improvement of regional myocardial metabolism after coronary thrombosis induced with tissue type plasminogen activator or streptokinase. Circulation 69: 983–990

19. Matsuo O, Rijnen DC, Collen D (1981) Comparison of the relative fibrinogenolytic, fibrinolytic and thrombolytic properties of tissue plasminogen activator and urokinase in vitro. Thromb. Haemostas. 45: 225–229

20. Smith RAG, Dupe RJ, English PD, Green J (1981) Fibrinolysis with acyl-enzymes: a new approach to thrombolytic therapy. Nature, 290: 505–508

21. Gurewich V, Parnell R, Louie S, Kelley P, Suddith RL, Greenlee R (1984) Effective and fibrin-specific clot lysis by a zymogen precursor form of urokinase (pro-urokinase). J. Clin. Invest. 73: 1731–1739

22. Kasper W, Erbel R, Meinertz T (1984) Intracoronary thrombolytis with an acylated streptokinase-plasminogen activator (BRL 26921) in patients with acute myocardial infarction. J. Am. Cardiol. 4: 357–363

Coronary thrombolysis with tissue-type plasminogen activator (t-PA)

D. COLLEN

Rationale for thrombolytic therapy of acute myocardial infarction

Coronary thrombolysis is presently under intensive investigation as a treatment for acute myocardial infarction for two main reasons. Firstly it is now well established that acute myocardial infarction is often associated with thrombotic occlusion of an atherosclerotic coronary artery [1]. Secondly it has been shown that administration of thrombolytic agents can reopen an occluded coronary artery in the majority of patients [2, 3] and that reperfusion of ischemic myocardial tissue is generally well tolerated. Coronary thrombolysis is however not a goal in itself but is employed to prevent necrosis and dysfunction of jeopardized myocardial cells. There is ample evidence in animals that the infarct size is smaller and the myocardial function better when an occluded coronary artery is reopened within at most a couple of hours [4]. The proof that coronary reperfusion is of real benefit to patients with acute myocardial infarction in terms of morbidity or mortality is however still lacking [5–7]. To this end several large-scale trials are currently in progress.

If the assumption that early reperfusion of a thrombosed coronary artery may be of benefit to the patient is correct, practical therapeutic schemes should fulfill or approach the following requirements: (1) coronary catheterization with its unavoidable morbidity, delay, and cost should be circumvented; (2) the thrombolytic agent should be effective and specific and should not produce a generalized breakdown of the hemostatic system; and (3) the agent should be widely applicable and safe, and should not require specific laboratory monitoring.

Several thrombolytic agents including urokinase [8], acylated streptokinase-plasminogen complex [9], tissue-type plasminogen activator [10] and pro-urokinase (unpublished) are presently evaluated with a view toward achieving therapeutic coronary thrombolysis with a better clot selectivity and more safety than can presently be obtained with streptokinase.

Human tissue-type plasminogen activator (t-PA) exhibits considerable fibrin-specificity [11]; it induced thrombolysis without systemic fibrinogenolysis in experimental animals with thrombosis [12, 13] and in a pilot study in patients [14]. Until recently, extensive studies of the potential clinical utility of t-PA were hampered by the lack of availability of the enzyme from natural sources [15] but this obstacle has now been overcome by the cloning and expression of the human t-PA gene [16].

Here we will briefly summarize the studies performed to date in animal models and in patients with acute myocardial infarction.

Studies with t-PA in animals with experimental coronary thrombosis

At present, four studies with t-PA in animal models for myocardial infarction have been completed [17–20].

Bergmann et al. [17] produced a thrombus in the left anterior descending (LAD) coronary artery with a copper coil. Intravenous or intracoronary infusion of t-PA, obtained from cell culture fluid, at a rate of 10,000 IU/min produced coronary reperfusion of 1–2 hours old occlusions within 10 min. In addition intermediary metabolism and nutritional myocardial blood flow were restored and thrombolysis was obtained without inducing a systemic fibrinolytic state.

Van de Werf et al. [18] compared the thrombolytic effect of recombinant t-PA with that of urokinase in dogs with a 1-hour old LAD occlusion introduced with a copper coil. Infusion of 1,000 IU (10 μg)/kg/min intravenous rt-PA in 9 dogs elicited reperfusion within 14 min without producing systemic fibrinolysis or distal coronary embolization. Infusion of urokinase at the same rate elicited thrombolysis in seven of 10 dogs within an average of 19 min. However, distal coronary embolization occurred in two dogs and systemic fibrinolysis was observed in all. In three dogs treated with urokinase thrombolysis was obtained only with subsequent intracoronary infusion. Restoration of myocardial perfusion and metabolism assessed with positron-emission tomography was consistently noted in dogs treated with rt-PA.

Gold et al. [19] studied the thrombolytic potency and infarct sparing potential of recombinant t-PA (rt-PA) in open chested, anesthetized dogs. Localized coronary thrombosis was produced in the LAD by endothelial injury and instillation of thrombin and fresh blood. After 2 hours of stable thrombotic occlusion, rt-PA was infused intravenously. At 5 μg/kg/min, time-to-reperfusion was greater than 40 min. However, at higher infusion rates a linear, dose-dependent time to coronary reperfusion was obtained (r = 0.88): at 10 μg/kg/min reperfusion occurred after 31 min; at 15 μg/kg/min it was 26 min; and at 25 μg/kg/min, lysis was obtained within 13 min. Thrombolysis was not associated with alterations in either plasma hemostatic factors (fibrinogen, plasminogen and α_2-antiplasmin) or in systemic blood pressures. Epicardial electrographic measurements revealed a significant reduction in ST elevation in all reperfused hearts.

Gold et al. [19] also performed a randomized-blinded study using 15 μg/kg/min of rt-PA versus saline in 18 dogs with 30 min of coronary thrombosis. Reperfusion in the treated group occurred after 28 min. No evidence of thrombolysis occurred in the saline treated group within 240 minutes. Myocardial infarct size was determined by triphenyl tetrazolium chloride staining and planimetry. Infarction involved 2.5% of the left ventricular wall in the rt-PA group, but 16% of the left ventricle in the saline group.

Flameng et al. [20] produced occlusive thrombi in the LAD of sixteen open chest baboons. In six control animals, occlusive thrombosis persisting over a period of 4 hours as evidenced by coronary arteriography, resulted in large transmural infarction (63% of the perfusion area). In ten animals rt-PA was infused systemically at a rate of 1,000 IU (10 μg) per kg per min for 30 minutes after 30 to 80 min of coronary thrombosis. Reperfusion occurred within 30 min in nine animals. In the rt-PA group mean duration of occlusion before reperfusion was 77 min. Recanalization resulted in an overall reduction of infarct size to 38%. Residual infarction was related to the duration of occlusion ($r = 0.80$). Reperfusion was associated with reduced reflow: myocardial blood flow in the perfusion area of the LAD was only 70% of normal after 4 hours in spite of perfect angiographic refilling. The infusion of rt-PA was not associated with systemic activation of the fibrinolytic system, fibrinogen breakdown or clinically evident bleeding.

From all these studies it is concluded that intravenous injection of t-PA may recanalize thrombosed coronary vessels without inducing a systemic fibrinolytic state. Timely reperfusion results in infarct sparing and restoration of nutritional blood flow.

Studies with t-PA in patients with acute myocardial infarction

Van de Werf et al. [9] performed a pilot study with t-PA obtained from cell culture fluid in seven patients with acute myocardial infarction. Coronary thrombolysis, confirmed angiographically, was induced within 19 to 50 minutes with intravenous or intracoronary t-PA in six of the seven patients. Circulating fibrinogen, plasminogen, and α_2-antiplasmin were not depleted by t-PA, in contrast to the case in the two patients subsequently given streptokinase. In the one patient in whom lysis was not inducible with t-PA, it was also not inducible with streptokinase. These observations indicate that clot-selective coronary thrombolysis can be induced in patients with evolving myocardial infarction by means of t-PA, without concomitant induction of a systemic lytic state. In two of these patients positron emission tomography revealed an improved regional palmitate accumulation following coronary reperfusion with t-PA [21].

At present three large scale studies with recombinant t-PA are in progress. The first study is a prospective, randomized placebo controlled trial of intravenous rt-PA in 50 patients with acute myocardial infarction. It was carried out in Johns Hopkins and Baltimore City Hospitals (Baltimore) Washington University – Barnes Hospital (St. Louis) and Massachussetts General Hospital (Boston). This study is completed and will be reported at the 57th Scientific Sessions of the American Heart Association, Miami, November 1984. The second study is a pilot study in 50 consecutive patients, as a preliminary to the N.I.H. sponsored multicenter randomized comparison of t-PA with streptokinase. The pilot study is completed but the results have not been made available yet. The third study is a multicenter European dual trial of rt-PA versus placebo and rt-PA versus streptokinase in 60 patients each. This study is in progress.

It can be anticipated that the potential clinical utility of rt-PA will at least to some extent be revealed by these studies and that the results will become available in a not too distant future.

References

1. DeWood MA, Spores J, Notske R (1980) Prevalence of total coronary occlusion during the early hours of transmural myocardial infarction. N Engl J Med 303: 897–902
2. Rentrop P, Blanke H, Karsch KR, Kaiser H, Kösterling H, Leitz K (1981) Selective intracoronary thrombolysis in acute myocardial infarction and unstable angina pectoris. Circulation 63: 307–317
3. Schröder R, Biamino G, von Leitner ER (1983) Intravenous short-term infusion of streptokinase in acute myocardial infarction. Circulation 67: 536–548
4. Bergmann SR, Lerch RA, Fox KAA (1982) Temporal dependence of beneficial effects of coronary thrombolysis characterized by positron tomography. Am J Med 73: 573–581
5. Anderson JL, Marshall HW, Bray BE (1983) A randomized trial of intracoronary streptokinase in the treatment of acute myocardial infarction. N Engl J Med 308: 1312–1318
6. Khaja F, Walton JA, Brymer JF (1983) Intracoronary fibrinolytic therapy in acute myocardial infarction. Report of a prospective randomized trial. N Engl J Med 308: 1305–1311
7. Kennedy JW, Ritchie JL, David KB, Fritz JK (1983) Western Washington randomization trial of intracoronary streptokinase in acute myocardial infarction. N Engl J Med 309: 1477–1482
8. Tennant SN, Dixon J, Venable TC (1984) Intracoronary thrombolysis in patients with acute myocardial infarction: comparison of the efficacy of urokinase with streptokinase. Circulation 69: 756–760
9. Walker ID, Davidson JF, Rae AP, Hutton I, Lawrie TDV (1984) Acylated Streptokinase-plasminogen complex in patients with acute myocardial infarction. Thromb. Haemost 51: 204–206
10. Van de Werf F, Ludbrook PA, Bergmann SR (1984) Coronary thrombolysis with tissue-type plasminogen activator in patients with evolving myocardial infarction. N Engl J Med 310: 609–613
11. Matsuo O, Rijken DC, Collen D (1981) Thrombolysis by human tissue plasminogen activator and urokinase in rabbits with experimental pulmonary embolus. Nature 291: 590–591
12. Korninger C, Matsuo O, Suy R, Stassen JM, Collen D (1982) Thrombolysis with human extrinsic (tissue-type)plasminogen activator in dogs with femoral vein thrombosis. J Clin Invest 69: 573–508
13. Collen D, Stassen JM, Verstraete M (1983) Thrombolysis with human extrinsic (tissue-type) plasminogen activator in rabbits with experimental jugular vein thrombosis. Effect of molecular form and dose of activator, age of the thrombus, and route of administration. J Clin Invest 71: 368–376
14. Weimar W, Stibbe J, Van Seyen AJ, Billiau A, De Somer P, Collen D (1981) Specific lysis of an iliofemoral thrombus by administration of extrinsic (tissue-type) plasminogen activator. Lancet, ii: 1018–1020
15. Collen D, Rijken DC, Van Damme J, Billiau A (1982) Purification of human tissue-type plasminogen activator in centrigram quantities from human melanoma cell culture fluid and its conditioning for use in vivo. Thromb Haemost, 48: 294–296
16. Pennica D, Holmes WE, Kohr WJ et al. (1983) Cloning and expression of human tissue-type plasminogen activator cDNA in E Coli Nature 301: 214–221
17. Bergmann SR, Fox KAA, Ter-Pogossian MM, Sobel BE, Collen D (1983) Clot-selective coronary thrombolysis with tissue type plasminogen activator. Science 220: 1181–1183

18. Van de Werf F, Bergmann SR, Fox KAA (1984) Coronary thrombolysis with intravenously administered human tissue-type plasminogen activator produced by recombinant DNA technology. Circulation 69: 605–610
19. Gold HK, Fallon JT, Yasuda T (in press). Coronary thrombolysis with recombinant human tissue-type plasminogen activator. Circulation
20. Flameng W, Van de Werf F, VanHaecke J, Verstraete M, Collen D (in press). Coronary thrombolysis and infarct size reduction following intravenous infusion of recombinant tissue-type plasminogen activator in non-human primates. J Clin Invest
21. Sobel BE, Geltman EM, Tiefenbrunn AJ, Jaffe AS, Spadaro JJ, Collen D, Ludbrook PA (1984) Improvement of regional myocardial metabolism after coronary thrombolysis induced with tissue type plasminogen activator (t-PA) or streptokinase. Circulation 69: 983–990

Financial background of PTCR and PTCA and regional distribution of cardiac catheterization laboratories in the Federal Republic of Germany

R. DÖRR, R. VON ESSEN, S. EFFERT, F. AHNERT and T. TOLXDORFF

Introduction

In comparison with percutaneous transluminal coronary recanalization (PTCR) [1, 2, 3] intravenous administration of a thrombolytic agent [4, 5, 6] has many potential advantages. The former requires only the placement of a peripheral intravenous line and can be initiated any where immediately after the diagnosis of acute myocardial infarction. On the other hand intracoronary reperfusion procedures require an expensive cardiac catheterization laboratory and an emergency team being on call 24 hours a day. Although there may be a possible delay until the initiation of the intracoronary thrombolysis due to the mobilization of experienced personel, reperfusion rates have been reported to be higher in intracoronary than in intravenous thrombolysis (75%–90% versus 50%–65%), and in addition, the time from the onset of therapy to recanalization was shorter with the intracoronary route [7].

Because of a high-degree residual coronary lesion, that is frequently seen at the site of a thrombotic occlusion, there remains a considerable hazard of coronary reocclusion after successful recanalization. In most studies, the incidence of clinically apparent rethrombosis was in the range between 15% and 35% within 48 hours [2, 8]. Thus, further measures to prevent reocclusion seem to be mandatory. Presumptive methods of subsequent treatment are percutaneous transluminal coronary angioplasty (PTCA) [9] within the same session or early coronary artery bypass surgery [10, 11, 12].

The aims of this study were the calculation of costs for PTCR and PTCA in acute myocardial infarction and an attempt to estimate the population of the Federal Republic of Germany, living within the 25 km-radius of at least one left heart catheterization laboratory.

PTCR in acute myocardial infarction

Figure 1 shows the catchment area of our hospital. From 14 community hospitals at present, patients with acute myocardial infarction are transferred to our catheterization laboratory. Fifty % of our patients were initially admitted to another hospital. Intracoronary thrombolysis was performed up to 8 hours after the onset of chestpain.

58

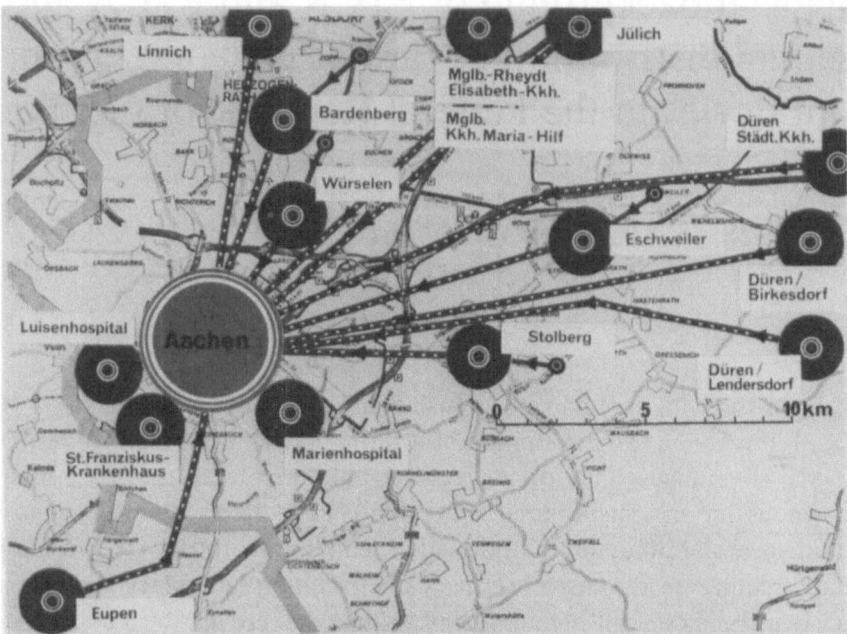

Figure 1. Catchment area of our hospital including 14 community hospitals, from which patients are transferred for intracoronary thrombolysis. The scale on the right side is 10 km.

From March 1980 until February 1984 400 patients, suffering from acute myocardial infarction were treated with PTCR. The mean age was 57 ± 12 years (range 21–83 years). 312 patients (78%) revealed, at first angiography, a totally occluded infarct related vessel, which was successfully recanalized within 1 hour in 86% (Figure 2). The average time of total coronary occlusion in successfully reperfused patients was 215 ± 87 minutes, and reperfusion was achieved within

PTCR IN ACUTE MYOCARDIAL INFARCTION
RWTH AACHEN, FEBRUARY 1984

```
                SUBTOTAL      ┌──────┐
                STENOSIS  ──── │ 22 % │
                              └──────┘
  ┌──────┐                              PTCR UN−      ┌──────┐
  │ N=400│                              SUCCESSFUL ── │ 14 % │
  └──────┘                                            └──────┘
                TOTAL        ┌──────┐
                OCCLUSION ── │ 78 % │
                             └──────┘
                                       PTCR          ┌──────┐
                                       SUCCESSFUL ── │ 86 % │
                                                     └──────┘
```

Figure 2. Incidence of total coronary occlusion and primary success rate of percutaneous transluminal coronary recanalization (PTCR) in acute myocardial infarction at our hospital.

28 ± 24 minutes after onset of intracoronary thrombolysis.

In successfully treated patients 28% underwent immediate balloon angioplasty [9], preferably within the same session, 22% underwent early bypass surgery within 10 days [10, 11, 12], and 50% had medical follow-up treatment.

The average 30-day mortality in our patients was 5.2%, which was remarkably low compared with literature. The fatality rate was 8.0% in patients treated medically, 3.1% within the PTCA group, and only 1.5% in patients, who underwent subsequent surgical treatment. Comparable data from the Western Washington Randomized Trial on intracoronary streptokinase in acute myocardial infarction have been published [3]. A statistically significant reduction of 30-day mortality from 11.2% to 3.7% was found for intracoronary thrombolytic therapy.

Calculation of costs for non-surgical interventions in acute myocardial infarction

In collaboration with our hospital management we calculated our present expenses for PTCR and PTCA in acute myocardial infarction (Figure 3). Specified are only additional charges, depreciation costs for a complete cath lab installation are not included. All calculations are based on US-$ exchange rates used in May 1984.

The basic expenditure for the exclusive PTCR intervention was summed up to US$ 1166.—. This amount consists of:

CALCULATION OF COSTS FOR NON-SURGICAL INTERVENTIONS IN ACUTE MYOCARDIAL INFARCTION RWTH AACHEN, MAY 1984	PTCR	ELECTIVE PTCA	COMBINED PTCR+PTCA
1. LEFT HEART CATHETERIZATION	US-$ 740.-	US-$ 1429.-	US-$ 1580.-
2. DRUGS	42.-	7.-	42.-
3. SALARIES	317.-	304.-	363.-
4. MISCELLANEOUS	67.-	63.-	72.-
Σ	US-$ 1166.-	US-$ 1803.-	US-$ 2057.-
		US-$ 2969	

Figure 3. Costs for PTCR and PTCA in acute myocardial infarction, calculated in collaboration with our hospital management in May 1984.

1) Costs for the left heart catheterization- catheters, contrast medium and cinefilms
2) Costs for drugs – premedication and thrombolytic agent (streptokinase)
3) Salaries for 2 physicians, 1 technician and 1 cath lab nurse
4) Miscellaneous amounts for one-way articles and laundry requirements.

The elective balloon angioplasty amounted to US-$ 1803.— and the combined PTCR plus immediate PTCA intervention within the same session was estimated at US$ 2057.—.

In case of a high degree residual coronary lesion, suitable for PTCA, our calculations show, that 31% of expenses can be saved, if PTCA is already performed during the initial catheterization. Without significant risk this approach can increase blood flow to the ischemic myocardium and will probably prevent early coronary reocclusion. Our average initial success rate ($\geq 20\%$ diameter increase) in patients, who underwent PTCA within the same session was 76%, including patients treated before the introduction of steerable guidewires. Only 2 patients suffered from coronary reocclusion during the attempted PTCA because of coronary dissection. Both patients survived.

Based on the amount of US$ 1166.— for the PTCR intervention only, the total additional expenditure for a hypothetical catheterization laboratory, treating 100 patients a year, would be about US$ 110,000.—.

Regional distribution of left heart catheterization laboratories in the Federal Republic of Germany

Because of a proposed draft of a bill for economic control of large medicotechnical installations by the German 'Bundesrat' it was published in 'Deutsches Ärzteblatt', that there were 100 left heart catheterization facilities in the Federal Republic of Germany in January 1984 [13]. Our corresponding investigations showed, that 14 of these laboratories belong to departments for pediatric cardiology, at least 12 cardiological departments are operating with two or more laboratories. Thus, the total number of adult left heart catheterization laboratories should be in the range of 75 to 80.

Concerning the total number of 100 laboratories there was a statistical relation of 616,000 people per cath lab, ranging from 313,000 to 873,000 [13]. The comparable rates for the United States of America are 189,000 to 313,000 people per cath lab, showing a coverage being twice to three times better than in the Federal Republic of Germany [14].

Based on information from two major companies, engaged in cardiac x-ray equipment, completed by our own inquiries and by data from the 'Deutsche Gesellschaft für Herz- und Kreislaufforschung', we could identify the following adult left heart catheterization laboratories in the FRG (Figure 4). Black circles represent general hospitals for emergency care, and grey circles represent re-

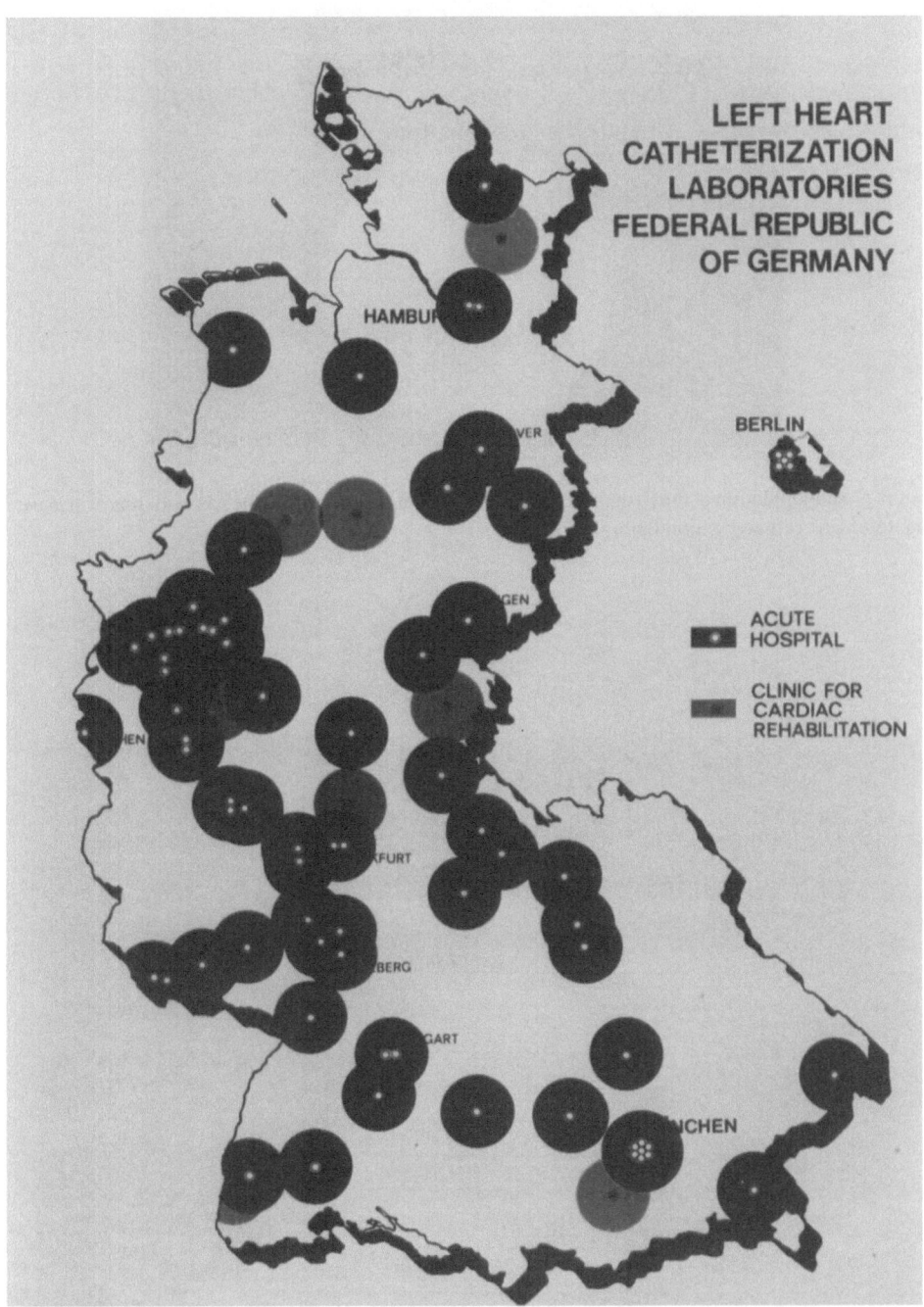

Figure 4. Adult left heart catheterization laboratories in the Federal Republic of Germany (January 1984). Black circles represent general hospitals for acute medical care and grey circles indicate rehabilitation clinics. Each circle has a radius of 25 km.

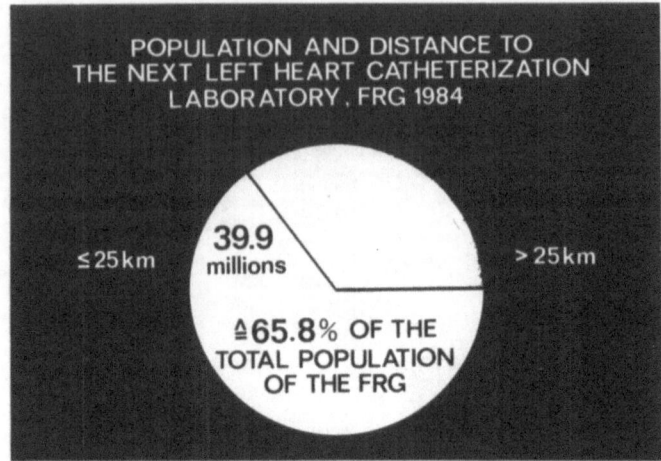

Figure 5. Subpopulation of the Federal Republic of Germany, living within the 25 km-radius of at least one left heart catheterization laboratory.

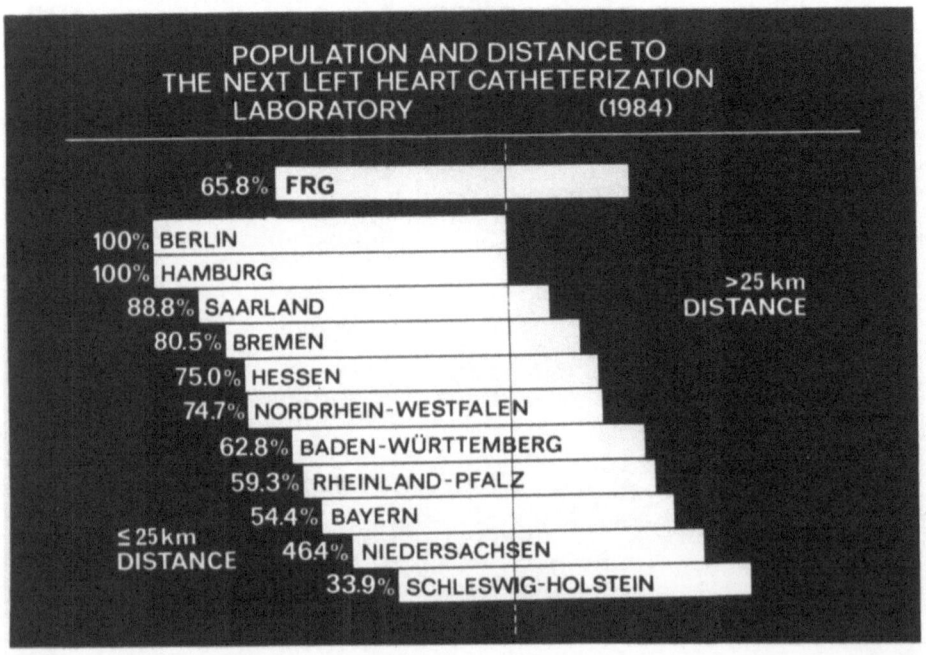

Figure 6. Regional coverage after further subdivision into Federal Countries, indicated as percentage of population, living next to at least one left heart catheterization laboratory.

habilitation clinics. Each circle has a radius of 25 km.

In collaboration with the Department of Physical Geography and the Department of Medical Statistics of the RWTH Aachen we were able to estimate the percentage of population, that lives within the 25 km-limit of these catheterization laboratories. The geographical coordinates of all laboratories and the population rates and geographical coordinates of 12,000 communities were investigated with the aid of a computer. The results are indicated in Figure 5. 39.9 million people or 65.8% of the total population of the Federal Republic of Germany live within the 25 km-radius of at least 1 left heart catheterization laboratory.

The further subdivision into Federal countries is shown in Figure 6. A 100% coverage is provided for Berlin and Hamburg, less than average facilities were found for Rheinland-Pfalz, Bayern, Niedersachsen and Schleswig-Holstein.

Conclusions

If PTCR should prove to be an advisable treatment of acute myocardial infarction, then, technical facilities for this treatment are already available for two thirds of the total population of the Federal Republic of Germany. Further large randomized trials are necessary to clarify the presumptive advantages of intracoronary thrombolytic treatment over intravenous thrombolysis, to find the optimal thrombolytic agent, to define the ultimate time limit after the onset of an acute myocardial infarction and to find the suitable subgroup of patients, that will probably derive the greatest benefits from thrombolytic therapy.

References

1. Rentrop P, Blanke H, Karsch KR, Kaiser H, Köstering H, Leitz K (1981) Selective intracoronary thrombolysis in acute myocardial infarction and unstable angina pectoris. Circulation 63: 307
2. Merx W, Dörr R, Rentrop P, Blanke H, Karsch KR, Mathey DG, Kremer P, Rutsch W, Schmutzler H (1981) Evaluation of the effectiveness of intracoronary streptokinase infusion in acute myocardial infarction: postprocedure management and hospital course in 204 patients. Am Heart J 102: 1181
3. Kennedy JW, Ritchie JL, Davis KB, Fritz JK (1983) Western Washington randomized trial of intracoronary streptokinase in acute myocardial infarction. N Engl J Med 309: 1477
4. Schröder R, Biamino G, von Leitner ER, Linderer T, Brüggemann T, Heitz J, Vöhringer HF, Wegschneider K (1983) Intravenous short-term infusion of streptokinase in acute myocardial infarction. Circulation 67: 536
5. Laffel GL, Braunwald E (1984) Thrombolytic therapy: a new strategy for the treatment of acute myocardial infarction (First of two parts). N Engl J Med 311: 710
6. Laffel GL, Braunwald E (1984) Thrombolytic therapy: a new strategy for the treatment of acute myocardial infarction (Second of two parts). N Engl J Med 311: 770
7. Schröder R (1983) Systemic versus intracoronary streptokinase infusion in the treatment of acute myocardial infarction. J Am Coll Cardiol 1: 1254

8. Gold HK, Leinbach RC, Palacios IF. Coronary reocclusion after selective administration of streptokinase. Circulation 68(2: Part 2): 1–50

9. Meyer J, Merx W, Schmitz H, Erbel R, Kiesslich T, Dörr R, Lambertz H, Bethge C, Krebs W, Bardos P, Minale C Messmer BJ, Effert S (1982) Percutaneous transluminal coronary angioplasty immediately after intracoronary streptolysis of transmural myocardial infarction. Circulation 66: 905

10. Messmer BJ, Merx W, Meyer J, Bardos P, Minale C, Effert S (1983) New developments in medical-surgical treatment of acute myocardial infarction. Ann Thorac Surg 35: 70

11. Dörr R, Merx W, Messmer BJ, von Essen R, Effert S, Schmidt WG, Mertes G (1984) Sofortige Bypass-Operation nach erfolgreicher intrakoronarer Thrombolyse beim akuten Myokardinfarkt. Intensivmed 21: 109

12. Dörr R, Merx W, Meyer J, Messmer BJ, von Essen R, Mertes G, Schmitz HJ, Effert S (1983) Early balloon dilatation or bypass surgery after successful selective thrombolysis in acute myocardial infarction. Circulation 68 (Supp III): III:326

13. Medizinisch-technische Grossgeräte in der Bundesrepublik Deutschland (1984) Dtsch Ärzteblatt 81: 1341

14. Kennedy RH, Kennedy MA, Frye RL, Guiliani ER, McGoon DC, Pluth JR, Smith HC, Ritter DR, Nobrega FT, Kurland LT (1982) Cardiac-catheterization and cardiac-surgical facilities. Use, trends, and future requirements. N Engl J Med 307: 986

Natural history of coronary artery stenosis

WOLF RAFFLENBEUL

Introduction

The natural history of coronary artery stenosis has to be studied by comparison of coronary angiograms of the same patient taken at different times. Unfortunately, although thousands of coronary angiograms are performed each year, only a limited number of *repeated* studies is available, particularly in patients who are medically treated over an interval of more than one year.

However, conclusions from repeated angiographic studies might be fraught with substantial errors because of inherent pitfalls, some of which are:

1. Since patients selection mostly entails persistance or progression of clinical symptoms the study population might be short on patients with stable disease and obviously excludes all patients whose disease progression had a fatal course.

2. Furthermore, to include patients with differing severity of coronary artery disease might be inappropriate, because the speed of anatomical changes might be variable according to the stage of the disease or might be judged differently by the observer.

3. Because in most instances the second angiogram is only performed to reassess suitability for bypass surgery most studies:

a) are designed retrospectively,

b) show a highly variable time interval between angiograms and

c) are mostly poorly controlled.

4. Another problem when the observation interval is long is the use of new and upgrades x-ray-equipment for the second study. In addition, exposure conditions should be controlled precisely as well as film quality and film processing. Consistent interpretation includes matching angle and sequence of views to facilitate simultaneous reading of both angiograms. In most studies severity of the coronary artery disease is assessed by qualitative criteria which are – despite sophisticated scoring systems – too often fraught with both intra- and interobserver variability [15, 16, 21, 54, 56, 63]. But even when quantitative measurements are taken – as we have done for several years – the physiologic state of the patient during coronary angiography may substantially influence the results. Dynamic changes in luminal diameter due to different vasomotor tone, platelet aggregation or thrombolysis may alter the angiographic appearance of the disease.

Although it is difficult to eliminate the bias introduced by these pitfalls completely, a reasonable number of follow-up studies give valuable information concerning the evolution of coronary artery disease by angiography [3, 4, 10, 20, 22, 26, 28, 29, 33, 38, 40, 42, 45, 50, 52, 56, 60].

Figure 1 represents the data reported in 17 studies published between 1972 and 1984 overlooking a total of 1922 patients who underwent a second angiogram between 2 and 182 months. Because in most studies the time interval between the two angiograms was highly variable, these studies were subdivided according to their *average* time interval and for each time interval the percentage of patients with progressive coronary artery disease found in each study was plotted. The open circles indicate results of quantitative studies performed in our own lab.

Progression and time interval

Figure 1 indicated that most interval angiograms were performed already after 1 to 3 years, i.e. a relatively short interval with regard to the time coronary artery disease needs to become symptomatic. However, even after such short time intervals profound differences of the percentage of patients with progressive coronary artery disease are obvious.

Despite a substantial overlap of the number of patients showing progression in

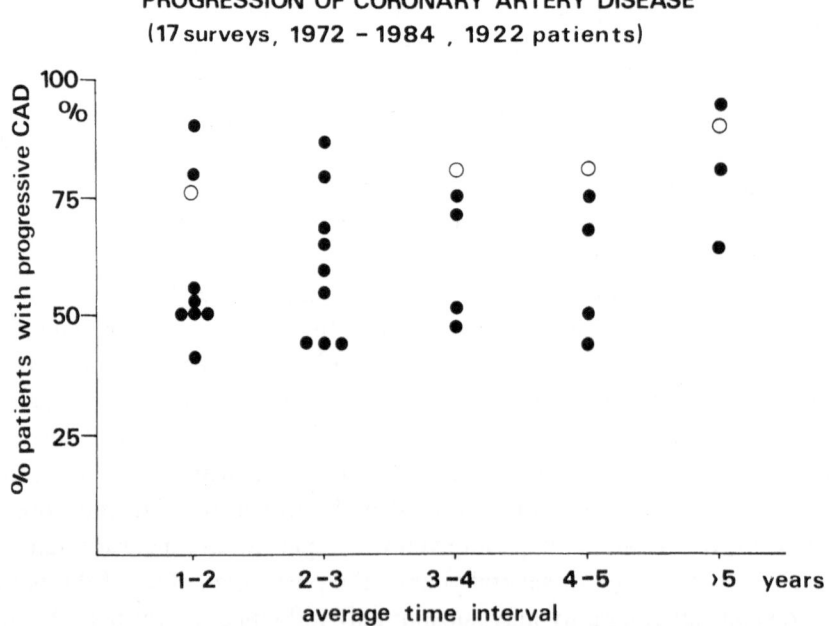

Figure 1. Progression of coronary artery disease as judged from repeated coronary angiograms published in 17 studies between 1972 and 1984. Open circles represent data of quantitative studies performed in our own lab (W. Rafflenbeul et al., Circ. 70 (Suppl II) II-410, 1984). See text for details.

general there is a tendency towards more progression with increasing time interval. After 1–2 years an average of 58% of patients, between 2 and 5 years about 65% and after more than 5 years 85% of patients had progressive coronary artery disease. This tendency is supported by the findings of others [10, 28, 29], who computed a regression line from their data and found about 50% of patients after 2 years and about 80% of patients after 5 years with progressive coronary artery disease at angiography.

However, this statistical analysis might be misleading regarding those patients who suffer from rapid progression during the first months following their initial angiogram mostly associated with rapid deterioration of clinical symptoms.

Based on this experience we assume that basically two distinctively different types of progression exist (Table 1) [34]: *Primary* progression represents the formation or growth of a plaque by the basic atherosclerotic process, taking place over years – possibly in bouts – and is characterized clinically by a slowly progressive exertional angina pectoris. On the other hand, *secondary* progression describes more rapid changes in stenosis severity elicited by the formation of platelet thrombus, intramural hemorrhage or sudden increase of vasomotor tone, leading to unstable angina pectoris or acute myocardial infarction.

Progression and risk factors

Most of the studies published on this subject reported a significant higher incidence of abnormal lipid levels at the time of the first angiogram in patients with progressive disease [3, 4, 24, 42, 50]. In addition, the observation of Moccetti et al. [38] and Marchandise and coworkers [35] that obese patients had a significant prevalence of progressive disease, might be related to their lipid levels. Only recently, Kuo and coworkers [31] confirmed stagnation of angiographically visi-

Table 1. Characteristics of primary and secondary progression of coronary artery disease [after 34].

	Primary progression	Secondary progression
Pathophysiology	Formation or 'growth' of the atherosclerotic plaques by: • Lipid accumulation • Cellular proliferation • Necrosis/fibrosis • Calcification	Rapid enlargement of the plaque by: • Thrombus formation • Hemorrhage • Vasoconstriction
Time interval	Years (with variable speed)	Minutes – hours
Clinical symptoms	Slowly progressive angina pectoris (stepwise)	Sudden deterioration of angina pectoris (unstable angina pectoris, acute myocardial infarction)

ble narrowings with effective combined drug treatment in patients with type II hyperlipidemia.

Except hyperlipoproteinemia, significant differences in the prevalence of a family history of cardiovascular disease, hypertension, diabetes or cigarette smoking could not be found [10, 28, 40, 49, 56].

According to the reviewed papers even the effective treatment of these risk factors during the interval between angiograms does not influence the progression of the disease. In essence, that means that factors which are regarded responsible for the formation of the atherosclerotic plaque exert obviously only minor influence on the progression of the disease if it once has become symptomatic. However, relatively short time intervals between the first and second angiographic study may obscure a positive correlation between progression and single risk factors as reported in clinical studies over a prolonged time interval.

Progression and clinical symptoms

From clinical symptoms a decreasing threshold of angina pectoris was not uniformly found associated with subsequent angiographic demonstration of progression; some studies could demonstrate a positive correlation [8, 17], others not [3, 10, 13]. If patients were included into progression studies *after* a phase of unstable angina, the interval angiogram did not show any significant progression. However,if the angiogram during the period of unstable angina could be compared *retrospectively* with a previous one, unstable angina was clearly associated with progression of coronary artery disease [39].

ECG-changes also could not be related to progression, except myocardial infarction. In most cases with an interval myocardial infarction there was evidence of progression at angiography, at least at the site appropriate for the infarct [3, 10, 13, 17, 29, 30, 51, 56, 60].

Progression and coronary anatomy at angiography

The number of diseased vessels at the time of the first angiogram could not be related to progressive disease [29]. The severity of coronary artery disease at the time of the first angiogram – coded in different scoring systems – could not uniformly correlated to progressive disease depending on the score used. If the number of diseased vessels was included into the score there was no correlation. A positive correlation could be found often if the score was predominantly based on the severity of the individual stenosis.

Regression of coronary artery disease

A growing number of studies in experimental animals as in humans as well indicate, that the process of atherosclerosis is almost completely preventable and that it is reversible if already present. Perhaps the most encouraging evidence for substantial regression of advanced atherosclerosis come from the work in the non-human primate. The prospective studies [1, 58, 62] demonstrated that a 40 months period of feeding either a low fat, low cholesterol ratio or a high-fat (corn oil) low-cholesterol diet resulted in a remarkable improvement in luminal narrowings in all of the main coronary arteries of severely atherosclerotic rhesus monkey.

Although human atherosclerotic lesions have components different from those of the experimental lesion it might be conceivable that they too can regress. However, convincing evidence that substantial regression of advanced lesions can be induced in man is difficult to obtain. Only recently, repeated angiography proved to be a most promising tool to study changes in the atherosclerotic lesions already intravitaly [2, 11, 12, 27, 57]. Some of these papers are anecdotal case reports, others demonstrate a rather extensive experience in measuring atherosclerotic plaques size and luminal diameter of coronary and femoral arteries from successive coronary angiograms [5–7, 14]. The results of various kinds of treatments, including cholesterol lowering diets, exercise and drugs, were quantitatively evaluated and substantiated definite regression of coronary artery disease even in brief intervals of study and without necessarily lowering the serum cholesteril to normal values.

Beside these, several other papers documented so-called 'regressive' coronary lesions. This is most likely due to a resolving thrombus or spasm, i.e. events which – as emphasized also by Roskam et al. [52] – are of secondary nature and should be separated from real regression of an atherosclerotic plaque.

According to Blankenhorn [6] atherosclerotic plaques are only reversible at a very early stage which he called the 'latent phase' of atherosclerosis, a period in which the plaque already visibly enchroaches into the vascular lumen but is still not clinically symptomatic.

This indicates that in particular the process of regressive disease is more a feature of the individual lesion than of the overall coronary artery disease. Factors, like age, composition, remodelling and healing processes of the single stenosis may determine the angiographic appeerence.

Summary

The evolution of coronary artery disease has to be studied by comparing coronary angiograms of the same patient taken at different times. However, conclusions from repeated angiographic studies are fraught with substantial errors mainly because of:

1. patients selection,
2. variable time interval and
3. technical pitfalls.

Despite this bias published interval studies demonstrate that coronary athe rosclerosis predominantly is a progressive disease: after 2–3 years 50% to 60% after 3–4 years 60% to 70% and after 5 years more than 80% of patient demonstrate progressive coronary artery disease at angiography. In addition quantitative evaluation of coronary angiograms reveals that progression of coro nary artery disease (1) has a variable pattern and pace in each coronary artery an((2) predominantly involves initially normal coronary artery segments.

From all clinical and angiographic parameters under scrutiny progressive coro nary artery disease is significantly correlated to:
1. abnormal lipid levels at the time of the first angiogram,
2. a period of unstable angina pectoris,
3. interval myocardial infarction and
4. initial severity of coronary artery obstruction.

It has to be emphasized, however, that in the individual patient the speed o progression is highly variable supporting the concept of different underlyin; pathophysiological mechanisms (primary/secondary progression).

Regression of coronary artery stenosis is a rare phenomenon which may occu spontaneously and is anecdotally reported in patients after vigorous treatment o severe hyperlipoproteinemia.

Therefore, natural history of symptomatic coronary artery disease is charac terized nearly exclusively by further deterioration focusing our interest on th(major problem of primary or secondary prevention of progressive coronar' artery disease.

References

1. Armstrong ML, Megan MB (1975) Arterial fibrous proteins in cynomolgus monkeys after athe rogenic and regression diets. Circ Res 36: 256
2. Basta LL, Williams C, Kioschos JM, Spector AA (1976) Regression of atherosclerotic stenosin; lesions of the renal arteries and spontaneous cure of systemic hypertension through control o hyperlipidemia. Am J Cardiol 61: 420
3. Bemis CE, Gorlin R, Kemp HG, Herman MV (1973) Progression of coronary artery disease. / clinical arteriographic study. Circulation 47: 455.
4. Ben-Zvi J, Hildner PJ, Javier RP, Fester A, Samet P (1974) Progression of coronary arter' disease. Cinearteriographic and clinical observations in medically and surgically treated patients Am J Cardiol 34: 295
5. Blankenhorn DH, Brooks SH, Selzer RH, Crawford DW, Chin HP (1974) Assessment o atherosclerosis from angiographic images. Proc Soc Exp Biol Med 145: 1298
6. Blankenhorn DH, Sanmarco ME (1979) Editorial: angiography for study of lipid-lowerin; therapy. Circulation 59: 212
7. Blankenhorn DH, Sanmarco ME (1979) Angiography for study of lipid-lowering therapy (edi torial). Circulation 59: 212

8. Bourassa MG, Lespérance J, Corbara F, Saltiel J, Campeau L (1979) Progression of obstructive coronary artery disease 5 to 7 years after aoroto-coronary bypass surgery. Circulation 58 (suppl I) I: 100

9. Bourassa MG, Ryan TJ, Coulet C, Abramowitz BA, Lespérance JP, Faxon DP, Enjalbert M, McCabe CH (1981) Early progression of coronary disease in patients assigned to medical therapy (abstr). Circulation 64 (suppl IV) IV: 83

10. Bruschke AVG, Wijers TS, Kolsters W, Landmann J (1981) The anatomic evolution of coronary artery disease demonstrated by coronary arteriography in 256 nonoperated patients. Circulation 63: 527

11. Buchwald H, Moore RB, Varco RL (1974) Surgical treatment of hyperlipidemia. Circulation 49 (Suppl. I): 1

12. Buchwald H, Moore RB, Varco RL (1974) The partial ileal bypass operation in treatment of hyperlimpemias. Advan Exp Med Biol 63: 221

13. Buda AJ, Macdonald H, Kwok KL, Orr SA (1982) Coronary disease progression and its effect on left ventricular function. Chest 82: 285

14. Crawford DW, Beckenbach ES, Blankenhorn DH, Selzer RH, Brooks SH (1974) Grading of coronary atherosclerosis: comparison of a modified IAP visual grading method and a new quantitative angiographic technique. Atherosclerosis 19: 231

15. De Rouen TA, Murray JA, Owen W (1977) Variability in the analysis of coronary arteriograms. Circulation 55: 324

16. Detre KM, Wright E, Murphy ML, Takaro T (1975) Observer agreement in evaluating coronary angiograms. Circulation 52: 979

17. Dyrda I, Petitclerc R, Saltiel J, Bourassa MG (1973) Clinical indices of angiographic progression in coronary artery disease (abstr). Circulation 48 (suppl IV) IV: 58

18. Engel HJ, Kaltenbach M, Rafflenbeul W, Kober G, Scherer D, Simon R, Lichtlen PR (1982) Changes of coronary obstructions in the months following transluminal coronary angioplasty. In: M. Kaltenbach, A Grüntzig, K. Rentrop, W.-D. Bussmann (Hrsg.): Transluminal coronary angioplasty and intracoronary thrombolysis. Springer-Verlag, Berlin, Heidelberg, New York, S. 102

19. Fleckenstein A (1983) Calcium-antagonism in heart and smooth muscle. Experimental facts and therapeutic prospects. Wiley-Interscience Publ., New York, S. 109

20. Frick MH, Valle M, Harjola PT (1983) Progression of coronary artery disease in randomized medical and surgical patients over a 5 year angiographic follow-up. Am J Cardiol 52: 681

21. Galbraith JE, Murphy ML, de Soyza N (1978) Coronary arteriogram interpretation: interobserver variability, JAMA 240: 2053

22. Gensini GG, Kelly AE (1972) Incidence and progression of coronary artery disease. An angiographic correlation in 1263 patients. Arch Intern Med 129: 814

23. Gohlke H, Sturzenhofecker P, Gornandt L, Haakshorst W, Roskamm H (1980) Progression und Regression der koronaren Herzerkrankung im chronischen Infarktstadium bei Patienten unter 40. Schweiz Med Wochenschr 110: 1663

24. Henderson RR, Rowe GG (1973) The progression of coronary atherosclerotic disease as assessed by cine-angiography arteriography. Am Heart J 86: 165

25. Henry PD (1983) Nifedipine suppresses atherogenesis in cholesterol-fed rabbits. 5th International Adalat Symposium, Excerpta Medica, Amsterdam, Oxford, Princeton, S. 55

26. Kimbiris D, Lavine P, Van Den Brock H, Najmi M, Likoll W (1974) Devolutionary pattern of coronary atherosclerosis in patients with angina pectoris. Coronary arteriographic studies. Am J Cardiol 33: 7

27. Knight L, Scheibel R, Amplatz K, Varco RL, Buchwald H (1972) Radiographic appraisal of the Minnesota partial ileal bypass study. Surg Forum 23: 141

28. Kramer JR, Matsuda Y, Mulligan JC, Azonow M, Proudfit WL (1981) Progression of coronary atherosclerosis. Circulation 63: 519

29. Kramer JR, Kitazume H, Proudfit WL, Matsuda Y, Williams GW, Sones FM Jr. (1983) Progression and regression of coronary atherosclerosis: relation to risk factors. Am Heart J 105: 134

30. Kramer JR, Kitazume H, Proudfit WL, Matsuda Y, Goormastic M, Williams GW, Sones FM (1983) Segmental analysis of the rate of progression in patients with progressive coronary atherosclerosis. Am Heart J 106: 1427

31. Kuo PT, Hayase K, Kostis JB, Moreyra AE (1979) Use of combined diet and colestipol in long-term (7–7½ years) treatment of patients with type II hyperlipoproteinemia. Circulation 59: 199

32. Landmann J, Kolsters W, Bruschke AVG (1976) Regression of coronary artery obstructions demonstrated by coronary arteriography. Eur J Cardiol 4: 475

33. Landmann J, Kolsters W, Bruschke AVG (1978) Progression der obstruktiven koronaren Herzkrankheit, dargestellt anhand wiederholter Koronarangiographie. Schweiz Med Wschr 108: 55

34. Lichtlen PR, Rafflenbeul W (1983) Progression of coronary artery disease as judged from segmential angiography. In: Second Münster International Arteriosclerosis Symposium (Abhandlung Band 70), Westdeutscher Verlag, S 101

35. Marchandise B, Bourassa MG, Chaitman BR, Lespérance J (1978) Angiographic evaluation of the natural history of normal coronary arteries and mild coronary atherosclerosis. Am J Cardiol 41: 216

36. Markis JE, Joffee CD, Roberts BH, Rasnil BJ, Cohn PF, Herman MV, Gorlin R (1980) Evolution of left ventricular dysfunction in coronary artery disease. Serial cineangiographic studies without surgery. Circulation 62: 141

37. McLaughlin PR, Berman ND, Morton BC, Schwartz L, Morch JE (1977) Long-term angiographic assessment of the influence of coronary risk factors on native coronary circulation and saphenous vein aortocoronary grafts. Am Heart J 93: 327

38. Moccetti T, Lichtlen P, Schönbeck M, Steinbrunn W (1976) Progression of coronary artery disease based on cineangiographic data. In: Coronary Angiography and Angina Pectoris. Stuttgart, Georg Thieme Publishers, p 88

39. Moise A, Theroux P, Taeymans Y et al. (1983) Unstable angina and progression of coronary atherosclerosis. N Engl J Med 309: 685

40. Moise A, Theroux P, Taeymans Y, Waters DD, Lespérance J, Fines P, Descoings B, Robert P (1984) Clinical and angiographic factors associated with progression of coronary artery disease. JACC 3/3: 659

41. Moraski E, Russell RO Jr., Kouchoukos NT, Mantle JA, Alison H, Rackley CE (1975) Progression of coronary artery disease in patients with unstable angina pectoris treated medically or surgically. Circ 51/52 (Suppl. II), II: 91

42. Nash DT, Gensini GG, Simon H, Arno I, Nash S (1977) The Erysichthon syndrome. Progression of coronary atherosclerosis and dietary hyperlipidemia. Circulation 56: 363

43. Nash DT, Gensini G, Escente P (1982) Effect of lipidlowering therapy on the progression of coronary atherosclerosis assessed by scheduled repetitive coronary arteriography. Int J Cardiol 2: 43

44. Oberman A, Jones WB, Riley CP, Reeves TJ, Sheffield LT, Turner ME (1972) Natural history of coronary artery disease. Bull NY Acad Med 48: 1109

45. Palac RT, Hwang MH, Meadows WR, Croke RP, Pifarre R, Loeb HS, Gunnar RM (1981) Progression of coronary artery disease in medically and surgically treated patients 5 years after randomization. Circulation 64 (Suppl II): 17

46. Petch MC (1981) The progression of coronary artery disease. Br Med J 283: 1073

47. Proudfit WL, Bruschke AVG, Sones FM Jr (1978) Natural history of obstructive coronary artery disease: ten-year study of 601 non-surgical cases. Prog Cardiovasc Dis 21: 53

48. Rafflenbeul W, Smith LR, Rogers WJ, Mantle JA, Rackley CE, Russell RO (1979) Quantitative coronary arteriography. Coronary anatomy of patients with unstable angina pectoris reexamined 1 year after optimal medical therapy. Am J Cardiol 43: 699

49. Robertson TL, Lee KK (1980) Failure to observe regression of coronary atherosclerosis following marked weight loss: A clinicopathologic study in a defined sample in Hiroshima and Nagasaki, Japan (abstr.). Circ 62 (suppl. III): 307

50. Rösch J, Antonovic R, Trenouth RS, Rahimtoola SH, Sim DN, Dotter CT (1976) The natural history of coronary artery stenosis. A longitudinal angiographic assessment. Radiology 119: 513

51. Rösch J, Rahimtoola SH (1977) Progression of angiographically determined coronary stenosis. Cardiovasc Clin 8: 55

52. Roskamm H, Stürzenhofecker P, Gornandt L, Gohlke H, Haakshorst W (1980) Progression and regression of coronary artery disease in postinfarction patients less than 40 years of age. Cleve Clin Q 47: 192

53. Roth D, Kostuk WJ (1980) Noninvasive and invasive demonstration of spontaneous regression of coronary artery disease. Circ 62: 888

54. Sanmarco ME, Brooks SH, Blankenhorn DH (1978) Reproducibility of a consensus panel in the interpretation of coronary angiograms. Am Heart J 96: 430

55. Schwartz JN, Kong Y, Hackel DB, Bartel AG (1975) Comparison of angiographic and post-mortem findings in patients with coronary artery disease. Am J Cardiol 36: 174

56. Shub C, Vlietstra RE, Smith HC, Fulton RE, Elveback IR (1981) The unpredictable progression of symptomatic coronary artery disease. A serial clinical angiographic analysis. Mayo Clin Proc 56: 155

57. Starzl TE, Chase HP, Putnam CW, Nora JJ (1974) Follow-up of patients with postocaval shunt for the treatment of hyperlipidemie. Lancet II: 714

58. Taylor CB, Cox GE, Manolo-Estrella P, Southworth J (1962) Atherosclerosis in rhesus monkeys: II. Arterial lesions associated with hypercholesteremia induced by dietary fat and cholesterol. Arch Path (Chicago) 74: 16

59. Thompson G, Kilpatrick D, Oakley C, Steinar R, Myant N (1978) Reversal of cholesterol accumulation in familial hypercholesterolemia by long-term plasma exchange. Circ 58 (suppl II), II: 71

60. Vanhaecke J, Piessens J, van de Werf F, Willems JL, de Geest H (1983) Angiographic evolution of coronary atherosclerosis in non-operated patients. Europ Heart J 4: 547

61. Viestra RE, Frye RL, Kronmal RA, Sim DA, Tristani FE, Killip T (1980) Risk factors and angiographic coronary artery disease: a report from the coronary artery surgery study (CASS). Circulation 62: 254

62. Wissler RW, Vesselinovitch D (1976) Studies of regression of advanced atherosclerosis in experimental animals and man. In: Atherogenesis (Proceedings of an International Symposium. Acapulco, December 1975), edited by RA Camerini-Davalos, A Kappert, F Numano, W Redisch, T Shimamoto. Ann NY Acad Sci 275: 363

63. Zir L, Miller SW, Dinsmore RE, Gilbert JP, Harthorne JW (1976) Interobserver variability in coronary angiography. Circulation 53: 627

ECG and reperfusion

R. VON ESSEN, W. SCHMIDT, R. UEBIS, B. EDELMANN, S. EFFERT,
J. SILNY* and G. RAU*

Introduction

The most important tool for the diagnosis of an acute myocardial infarction (a MI) is the ECG. ST segment elevation can be seen within a few seconds after complete occlusion of a coronary artery. During the next 6 to 8 hours there is a loss or reduction of R-waves and a development of pathological Q-waves [1, 2].

Though already in the sixties a rapid decrease of ST-elevation during intravenous streptokinase application (SK) in patients with aMI was described [3] and recently changes in the standard ECG leads after intracoronary SK have been published [4, 5], there are no detailed investigations available using ECG mapping to study the effectiveness of reperfusion. Therefore we looked at the ST-segment changes during reperfusion, documented angiographically, and at the change of Q- and R-waves in the subacute and chronic stages of MI.

Methods and patients

Since march 1980 all patients admitted to our hospital within 8 hours after onset of chest pain who had ECG changes consistent with an aMI (ST elevation in the lumb leads $\geq 0,2$ mV or in the chest leads $\geq 0,3$ mV) were treated with a 60 minute intracoronary SK infusion (3.000 Units per minute) into the infarct related vessel. Before, during and after infusion the influence of SK on the vessel and thrombus was documented by angiography performed every 20 minutes.

1. ST-segment changes in the acute stage of MI

1.1 In a consecutive series of 56 patients (47 m, 9 f, aged 41 to 81 years, 21 anterior and 35 inferior MI) ST segment elevation and depression in the limb leads I, II, III were summed up ($\sum$ ST) and compared to angiographic findings.

1.2 In 34 patients on-line monitoring of the ST-segment using up to 8 precordial leads was done during the 48 hours following SK infusion in order to detect the occurance of reischemia.

1.3 In 6 patients during percutaneous transluminal coronary angioplasty

(PTCA) of the remaining stenosis of the infarct related vessel after successful reperfusion we looked at the ST segment changes during the time of ballon inflation using a precordial on-line mapping system.

2. Changes of the Q- and R-waves during the following 6 months after aMI

In a consecutive series of 54 patients, not identical to 1.1 (45 m, 13 f, aged 27 to 79 years) with an anterior MI, standardized 48 electrode precordial mapping was performed immediately after SK infusion, at the 3rd day, 3rd week and 4 to 6 months later, when a follow-up coronary angiogram was carried out. Statistical analyses were done using the Student's t-test. Values are expressed as the mean ± standard deviation.

Results

1.1. During SK infusion in 43 of the 56 patients there was a significant decrease of $\sum ST$ from $0,68 \pm 0,32\,mV$ to $0,09 \pm 0,12\,mV$ (p<0,001). In all 43 patients the infarct related vessel was occluded at the start of SK infusion, thrombolysis was successful and reperfusion was achieved.

Figure 1 demonstrates one example with almost normalization of the ECG a few minutes after reperfusion.

In 10 patients the occluded vessel could not be opened and in 3 the vessel was already reperfused, when SK infusion started. In this group no significant changes of $\sum ST$ could be observed during SK infusion: $\sum ST$ before SK infusion was $0,40 \pm 0,29\,mV$ and after infusion $0,44 \pm 0,36\,mV$ (Figure 2).

In all patients with successful reperfusion a reduction of $\sum ST$ of more than 55% within one hour could be seen (Figure 3).

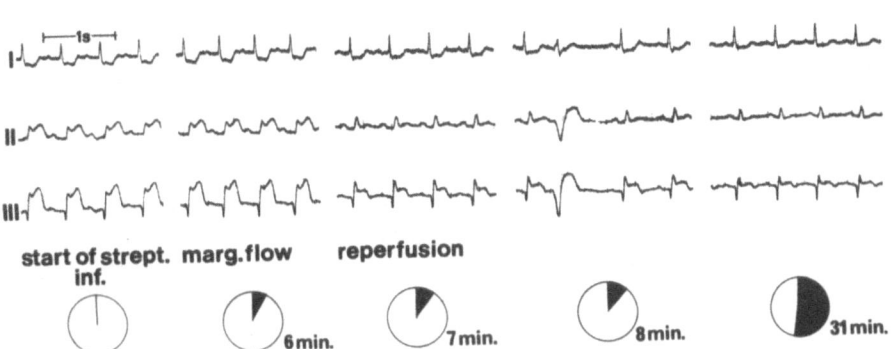

Figure 1. Rapid 'improvement' of ST-T changes after reperfusion.

ST-SEGMENTS BEFORE AND AFTER STREPTOKINASE INFUSION

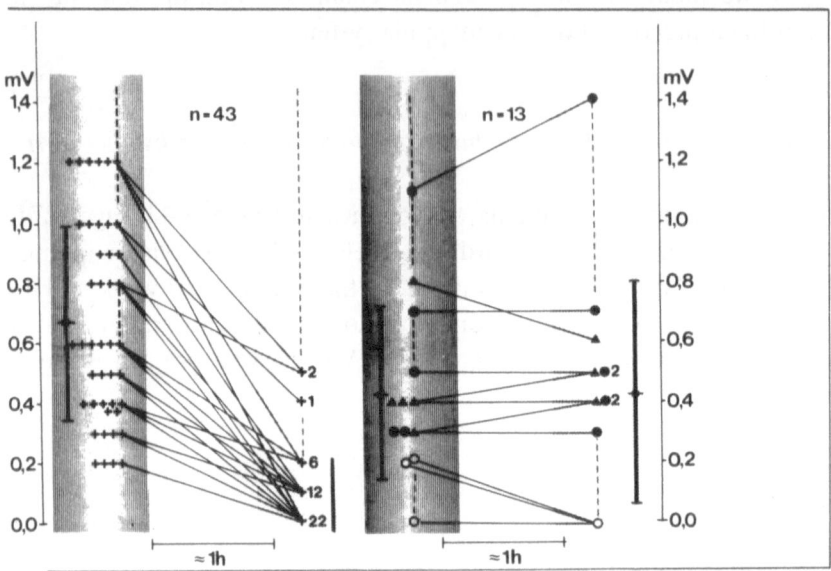

Figure 2. $\sum$ ST in lead I, II, III before and after intracoronary streptokinase infusion. Left: 43 patients with successful thrombolysis and reperfusion. Right: 10 patients with unsuccessful thrombolysis (● inferior, ▲ anterior MI) and 3 patients with initially already open infarct related vessel (○).

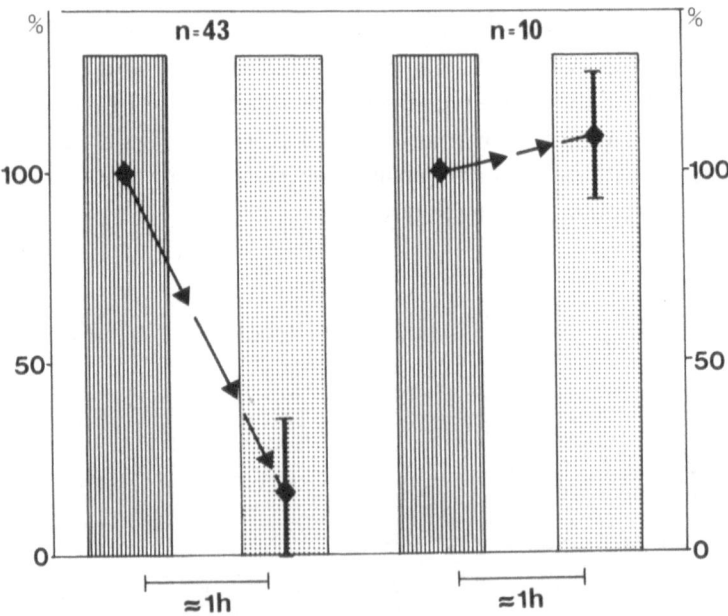

Figure 3. Changes of $\sum$ ST (ST elevation and depression in lead I, II, III) before and after SK infusion. Left: successful reperfusion. Right: unsuccessful thrombolysis.

1.2. The results of this study were recently reported [6].

1.3. During PTCA performed 3 days after successful thrombolysis in 4 of these patients the inflation of the balloon in the remaining stenosis of the infarct related vessel simulates reocclusion and was followed by a distinct new elevation of the ST segment in the precordial leads attached in and around the centre of initial ischemia. In 2 patients there were no ST segment changes seen. They had a long delay between onset of symptoms and reperfusion and severely depressed regional wall motion.

2. According to the angiographic findings at follow-up coronary arteriography 4 to 6 months after the infarction the 54 patients could be divided into 4 different groups:

Group A: 11 patients with spontaneous reperfusion before SK started and open infarct related vessel 4 to 6 months later.

Group B: 25 patients with successful thrombolysis in whom the infarct vessel was still open 4 to 6 months later at follow-up angiography.

Group C: 8 patients with reoccluded vessels 4 to 6 months later.

Group D: 10 patients with unsuccessful thrombolysis in whom the vessel remained occluded 4 to 6 months later.

In groups A and B there was a moderate but significant increase of precordial R waves 4 to 6 months after MI, whereas patients in group C and D showed a further loss of R waves (see Table 1). A simular course could be seen in the Q-waves: In group A and B the number of precordial leads with complete loss of R-waves (n QS) decreased but increased or remained stable in group C and D. Group A had the fewest number of Q waves in the 48 leads (n = 12,3) and group C the highest (n = 31) 4 to 6 months after MI (Table 2).

The increase in R-wave amplitudes in groups A and B could mostly be seen in the centre of the infarct area, whereas in group C with reocclusion a further loss of R-waves was found.

	n	ΣR acute after SK infusion	ΣR chronic 4-6 months later	$\Delta\Sigma$R	p
Ⓐ	11	18,1 ± 5,4	23,2 ± 7,0	+ 5,1 ± 7,5	0,04
Ⓑ	25	12,4 ± 10,9	16,2 ± 11,2	+ 3,9 ± 5,0	0,006
Ⓒ	8	14,0 ± 13,0	9,8 ± 11,0	−4,3 ± 2,8	0,003
Ⓓ	10	11,8 ± 12,8	10,7 ± 12,7	−1,1 ± 4,8	ns

Table 1. Precordial R-wave amplitudes [mV] in patients with spontaneous reperfusion Ⓐ, successful reperfusion using SK infusion and open vessel 4 to 6 months later Ⓑ, reocclusion of the infarct related vessel Ⓒ, and unsuccessful reperfusion Ⓓ. Comparison between the acute and chronic status.

	n	nQS acute after SK infusion	nQS chronic 4-6 months later	ΔnQS	p
Ⓐ	11	14,7 ± 10,8	12,3 ± 7,5	−2,4 ± 4,8	ns
Ⓑ	25	27,9 ± 13,1	21,2 ± 13,7	−6,6 ± 8,9	0,001
Ⓒ	8	26,5 ± 12,2	31,0 ± 12,2	+ 4,3 ± 3,2	0,007
Ⓓ	10	30,4 ± 12,2	30,7 ± 12,6	+ 0,3 ± 10,7	ns

Table 2. Number of precordial leads with complete loss of R-waves (n QS). Comparison between the acute and chronic status.

Conclusions

These data demonstrate that the ECG during and after reperfusion gives valuable information regarding whether or not sufficient reperfusion by thrombolysis was achieved and indicates reocclusion. PTCA of the infarct related vessels simulates reocclusion, and if it provokes new distinct ST elevation, proves there is viable myocardium in the reperfused area.

There is an increase of precordial R-wave amplitudes within a few months in patients in whom reperfusion can be achieved and whose vessels remain open, but a further loss of R-waves is seen if reocclusion occurs.

Thus, R-wave loss and development of pathological Q-waves in the early phase of MI does not necessarily mean dead myocardium and further loss of R waves after reocclusion indicates that the initial reperfusion salvaged myocardium.

References

1. von Essen R, Merx W, Effert S (1979) Spontaneous Course of ST-Segment Elevation in Acute Anterior Myocardial Infarction. Circulation 59: 105–112
2. von Essen R, Merx W, Dörr R, Effert S, Silny J, Rau G (1980) QRS Mapping in the Evaluation of Acute Myocardial Infarction. Circulation 62: 266–276
3. Lasch HG (1970) Die Therapie des Herzinfarktes. Therapiewoche 20: 107–114
4. Blanke H, Scherff F, Karsch KR, Levine RA, Smith H, Rentrop P (1983) Elekctrocardiographic changes after streptokinase-induced recanalization in patients with acute left anterior descending artery obstruction. Circulation 68: 406
5. Anderson JL, Marshall HW, Bray BF, Lutz JR, Frederick PR, Yanowitz FG, Datz FL, Klausner StV, Hagan AD (1983) A randomized trial of intracoronary streptokinase in the treatment of acute myocardial infarction. N Engl J Med 308: 1312–1318
6. von Essen R, Hinsen R, Louis R, Merx W, Silny J, Rau G, Effert S (1984) On-line monitoring of multiple precordial leads in high risk patients with coronary artery disease. European Heart Journal 5: 203–209

Intracoronary myocardial scintigraphy during intracoronary thrombolysis

J. SCHOFER, R. MONTZ, D.G. MATHEY and W. BLEIFELD

Abstract

Thirty-one patients with acute myocardial infarction underwent intracoronary thrombolysis. Intracoronary thallium scintigrams were obtained before and after thrombolysis. In 16 of the 31 patients intracoronary technetium pyrophosphate scintigraphy was performed simultaneously after thrombolysis. The scintigraphic results were compared with changes in regional ejection fraction in the area of infarction. Two patients had a normal left ventricular cine angiogram initially with no significant ventricular thallium defect before thrombolysis. In 8 patients regional ejection fraction normalized, all showed substantial new thallium uptake after thrombolysis. In 5 patients regional ejection fraction improved, 3 of these had new thallium uptake with a large residual defect after thrombolysis. Nine patients had no significant change in regional ejection fraction despite thrombolysis, and the initial thallium defect remained unchanged in 7. Four patients had a technetium pyrophosphate accumulation in the area of new thallium uptake. In these 4 patients regional wall motion did not change to an extent which was expected from the thallium scintigram.

In 18 patients with a complete occlusion of the right coronary artery who underwent intracoronary thrombolysis we performed intracoronary myocardial thallium scintigraphy. 15 of the 18 patients had a right ventricular thallium defect, and 17 of the 18 patients had a left ventricular thallium defect before thrombolysis.

All 15 patients with a right ventricular thallium defect initially but only 10 of the 17 patients with a left ventricular thallium defect initially showed new thallium uptake after thrombolysis.

It is concluded that combined intracoronary thallium-technetium pyrophosphate scintigraphy is helpful to predict myocardial salvage and areas of irreversible damage immediately after intracoronary thrombolysis. Moreover, intracoronary thallium scintigraphy seems to be a reliable method to study the incidence of right ventricular involvement in patients with inferior myocardial infarction and the effect of intracoronary thrombolysis on the right ventricular myocardium.

Introduction

Improvement in left ventricular function in the area of jeopardized myocardium seems to be the best way to document the benefit of thrombolysis in patients with acute myocardial infarction [1]. Full recovery of mechanical function of ischemic myocardium takes at least 10 days [2]. In order to prevent reinfarction, the immediate assessment of the effect of thrombolysis on ischemic myocardium however is required because in case a high grade residual stenosis after recanalization remains, balloon dilatation or coronary bypass surgery are needed early after thrombolysis to prevent reinfarction [3]. We used intracoronary thallium-201 and technetium pyrophosphate scintigraphy to select the appropriate patients for bypass surgery or PTCA [4].

In contrast to intravenous thallium scintigraphy after direct injection of thallium into the right coronary artery the right ventricular myocardium is clearly seen. This enabled us to study the incidence of right ventricular infarction and the effect of intracoronary thrombolysis on ischemic right ventricular myocardium in patients with inferior myocardial infarction.

Patients and methods

Patients

Thirty-one consecutive patients (27 men and 4 women with a mean age of 52 years) with acute transmural myocardial infarction were studied by comparing the results of intracoronary thallium scintigraphy and in some cases intracoronary technetium pyrophosphate scintigraphy with the change in left ventricular regional wall motion determined from an acute and follow-up left ventricular contrast cineangiogram.

Eighteen consecutive patients (14 men, and 4 women with a mean age of 54 years) with acute inferior myocardial infarction due to complete occlusion of the right coronary artery were included to study the incidence of right ventricular infarction and the effect of intracoronary thrombolysis on ischemic right ventricular myocardium. All patients had the onset of chest pain less than 3 hours before hospital admission and ST-elevation with no abnormal Q-waves in the leads with ST-elevation and no old transmural infarction. Patients with recent gastrointestinal hemorrhage, pectic ulcer, trauma, stroke or malignant neoplasm were excluded.

Protocol

Immediately after the diagnosis of acute myocardial infarction, the patient was transferred to the catheterization laboratory. Intracoronary thrombolysis was performed as previously described [5]. 0.3 to 0.5 mCi thallium-201 was injected into both coronary arteries. During intracoronary thrombolysis with strepto-kinase (2 000–4 000 units per minute) the initial scintigrams were obtained, using a mobile gamma camera (EDM, Searle). A second dose of 0.3 to 0.5 mCi thallium was injected into the infarct vessel 30 to 45 minutes after recanalization or after the maximal dose of streptokinase (250 000 units) had been given. In 16 of the 31 patients in addition 5 mCi technetium pyrophosphate was injected into the infarct vessel. A second series of simultaneously obtained thallium and technetium pyrophosphate scintigraphy were performed, followed by biplane left ventricular contrast cine-angiogram. Follow-up coronary and left ventricular contrast cineangiogram and an intracoronary thallium-201 scintigram were obtained 2 to 3 weeks after the acute infarct.

Analysis of scintigrams

The data were recorded in a 128 × 128 matrix and stored on a disk. The pictures were flood-corrected and slightly smoothed. Two independent observers classified these scintigraphic results as follows:

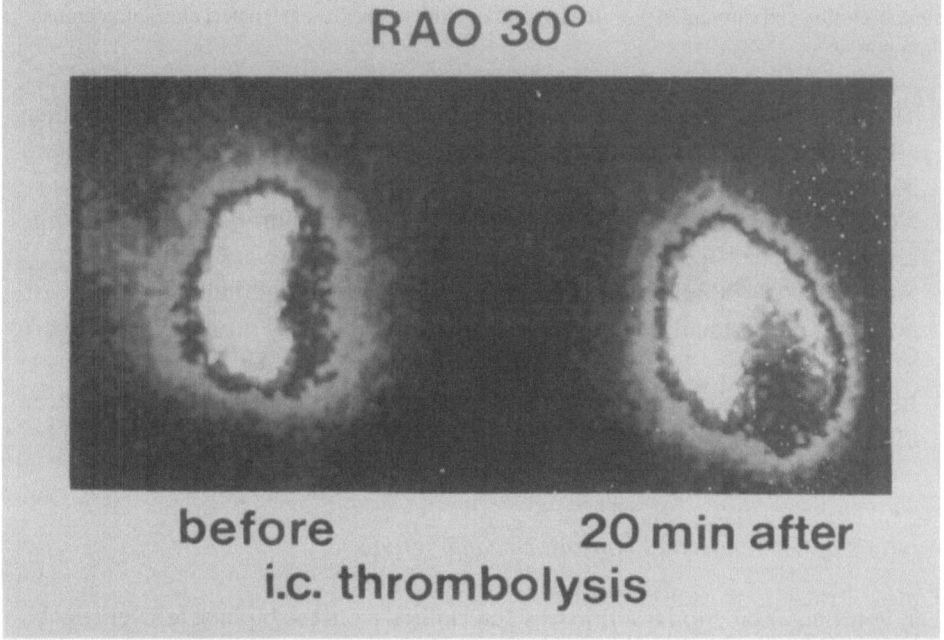

Figure 1. Intracoronary thallium-201 scintigram in a patient with left anterior descending coronary artery occlusion and new thallium-201 uptake with a large residual defect after intracoronary thrombolysis.

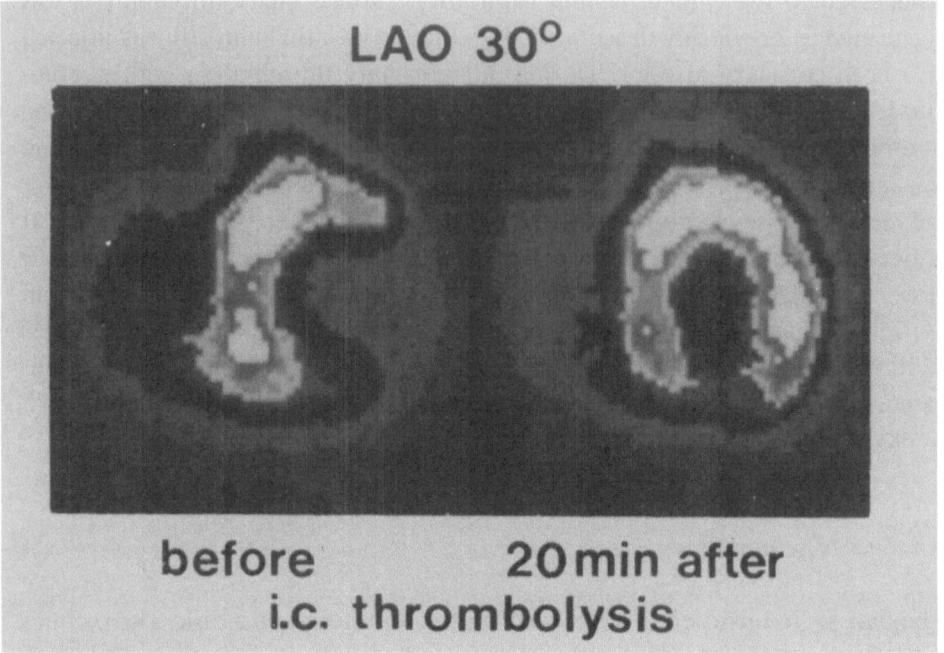

Figure 2. Intracoronary thallium-201 scintigram in a patient with left anterior descendinging coronary artery occlusion and substantial new thallium uptake with a small residual defect after intracoronary thrombolysis.

1. Thallium defect before intracoronary thrombolysis with no further change after intracoronary thrombolysis and intracoronary reinjection of thallium-201.
2. New thallium uptake in the area of the initial thallium defect with a large residual defect after intracoronary thrombolysis (Figure 1).
3. Substantial new thallium uptake in the area of the initial thallium defect with no or a small residual thallium defect after intracoronary thrombolysis (Figure 2).
4. Identification and localization of a technetium pyrophosphate accumulation after thrombolysis.

Analysis of left ventricular contrast cineangiograms

Left ventricular ejection fraction was determined from the biplane left ventricular angiogram and Simpson's rule was used for left ventricular volume measurements [6]. Regional left ventricular wall motion was analysed according to the following method [7]. The center point of the left ventricular enddiastolic projection was calculated and served as a reference point for both the enddiastolic and systolic frames. A triangular segment obtained by connecting the reference point with the corner points of the aortic annulus was excluded from analysis. The remaining area was devided into 5 segments, each of which had an identical angle around the left ventricular center point. The enddiastolic and endsystolic areas of each segments were measured and the difference expressed as percent change of the enddiastolic segment area (regional ejection fraction (%). Normal values for each segment were calculated from measurements of the left ventricle in 40 normal subjects. To determine the change in regional wall motion, we compared the segments within the perfusion area of the infarct vessel that initially showed an abnormal wall motion with the same segments at follow-up. The change in regional wall motion in the infarct area was expressed as the difference of the mean values of the regional ejection fraction of the involved segments between the acute and follow-up angiograms. A change in regional wall motion of more than 10% ejection fraction was defined as improvement; a change in regional wall motion from an abnormal value initially to the normal range was defined as normalization.

Results

A) Comparison of thallium/technetium pyrophosphate scintigraphic results with the change in regional wall motion

In 24 of the 31 patients the occluded coronary artery could be reopened and was patent at follow-up. After successful intracoronary thrombolysis we could divide the patients according to the scintigraphic results into 3 groups:

At best the initial thallium defect before thrombolysis almost completely disappeared after thallium reinjection into the recanalized infarct vessel (Figure 2). In a second group of patients we found significant thallium uptake after thrombolysis, but a large residual defect remained (Figure 1). In the worst case, the defect size after thrombolysis did not change despite recanalization of the infarct vessel. The change in regional left ventricular wall motion was determined from an acute and follow-up left ventricular contrast cineangiogram.

The mean values of the regional ejection fraction in the area of the infarct was reduced to a similar degree in all patients (Figure 3). At follow-up the regional wall motion became normal in 8 patients, in 5 patients wall motion improved, whereas in 9 patients with successful thrombolysis and in 7 patients with unsuccessful thrombolysis regional wall motion remained depressed.

In the 8 patients with a normalization of regional wall motion in the infarct area a substantial reduction of the initial LV thallium defect size was noted (Figure 4). In 5 of 3 patients with improvement of regional wall motion left ventricular thallium defect size was reduced, but a large residual defect remained. Similarly, in 7 out of the 9 patients with no change in regional wall motion the initial thallium

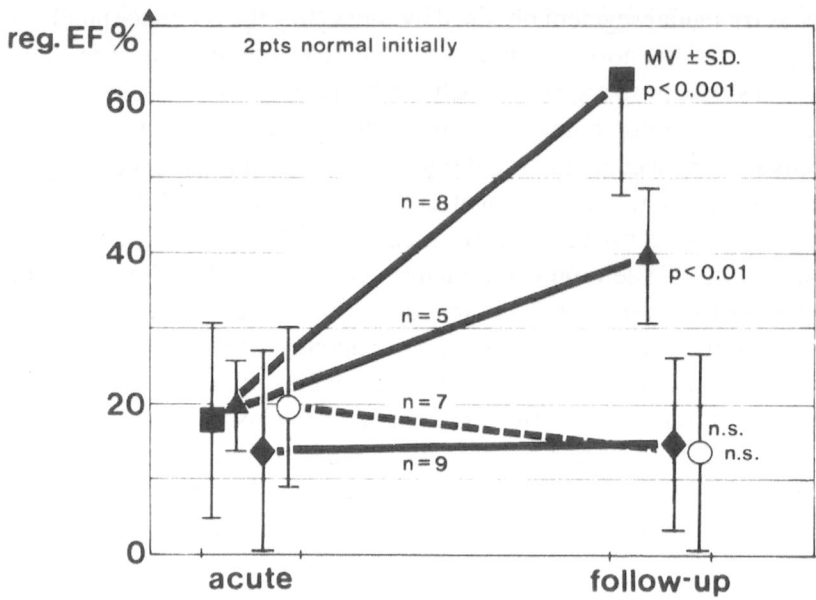

Figure 3. Mean values (± standard deviation) of regional ejection fraction (reg. EF) in the area of infarction obtained from the acute and follow-up left ventricular angiograms. See also text on page 9.

Number of pts.	Change in regional EF	LV TI-201 uptake a f t e r coronary artery recanalization
2	unchanged, but normal initially	no LV-defect initially
8	normalization	7 substantial reduction of LV-defect size with no or small residual defect 1 questionable LV-defect initially
5	improved	2* substantial reduction of LV-defect size with small residual defect 3 new TI-201 uptake with a large residual defect
9	no change	2 little TI-201 uptake in the basal segment 5 no change 2* new TI-201 uptake with a large residual defect

Figure 4. Relation between changes in left ventricular ejection fraction and new thallium-201 uptake after intracoronary thrombolysis. *These patients had a significant overlap of new thallium-201 uptake and technetium-99m pyrophosphate accumulation. See also text on page 87.

defect size did not change significantly after thrombolysis. In 4 patients, however, with new thallium-uptake regional wall motion did not change to the extent which was expected from the thallium scintigrams. In these 4 patients we found an accumulation of pyrophosphate in the area of new thallium uptake (Figure 5). In the remaining 10 patients in whom intracoronary pyrophosphate scintigraphy was performed the pyrophosphate spot corresponds to the thallium defect.

B) Incidence of right ventricular infarction and effect of intracoronary thrombolysis in patients with inferior infarction

A right ventricular thallium defect before thrombolysis was seen in 15 of 18 patients and a left ventricular defect was seen in 17. After thrombolysis thallium was taken up in the right ventricular defect area in all 15 patients, whereas left ventricular thallium-uptake in the defect area was seen only in 10 of the 17 patients (Figure 6).

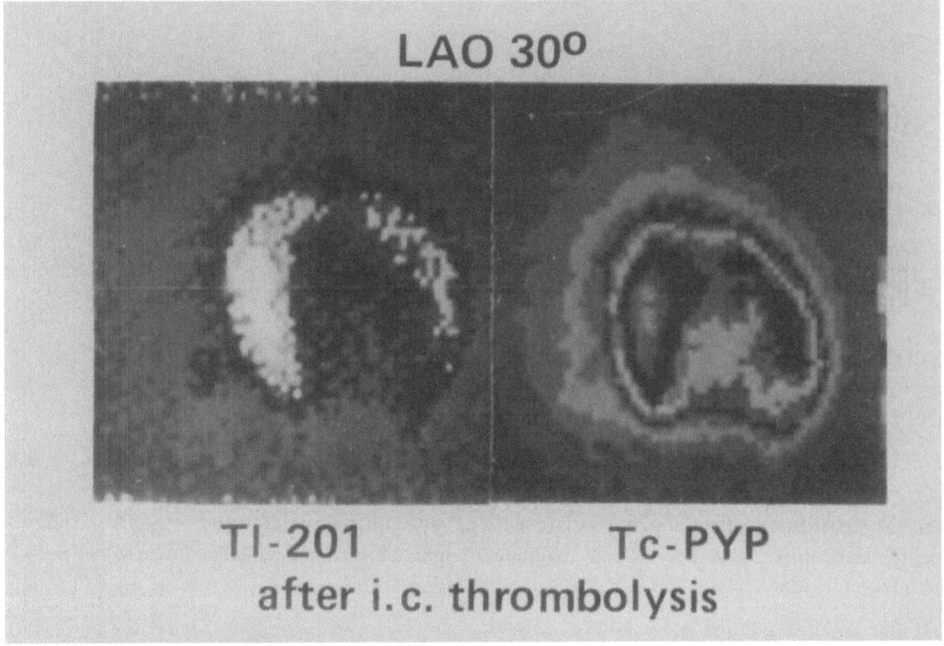

Figure 5. Intracoronary thallium-201 scintigram (left) and intracoronary technetium-99m pyrophosphate scintigram (right) of a patient with left anterior descending coronary artery recanalization and significant overlap of new thallium-201 uptake and technetium-99m pyrophosphate accumulation after intracoronary thrombolysis in the interventricular septum.

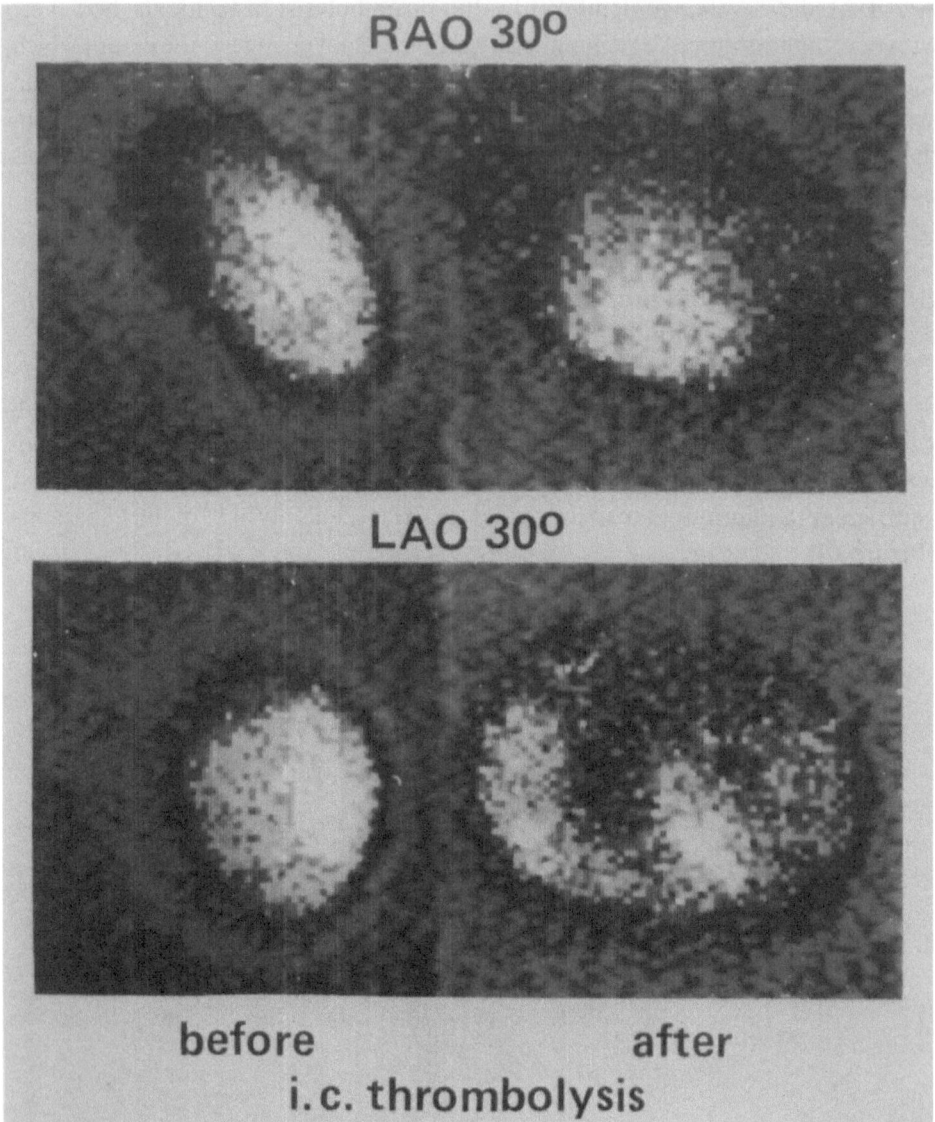

Figure 6. Intracoronary thallium-201 scintigram of a patient with inferior infarct before (left) and after (right) intracoronary thrombolysis. New thallium-201 uptake is seen in the right ventricle as well as in the interventricular septum.

Discussion

In contrast to the intravenous application of thallium after two intracoronary injections into the same coronary artery almost background free scintigrams were obtained, allowing the assessment of changes in myocardial thallium uptake in the reperfused area. Whether thallium uptake after intracoronary injection reflects viability of the myocardium immediately after intracoronary thrombolysis has not been validated. Therefore the acute changes in the thallium-201 defect sizes were compared with the change in regional left ventricular wall motion in the infarct area between the acute and follow-up left ventricular contrast cineangiograms.

In 27 of the 31 patients the relationship between new thallium uptake and recovery of mechanical function was evident. In 4 patients however, the intracoronary thallium scintigrams were considered false-positive. In these patients an accumulation of technetium pyrophosphate was found in the area of new thallium uptake. Technetium pyrophosphate was given intracoronarily because this route of administration results in a target to background ratio about twice as high as that after intravenous injection [8]. From experimental studies of Maddahi et al. [9] it is known that reperfusion results in an immediate technetium pyrophosphate accumulation exclusively in the area of the necrosis, while thallium-201 uptake occurs in non-necrotic myocardial cells. The thallium/technetium pyrophosphate overlap was seen experimentally [10] and also in patients with acute myocardial infarction [11]. We suggest that this scintigraphic overlap reflects areas of necrotic and viable myocardium laying close together.

Whereas after intravenous application the right ventricular myocardium is only seen in cases with abnormal right ventricular load after intracoronary injection of thallium-201 into the right coronary artery the right ventricular myocardium could be clearly seen in all cases. Using hemodynamic parameters [12, 13], technetium pyrophosphate scintigraphy [14, 15], radionuclide ventriculography [16, 17] and echocardiography [18] the right ventricular myocardium is involved in patients with inferior myocardial infarction in up to 40%. The high incidence of right ventricular infarction in our patients [15 of 18] in comparison to other studies may be caused by several factors. In all of our patients the right coronary artery was completely occluded, patients with subtotal occlusion or spontaneous recanalization or with an occlusion of the circumflex coronary artery were excluded.

All 15 patients who had a right ventricular thallium defect before thrombolysis had new thallium uptake in the right ventricular myocardium after thrombolysis, whereas in only 10 of the 17 patients with a left ventricular thallium defect thallium uptake was seen after thrombolysis. These findings may be of clinical relevance in patients with acute inferior myocardial infarction associated with right ventricular failure including cardiogenic shock. We would recommend to perform thrombolysis in these patients even after a time when salvage of the left ventricular myocardium is unlikely since the iscnemic right ventricular myocardium may still be viable [19].

References

1. Sheehan FH, Mathey DG, Schofer J, Krebber HJ, Dodge HT (1983) Effect of interventions in salvaging left ventricular function in acute myocardial infarction: a study of intracoronary streptokinase. Am J Cardiol 52: 431–438
2. Baughmann KL, Maroko PR, Vatner SF (1981) Effects of coronary artery reperfusion on myocardial infarct size and survival in conscious dogs. Circulation 63: 317–323
3. Merx W, Dörr R, Rentrop P, Blanke H, Karsch KR, Mathey DG, Kremer P, Rutsch W, Schmutzler H (1981) Evaluation of the effectiveness of intracoronary streptokinase infusion in acute myocardial infarction: post-procedure management and hospital course in 204 patients. Am Heart J 201: 1181–1189
4. Schofer J, Mathey DG, Montz R, Bleifeld W, Stritzke P (1983) Dual intracoronary scintigraphy with thallium-201 and technetium-99m pyrophosphate is helpful to predict improvement in left ventricular wall motion immediately after intracoronary thrombolysis in acute myocardial infarction. J of Am Coll of Cardiol 4: 737–744
5. Mathey DG, Kuck KH, Tilsner V, Krebber HJ, Bleifeld W (1981) Nonsurgical coronary artery recanalization in acute transmural myocardial infarction. Circulation 63: 489–97
6. Chapman CB, Baker O, Reynolds J, Bonte FJ (1958) Use of biplane cinefluorography for measurements of ventricular volume. Circulation 18: 1105
7. Rickards A, Seabra-Gomes R, Thurston P (1977) The assessment of regional abnormalities of the left ventricle by angiography. Eur J Cardiol 5: 167–176
8. Parkey RW, Kulkarni PV, Lewis SE, Datz FL, Dehmer GJ, Gutekunst DP, Bujy LM, Bonte FJ, Willseron J (1981) Effect of coronary blood flow and site of injection on technetium-99m pyrophosphate detection of early canine myocardial infarcts. The Journal of Nuclear Medicine 22: 133–137
9. Maddahi J, Geft J, Hülse J, Berman D, Swan HJC, Ganz W (1982) Intracoronary technetium-99m pyrophosphate immediately demonstrates necrosis in reperfused myocardium and complements post-reperfusion intracoronary thallium-201 imaging. Circulation 66: II-86 (abstr)
10. Buja LM, Parkey RW, Stokely EM, Bonte FJ, Willerson JT (1976) Pathophysiology of technetium-99m stannous pyrophosphate and thallium-201 scintigraphy of acute anterior myocardial infarcts in dogs. The Journal of Clinical Investigation 57: 1508–1520
11. Berger HJ, Gottschalk A, Zaret BL (1978) Dual radionuclide study of acute myocardial infarction. Comparison of thallium-201 and technetium-99m stannous pyrophosphate imaging in man. Annals of Internal Medicine 88: 145–154
12. Cohn JN, Guiha NH, Broder ML, Limas CJ (1974) Right ventricular infarction. Clinical and hemodynamic features. Am J Cardiol 33: 209–214
13. Lorell B, Leinbach RC, Pohost GM, Crold HK, Dinsmore RE, Hutter RM Jr, Pastore JO, De Sanctis RW (1979) Right ventricular infarction. Clinical diagnosis and differention from cardiac tamponade and pericardial constriction. Am J Cardiol 43: 465–471
14. Legrand V, Rigó P, Smeets JP, Demoulin JC, Collignon P, Kulbertus HE (1983) Right ventricular myocardial infarction diagnosed by 99m technetium pyrophosphate scintigraphy: Clinical course and follow-up. Eur Heart J 4: 9–19
15. Wackers FJ TH, Lie KJ, Sokole EB, Res J, Van der Shoot JB, Dürrer D (1978) Prevalence of right ventricular involvement in inferior wall infarction assessed with myocardial imaging with thallium-201 and technetium-99m pyrophosphate. Am J Cardiol 42: 358–363
16. Rigo P, Murray M, Taylor DR, Weisfeldt ML, Kelly DT, Strauss HW, Pitt B (1975) Right

ventricular dysfunction detected by gated scintigraphy in patients with acute inferior myocardial infarction. Circulation 52: 268–274

17. Reduto LA, Berger HJ, Cohen LS, Gottschalk A, Zaret BL (1978) Sequential radionuclide assessment of left and right ventricular performance after acute transmural myocardial infarction. Annals of Internal Med 89: 441–447

18. Sharpe DN, Botvinich EH, Shannes DM, Schiller NB, Massie BM, Chatterjee K, Parmley WW (1978) The noninvasive diagnosis of right ventricular infarction. Circulation: 483–490

19. Mathey DG, Kuck KH, Remmecke J, Tilsner V, Bleifeld W (1980) Transmural recanalization of coronary artery thrombolysis: a preliminary report of its application in cardiogenic shock. Eur Heart J 1: 207–210

20. Schofer J, Krebber HJ, Montz R, Spielmann R, Bleifeld W, Rodewald G, Mathey DG (1983) Decision for early post-thrombolytic coronary artery bypass-grafting based on intracoronary myocardial scintigraphy. Circulation 68: Suppl. III, 153

Opposite ends of the intervention spectrum: Effects of intracoronary thrombolysis on long-term survival and LV function – Detection of early CAD by non-invasive positron imaging

K.L. GOULD, R.W. SMALLING, N. MULLANI, R.A. GOLDSTEIN,
F. FUENTES, G. WONG and M. MATTHEWS

Introduction

In keeping with the theme of this conference, we report on the opposite ends of the spectrum involving intervention therapy for coronary artery disease. At the invasive end, we present our data on the effects of intracoronary thrombolysis during acute myocardial infarction on long-term survival and LV function. At the noninvasive end of the spectrum, we describe our approach using positron imaging for diagnosis of early asymptomatic CAD, thereby allowing early medical intervention to stabilize or reverse anatomically mild disease before symptoms or myocardial infarction require more invasive intervention. Since mild asymptomatic disease is more reversible than advanced symptomatic disease, the process of early diagnosis becomes an essential part of therapy aimed at regression – a process we call diagnostic therapeutics. We believe that the evolution of these two approaches at the opposite ends of intervention cardiology will radically and profoundly change the field by becoming routine clinical practice over the next five years.

Effects of intracoronary thrombolysis during acute myocardial infarction on long-term survival and LV function

Methods

Since 1980, we have studied 258 patients with acute myocardial infarction at The University of Texas Medical School at Houston and Hermann Hospital. One hundred eighty of these patients met appropriate criteria of the intracoronary streptokinase protocol (less than 18 hours from onset of chest pain, no cerebrovascular accident within previous two months, absence of major surgical intervention or trauma within the previous two weeks, absence of significant mitral valvular disease). Seventy-eight patients who were not eligible for the protocol or who refused the protocol were studied prospectively and served as a control group for comparison. All patients had a gated radionuclide angiogram within 24-hours from onset of chest pain and 10 days after myocardial infarction to assess changes in left ventricular function.

Those patients who accepted the streptokinase protocol after informed consent was obtained, were taken to the cardiac catheterization laboratory directly from the emergency center after the diagnosis of acute myocardial infarction was made by standard electrocardiographic and historical criteria. In general, patients were instrumented with a balloon tipped thermodilution catheter and pacemaker catheter, prior to coronary arteriography. Coronary arteriography was performed in the infarct related artery in an attempt to establish whether the artery was thrombosed or simply critically stenosed. After the infarct related artery was identified, intracoronary nitroglycerin was administered followed by intracoronary streptokinase therapy (10,000 to 20,000 unit bolus followed by a 2,000 to 4,000 unit per minute infusion). Coronary angiograms were repeated every 15 minutes, until arterial patency was achieved, or until 60–120 minutes of infusion were reached. Once arterial patency was established, the streptokinase infusion was continued for an additional 30 minutes or until evidence of intraluminal thrombus was eliminated. After intracoronary streptokinase infusion, the remaining coronary artery was then studied angiographically and if the patients were hemodynamically stable, a biplane left ventricular cine angiogram was performed. The catheter introducers were left in place for 24-hours or until the coagulation parameters had normalized. All patients received 10,000 units of intraarterial Heparin prior to beginning angiography. Heparin was continued only subcutaneously (5,000 units q12h) post catheterization. All patients were treated with aspirin 300 mg daily and Dipyridamole 75 mg b.i.d. Control patients were treated similarly with antiplatelet agents and subcutaneous Heparin. All patients received nifedipine 10 mg q8h, Propranolol 10–40 mg q6h, and Nitrates, if hemodynamically tolerated. The control population received the same medical therapy, excluding acute catheterization and streptokinase therapy.

The control patient population was identical to the streptokinase population in terms of infarct location, history of previous myocardial infarction, history of congestive heart failure and clinical class (Killip Class) on admission. Results are presented in terms of percent change of ejection fraction at hospital discharge, compared with ejection fraction obtained on admission during the acute phase of myocardial infarction. The mortality results are the current mortality rates of the entire population that we have studied. The follow-up ranges from 6 months to three years with the average follow-up being 14 months. Statistical techniques included the paired student T test, non-paired student T test and chi-square analysis with statistical significance being noted at $P \leq .05$.

Results

Reperfusion was successful in 83% of anterior myocardial infarctions and 61% of inferior or lateral infarctions. Total mortality in the entire streptokinase group was 12% which was significantly lower than the control group mortality of 28% (P<.002). Similarly, average left ventricular ejection fraction increased by 15% in the streptokinase group, compared to 2.7% in the control group (P<.001.). The in-hospital reinfarction rate was 8% in the streptokinase group including those patients with perioperative infarctions.

Effects of patient age

As might be expected, elderly patients have a much worse survival than those less than or equal to 65 years of age. However, left ventricular function appeared to improve with reperfusion irrespective of patient's age. The percent increase in ejection fraction in patients greater than 65 years of age treated with streptokinae was 16%, which was not significantly different from the 18% improvement seenin patients less than or equal to 65 years of age. Patients who had successful reperfusion and were less than 65 years of age had a much larger percent change in ejection fraction compared to the control patients in that age group (18% vs. 4%, P = .002). However, when examining the mortality in those patients greater than or equal to 65 years of age, the streptokinase and the control patients had an identical mortality of 38% and 39% respectively. Patients less than or equal to 65 years of age who were treated with streptokinase, demonstrated a striking improvement in mortality compared to similar control patients (7% vs. 19%, P = .02). Thus, it would appear that improved ventricular function during myocardial infarction is not directly correlated with improved survival in patients of advanced age.

Location of infarct

Forty-seven percent of the streptokinase patients had anterior myocardial infarctions which was similar to the 46% incidence seen in control patients. Reperfusion in patients with anterior myocardial infarctions, resulted in a 24% increase in average left ventricular ejection fraction, compared to a 4% increase in the control patients with anterior myocardial infarction (P<.001). Although patients with successful reperfusion in the setting of an inferior or lateral myocardial infarction had an 11% increase in ejection fraction, this increase was not significantly different from similar control patients who demonstrated a 2% increase in ejection fraction (P = .07, NS).

Mortality results were particularly striking in patients with anterior myocardial infarctions. Patients with anterior myocardial infarctions treated with streptokinase had a 12% mortality which was significantly less than the 33% occurring in the control patients with anterior myocardial infarctions (P = .05). The mortality in streptokinase patients with inferior MI's was 13% while control patients demonstrated a 24% mortality with inferior or lateral myocardial infarctions. Although the control group motality was twice as high as the mortality in similar streptokinase patients, this difference did not achieve statistical signifcance. Thus, patients with anterior myocardial infarctions appear to benefit more with striking reduction in mortality and significant improvement in left ventricular function than patients with inferior or lateral myocardial infarctions.

Time from onset of pain to reperfusion

It has been suggested that reperfusion must occur within six hours after onset of pain for significant benefit to occur. We found that patients who achieved successful reperfusion 0–6 hours after onset of pain demonstrated a 16% improvement in left ventricular ejection fraction compared to the entire control population which demonstrated only a 3% improvement in ejection fraction, a difference which almost achieved statistical significance at $P = .07$. Interestingly, however, those patients reperfused from 6–12 hours after onset of pain had a striking improvement in left ventricular function with a 20% increase in ejection fraction which was significantly higher than that seen in the control population ($P < .001$).

Similarly, there were no significant differences in the improved mortality seen in the streptokinase patients admitted 0–6 and 6–12 hours after onset of pain as compared to the controls which had a significantly higher mortality. However, each streptokinase group had a lower mortality than the control population. The mortality rate in the patients admitted 0–6 hours after onset of pain was 9% compared to the mortality in the patients reperfused 6–12 hours after onset of pain, which was 15%. These mortality rates were significantly less than 28% observed in the control population ($P = .005$ to $.003$). Thus, there appeared to be little correlation between time from onset of pain to reperfusion and objective improvement in left ventricular function and improved survival.

Electrocardiographic findings

Q waves have been considered a sign of completed transmural infarction. If the presence of Q waves on the admission electrocardiogram signified a completed infarct, one would expect that successful thrombolytic therapy would have little effect. However, left ventricular function improved similarly in patients with or without Q waves on hospital admission (15% vs. 21%, $P = NS$). The improvement in ejection fraction in patients with Q waves who had successful reperfusion was 15% compared to control patients with a 3% improvement ($P = .001$).

Mortality also seemed to be little effected by the presence of Q waves on the admission electrocardiogram. Patients with Q waves who were treated with streptokinase demonstrated a 9% mortality compared to 15% in those who had persistent ST elevation only prior to entry into the protocol. The mortality in patients with Q waves on admission who underwent streptokinase therapy was significantly less than the 28% seen in the control patients (P = .002). Since coronary reperfusion is often accompanied by rapid evolution of the electrocardiogram from ST elevation to Q wave formation with T wave inversion, the presence of Q waves on the admission electrocardiogram, early in the course of acute myocardial infarction may actually be a good prognostic sign signaling early evolution of the infarct secondary to significant collateral in-flow or partial reperfusion.

Effect of left ventricular function on admission

Although global left ventricular function often correlates with survival, it is difficult to equate changes in left ventricular function with successful outcome of an infarct intervention if the patient's left ventricular ejection fraction is normal at study entry. In other words, patients with normal left ventricular function would be expected to show little improvement in global left ventricular function even with successful reperfusion. Our data confirms this hypothesis since patients admitted with ejection fractions greater than 45% had an average improvement in ejection fraction of only 2% which was much less than that seen in patients who had a successful thrombolysis who were admitted with an ejection fraction less than 45%. These patients with relatively poor left ventricular function on admission, demonstrated a 26% improvement in left ventricular function with reperfusion regardless of location of the infarction. Patients admitted with ejection fractions less than 45% who had successful reperfusion, had a much larger increase in ejection fraction (26% vs. 5%) than those patients admitted in the control group with ejection fractions less than 45% (P<.001). No significant differences were demonstrated between change in ejection fraction in the reperfusion group with normal left ventricular function and similar controls.

Interestingly, patients in the streptokinase group with normal left ventricular function demonstrated a mortality rate of 4% which was significantly less than the 19% seen in similar control patients with normal left ventricular function (P = .02). Patients with ejection fractions less than 45% in the control group had a 47% mortality which was approximately two times the mortality in the streptokinase patients with poor ventricular function, but this difference did not achieve statistical significance. Patients in Killip Class I and II in the streptokinase group had a 7% mortality which was less than the 21% seen in the similar control patients (P = .002). In patients admitted in Killip Class III or IV, the differences were much less striking with the streptokinase group demonstrating a

52% mortality which was not significantly different than the 67% observed in the control group.

Reperfusion success

A major determinate of success of thrombolytic therapy is reperfusion with significant restoration of blood flow to the ischemic myocardium. The greater percentage of patients with successful reperfusion, the better the expected outcome of the therapy. Reperfused patients demonstrated an 18% increase in ejection fraction which was much greater than the 3% change seen in patients failing reperfusion (P = .03). Similarly, patients with successful reperfusion had a significantly greater improvement in ejection fraction than the cotrol group which demonstrated only a 3% increase in ejection fraction (P<.001). The percent increase in ejection fraction in the streptokinase patients not reperfused was identical to that seen in the control patients.

The mortality in reperfused patients was only 6% compared to 37% in patients failing reperfusion (P = .001). After streptokinase therapy the mortality in patients without successful reperfusion was insignificantly higher than the mortality rate of 28% observed in control patients (P = NS). However, the mortality rate in all patients treated with streptokinase (12%) and in patients with successful reperfusion (6%) was significantly less than the 28% mortality rate in the control patients (P = .001 and .002 respectively).

Complications

Two deaths could have been directly associated with the procedure (1% of intracoronary streptokinase group). One was secondary to an embolic cerebrovascular accident occuring during catheter manipulation. Another was associated with left main coronary spasm which could have been aggravated by catheter manipulation. In the second patient all vessels were patent at post mortem and no dissection was present. Bleeding was not infrequent with 14% of intracoronary streptokinase patients requiring transfusion. However, there were no deaths secondary to bleeding. Most bleeding occurred at the catheter insertion site or from traumatic nasogastric or endotracheal tube insertions.

Discussion

Although this study was not randomized, patients were studied consecutively and treated by the same physicians in the same facility. The characteristics of both the streptokinase patients and the control patients were similar. Thrombolytic therapy and especially intracoronary thrombolytic therapy, is not a completely benign procedure. As we have previously published [1], significant bleeding may occur, as well as potential deaths which are directly attributable to the therapy. Nonetheless, the benefits of this therapy appear to substantially outweigh the risks of bleeding and other risks attendant with catheterization.

Several randomized studies of intracoronary streptokinase therapy have been published with mixed results. Khaja et al, demonstrated no significant improvement in ventricular function in patients treated with streptokinase, compared to patients treated with placebo when both groups were subjected to acute catheterization during evolving myocardial infarction [2]. Their study reported a 60% reperfusion rate, compared to 75% achieved in most centers. In addition the average admission radionuclide ejection fraction in the streptokinase group was 45% which is very close to normal [2]. Therefore, one might not expect striking results with low reperfusion success in patients having close to normal LV function at hospital admission. In a similar study by Anderson et al. [3], 79% of patients were reperfused and the average left ventricular ejection fraction did improve significantly. Thus, reperfusion success as demonstrated in this study and as suggested by the disparate results in the studies discussed above, is an important factor.

Patients older than 65 years of age appear to benefit little in terms of mortality from intracoronary thrombolytic therapy and hence, its use in these patients especially if they are physiologically older than their apparent ages, may be unwarrented. Although the left ventricular function does appear to improve in this subgroup of patients, their mortality clearly is not improved by intracoronary thrombolytic therapy.

Patients with anterior myocardial infarctions appear to benefit more than those patients with inferior myocardial infarction, probably secondary to the larger area of myocardium supplied by the responsible infarct related artery. The extent rather than location, per se, of the infarction appears to be the most important factor. Patients with large inferior wall myocardial infarctions which depress the global ejection fraction show improvement in proportion to the severity of the initial ejection fraction.

The time from onset of pain to reperfusion appears to have minimal influence, if any, on outcome in terms of either return of left ventricular function or mortality. Many of our patients were referred from outlying hospitals on a helicopter air transport system. These patients tend to be relatively more ill than the average patient who presents to the emergency center, primarily. We have elected to offer therapy to those patients, upto 18 hours after onset of pain and have not been able to demonstrate differences in those patients treated early compared to those patients treated late either in terms of the return of left ventricular function or mortality. Those patients presenting later than 6 hours of chest pain may have significant collateral flow allowing a wider time window for successful myocardial salvage.

Neither has the electrocardiogram been particularly helpful in patient selection. Early evolution of Q waves appears to be a good sign and may relate to collateral blood flow or spontaneous reperfusion of the infarct related vessel. Thus, Q waves on the admitting electrocardiogram should not be a deterent to treatment with thrombolytic therapy.

Patients with normal left ventricular function will not demonstrate substantial increase in ejection fraction, after successful thrombolytic therapy. Nonetheless, the mortality is improved in this subgroup of patients with good left ventricular function. Thus, there is an effect of thrombolytic therapy on survival which is independent of changes in LV function. A measurable difference in left ventricular function will be achieved in the majority of patients who undergo successful reperfusion, if their admission left ventricular function is abnormal. However, due to concurrent hyperfunction in adjacent myocardial segments patients admitted with normal left ventricular function may demonstrate only regional changes in left ventricular function. Thus, using left ventricular function to determine which patient should be subjected to thrombolytic therapy would delay onset of therapy and appears to have little impact on overall outcome.

Reperfusion success is correlated with improved left ventricular function and survival. Hence, all efforts at improving the reperfusion rate, may be beneficial including vigorous administration of vasodilators, if the patients are hemodynamically stable and liberal use of antiplatelet therapy post reperfusion. Full anticoagulation does not appear to be necessary in the peri-infarct period in our hands but antiplatelet drugs do appear to be important, as might be expected in the arterial circulation.

Detection of early CAD by noninvasive positron imaging using affordable, clinical tomographic systems without a cyclotron

In order to provide appropriate perspective for this presentation, it is necessary to review the fundamental steps of perfusion imaging and the essential criteria for a satisfactory perfusion imaging method. A basic assumption underlying this discussion is that the goal of perfusion imaging is to maximize diagnostic sensitivity and specificity applied to any population of subjects, either as a screening test in asymptomatic populations with low prevalence of disease or for specific diagnosis in symptomatic patients.

The most useful noninvasive test widely used for localizing abnormal myocardial perfusion due to coronary artery disease utilizes thallium-201 injected during treadmill exercise. Diagnostic sensitivity has ranged from 70% to 90% and specificity has ranged from 86% to 100% [4]. Thallium exercise imaging has been associated with 10% to 30% false negative and up to 14% false positive results. There is an inverse relation between sensitivity and specificity. Those publications reporting high sensitivity are associated with a lower specificity and those publications reporting lower sensitivity are associated with higher specificity. These results are typical of receiver operating curves for an imperfect test [5, 6] in which an observer who overinterprets borderline images as being positive will also thereby read as positive a number of studies which are, in fact, negative, thereby resulting in a larger number of false positives, i.e. a lower specificity. Conversely, conservative interpretation will increase the specificity but decrease the sensitivity. Quantitative kinetic analysis has provided much needed objectivity to the utility of thallium [4] but not the radical improvement required. Identification of specific coronary arteries affected or of one, two or three vessel disease has also been unreliable with thallium imaging.

A sensitivity and specificity of approximately 85% might suggest that the test could be adequate as a screening procedure for detecting coronary artery disease in asymptomatic patients. However, this sensitivity and specificity does not account for the effect of disease prevalence on the diagnostic accuracy and utility of thallium imaging when it is applied to asymptomatic populations. A number of papers utilizing Bayesian analysis have indicated that the sensitivity and specificity of thallium stress testing is grossly inadequate as a screening test in populations with a low prevalence of coronary artery disease ranging from 5–10% of the population studied [5, 6]. An abnormal exercise thallium test in an asymptomatic subject in this population is associated with only a 10–20% probability of having coronary artery disease. Thus, in order for a diagnostic test to be useful in an asymptomatic population, the sensitivity and specificity must be much higher than that obtainable with current convention thallium imaging.

Early mild coronary atherosclerosis appears to be reversible in man based upon data from both primate experimentation and limited human studies. However, symptomatic coronary artery disease in humans is usually associated with anatomically advanced coronary plaques that are often calcified with little potential for reversal. Early diagnosis in asymptomatic man five to ten years before clinical events or symptoms therefore becomes an integral part of potential regression or arrest of progression. Current non-invasive tests have not proven adequate to reliably detect or quantify even advanced clinical disease, much less early, mild asymptomatic disease.

The reader may appropriately ask whether such early diagnosis of mild disease is useful clinically. There are two answers to this question. The first is that the early diagnosis approach would have a profound impact on cardiology by changing our current therapy of antianginal drugs, bypass surgery and angioplasty to one of specific selective prevention of progression in specific asymptomatic individuals. The second answer is that a diagnostic imaging test adequate to detect early mild disease with relatively high certainty will be even more accurate for identifying and quantifying severity of more advanced symptomatic disease.

Experimentally, the difference in regional perfusion between abnormal and normally perfused areas of myocardium must be at least 200% to 250% before being detected by thallium imaging [7], a difference corresponding to a 70–80%

diameter stenosis, which is advanced, clinical disease. The use of the seven pinhole collimator with thallium imaging has not improved this sensitivity. Single photon emission tomography of thallium images has likewise not yet been demonstrated to provide a solution although it shows some borderline improvement. The specificity of exercise gated blood pool imaging and regional left ventricular dysfunction during exercise as a means of detecting coronary artery disease has been sufficiently low that its value as a screening test is not useful due to many false positive tests.

The problem is further complicated by the lack of a 'gold standard' or a reference for defining severity of coronary artery stenosis. Coronary arteriography has several limitations. Interpretation of coronary arteriograms is complicated by marked interobserver and intraobserver variability. The universal use of relative percent diameter narrowing as a measure of severity ignores other critical geometric characteristics of stenoses such as length, absolute diameter, multiple lesions in series, eccentric lesions which are worse in one view than another view or dynamic lesions which change severity due to coronary artery spasm [8, 9]. Thus, determination of percent stenosis alone has limited theoretical and experimental validity for assessing the significance of a stenosis. For all of these reasons, it is difficult to know with visually interpreted coronary arteriography whether the imaging technique has failed to identify a stenosis or whether stenosis severity has been erroneously determined by the visual interpretation. Quantitative coronary arteriography provides the best gold standard for determining stenosis severity in either animals or man. It is, therefore, the most accurate, objective basis from which the adequacy of an imaging technique can be measured.

Within the context of these limitations, the sensitivity and specificity of a diagnostic imaging technique depends upon three categorical parts of the method: The quality of the myocardial *perfusion imaging agent,* the power of the *imaging camera* and the adequacy of the *stimulus for increasing myocardial perfusion* [7, 10–15]. These factors individually as well as their interaction markedly influence sensitivity and specificity. For example, the degree of exercise stress, namely the quality of the stimulus for increasing coronary flow has been demonstrated to be important with submaximal stress leading to diminished sensitivity and specificity [2]. A stronger stimulus for increasing coronary blood flow will increase myocardial uptake relative to background thereby resulting in improved images and diagnostic accuracy even with suboptimal tracers. On the other hand, as compared to a poorly extracted tracer, a highly extracted one will produce good myocardial to background ratios and good images despite suboptimal stress. Even with radiotracers that are fairly poorly extracted in the myocardium, e.g. 20% to 50%, rapid data acquisition and appropriate modeling allows determination of extraction thereby providing quantitative measures of myocardial perfusion [16, 18]. Thus, appropriately designed, quantitative cameras, hardware and software can provide good images and measurements even with suboptimal tracers. In order to obtain first pass extraction, the camera must be 'fast', i.e. sufficiently sensitive that statistically reliable data can be obtained at five second intervals which is the necessary sample rate for making extraction or flow measurements with a monovalent cation [17].

Thus, the 'speed' of the camera becomes essential for quantitative metabolic or perfusion measurements even for non-moving static targets such as the brain, an approach we refer to as 'dynamic imaging'. By contrast, 'static imaging' refers to imaging the final deposition of radiotracer in an organ at more or less steady state conditions relative to the data collection or sample times and does not provide information on the tracer kinetics leading to its final tissue concentration. Such rapid sequence dynamic imaging is not intended to freeze the motion of the heart since that would require much faster frame rates. Heart motion is handled by EKG gating even with rapid sequence imaging. It is not widely recognized that the value of a fast nuclear camera resides primarily in its ability to measure first pass extraction as a basis for quantitative flow or metabolic measurements. Thus, it is apparent from this brief discussion that the adequacy of a new myocardial perfusion methods agent depends not only upon optimizing each of the three essential characteristics required but also upon their interaction. To this observer, cardiovascular imaging is evolving toward quantitative improvements in diagnostic sensitivity and specificity not through upgrading of standard and single photon imaging systems but through development of affordable clinical positron cameras specifically designed for dynamic cardiovascular imaging. Unlike the x-ray CAT scan which evolved in the market place, positron cameras have undergone a prolonged, extensive evolution through many generations and have progressed beyond instrumentation for instrumentation's sake to a period of 'down design' for lower price and complexity.

There are two essential capabilities of a positron camera necessary for widespread applications and for quantitative improvements in diagnostic accuracy. While such cameras also require mechanical simplicity, dedicated tested clinically oriented software, efficient inexpensive construction, etc., there are two functional characteristics that are crucial for significant improvement in diagnostic accuracy from this author's point of view. They are 'speed' or the capacity to provide rapid sequential (five-second) images and, at the same time, three-dimensional imaging. The rationale for 'fast' positron cameras sufficiently sensitive to obtain five second sequential images with adequate statistics (true coincidence count rate capability) has been outlined above. Rapid sequence imaging provides measurements of first pass extraction and of the kinetics of radiotracers which is the basis for quantitative imaging.

The second criteria, three-dimensional imaging, is not simply to produce pretty pictures. Quantitative accuracy with even the best one, two or even three-ring positron camera is severely limited by partial volume problems. In addition, virtually all investigators in tomography have discovered that displacement of the imaging plane by even one centimeter in sequential tomograms of an organ may produce a markedly different image due to displacement of the slice location on followup tomograms rather than a change in regional metabolism of perfusion. Furthermore, with myocardial ischemia or infarction, the dynamics of cardiac contraction and heart motion change markedly thereby altering cardiac translation and rotation such that even if the body of the subject does not move, the heart clearly changes location and pattern of contraction sufficiently to produce changes in tomographic images by displacement of the imaging plane alone. Three-dimensional imaging utilizing multi-ring positron cameras with cubic resolution offers a solution to these problems. Thus, it is our opinion that major advances in the diagnostic sensitivity and specificity of functional cardiac imaging will occur only with fast multi-ring positron cameras utilizing three-dimensional reconstruction by affordable, simplified, clinically oriented systems which can be run by a technician under supervision of an experienced physician.

What about positron radionuclides? Can everyone afford a cyclotron? Currently, a number of major university centers are actively developing cyclotron-positron tomographic systems for basic and clinical investigation. Because of their expense and technical complexity, it is not likely that fully developed cyclotron-camera systems will become wide-spread for routine clinical care. However, with the development of generator-produced positron isotopes, such as rubidium-82, a cyclotron is no longer necessary in order to accomplish much of the major cardiovascular imaging required [15–20]. For example, with a fast camera, first pass gated blood pool function can be obtained by following the bolus of intravenously injected rubidium through the cardiac chambers, through the period of myocardial perfusion [19] and through the subsequent time of either washout from the myocardium or continuing uptake which provides an index of viability [20]. Thus, with a single injection of a short-lived isotope, cardiac function, myocardial perfusion and viability can be evaluated, because the half-life of rubidium-82 is short, rapeated studies can be done sequentially with acceptable radiation doses to the patient. Although the extraction of rubidium into myocardium under resting conditions is only 60–70% and falls to 20 or 30% at high coronary flows, with appropriate imaging process and modeling, all the required information can be obtained quantitatively [16–18].

This overview serves to focus our attention again on the essential elements of the interdependent imaging processes beginning with chemical manipulations of radiotracers and ending with a clinical or scientific conclusion in the mind of an observer mediated by an 'image transducer', the camera. It must be adequate to transduce a range of tracer kinetics quantitatively in three dimensions, it must be simple to operate mechanically; it must be clinically oriented with user friendly software and must be fundamentally designed for operational simplicity to serve a busy physician who has little time to play with complicated machinery. Based on current availability of such cameras and on the physiologic-clinical concepts outlined above, we believe that cardiology will evolve toward more vigorous non-invasive, early diagnosis and intervention in CAD.

Acknowledgements

The research related to this article was carried out as a joint collaborative research project with the Clayton Foundation for Research, Houston, Tx. We are indebted to Kathy Rainbird for manuscript preparation.

References

1. Smalling RW, Fuentes F, Matthews MW, Freund GC, Hicks CH, Reduto LA, Walker WE, Sterling RP, Gould KL (1983) Sustained improvement in left ventricular function and mortality by intracoronary streptokinase administration during evolving myocardial infarction. Circulation 68(1): 131
2. Khaja F, Walton Jr JA, Brymer JF, Lo E, Osterberger L, O'Neill WW, Colfer HT, Weiss R, Lee T, Kurian T, Goldberg AD, Pitt B, Goldstein S (1983) Intracoronary fibrinolytic therapy in acute myocardial infarction. The New England Journal of Medicine 308: 1305
3. Anderson JL, Marshall HW, Bray BE, Lutz JR, Frederick PR, Yanowitz FG, Datz FL, Klausner SC, Hagan AD (1983) A randomized trial of intracoronary streptokinase in the treatment of acute myocardial infarction. The New England Journal of Medicine 308(22): 1312
4. Gould KL (1982) Quantitative imaging in nuclear cardiology. Circulation 66: 1141–1146
5. Hamilton GW et al. (1978) Myocardial imaging with thallium-201. An analysis of clinical usefulness based on Baye's Theorem. Seminars in Nuclear Medicine 8: 358–364
6. Sisson JC (1981) What promise the premilinary tests of coronary artery disease. J Nucl Med 22: 303
7. Gould KL (1978) Noninvasive assessment of coronary stenoses by myocardial perfusion imaging during pharmacologic coronary vasodilation. I. Physiologic basis and experimental validation. Am J Card 41: 267–278
8. Gould KL, Kelley KO (1982) Experimental validation of quantitative coronary arteriography for determining pressure-flow characteristics of coronary stenoses. Circ 66: 930–937
9. Gould KL, Lee D, Lovgren K (1978) Techniques for arteriography and hydraulic analysis of coronary stenoses in unsedated dogs. Am J Physiol 235: H350–H356
10. Gould KL et al. (1974) A physiologic basis for assessing critical coronary stenosis: Instantaneous flow response and regional distribution during coronary hyperemia as measures of coronary flow reserve. Am J Card 33: 86–94
11. Gould KL et al. (1978) Noninvasive assessment of coronary stenoses by myocardial perfusion imaging during pharmacologic coronary vasodilatation. II. Clinical methodology and feasibility. Am J Card 41: 279–287
12. Albro PC, Gould KL (1978) Noninvasive assessment of coronary stenoses by myocardial imaging during pharmacologic coronary vasodilatation. III. Clinical trial. Am J Card 42: 751–760
13. Gould KL (1978) Assessment of coronary stenoses with myocardial perfusion imaging during pharmacologic coronary vasodilatation. IV. Limits of detection of stenosis with idealized experimental cross-sectional myocardial imaging. Am J Card 42: 761–768
14. Gould KL, Schelbert H, Phelps M, Hoffman E (1979) Noninvasive assessment of coronary stenoses by myocardial perfusion imaging during pharmacologic coronary vasodilatation. V. Detection of 47% diameter coronary stenosis with intravenous $^{13}NH_4$ andemission computed tomography in intact dogs. Am J Card 43: 200–208
15. Schelbert H et al. (1982) Noninvasive assessment of coronary stenoses by myocardial imaging during pharmacologic coronary vasodilation. VI. Detection of coronary artery disease in man with intravenous N-13 ammonia and positron computed tomography. Am J Cardiol 49: 1197–1207
16. Mullani NA, Gould KL (1983) First pass regional blood flow measurement with external detectors. J Nucl Med 24: 577–581

17. Mullani NA, Goldstein RA, Gould KL, Marani SK, Fisher DJ, O'Brien HA Jr, Loberg MD (1983) Perfusion imaging with rubidium-82: I. Measurement of extraction and flow with external detectors. J Nucl Med 24: 898–906
18. Goldstein RA, Mullani NA, Fisher DJ, Marani SK, Gould KL, O'Brien HA (1983) Perfusion imaging with rubidium-82: II. Effects of pharmocologic interventions on flow and extraction. J Nucl Med 24: 907–915
19. Mullani NA, Gould KL (1984) Flow, function and viability of myocardium using fast 3D cardiac positron tomography without a cyclotron. Presented at the Scientific Sessions of the Council on Circulation and Basic Science of the American Heart Association, August 9–12, 1984, Snowmass, Colorado.
20. Goldstein RA, MacLean JA (1984) Noninvasive marker of myocardial viability after reperfusion based on leakage of Rb-82. J Am Col Card 3: 475

Improvement of myocardial perfusion by thrombolysis evaluation of left-ventricular function by two-dimensional echocardiography

K.J. HENRICHS, R. ERBEL, C. STEUERNAGEL and J. MEYER

Introduction

Many studies have shown that intracoronary thrombolysis is effective to achieve coronary reperfusion in patients with acute myocardial infarction [1, 2, 3]. Coronary reperfusion may relieve chest pain and improve the general condition of the patient, but there is controversy whether the intervention induces a favourable effect on left ventricular function [3, 4].

Since two-dimensional echocardiography has been shown to be a useful tool for the assessment of left ventricular volumes and ejection functions [5] we applied two-dimensional echocardiography to assess repeatedly left ventricular function in patients who presented themselves with acute myocardial infarction and who were subjected to intravenous and intracoronary thrombolysis.

Methods

Patients without prior myocardial infarction with persistent chest pain unrelieved by nitroglycerin, associated with ST-segment elevation within 6 hours after onset of symptoms were subjected to combined intravenous-intracoronary thrombolytic therapy. Criteria for exclusion were contraindication to anticoagulative therapy or refusal of the patient. The regimen of thrombolytic therapy and cardiac catheterization procedure are described in detail elsewhere [6].

Two-dimensional echocardiography was performed as soon as possible after admission to the hospital, immediately after the end of the catheterization procedure, on the first and second day of hospital stay and at discharge from the hospital which was usually 3–4 weeks after admission.

Between April 1983 and July 1984 in 126 patients (105 males, 21 females) combined intravenous and intracoronary thrombolysis was performed. The patients age was between 33 and 72 (mean 56 ± 11).

Seventy patients where reflow of a totally or subtotally occluded vessel could be achieved, were subjected to successive echocardiographic assessments before, immediately after, on the 1st, 2nd day and at the end of the hospital stay.

Apical two-dimensional echocardiograms (2dE) were recorded with an electronic sector scanner with 2,25 MHz and a sector of 84° in the 4-chamber- and RAO equivalent view.

All echocardiographic views were recorded in held, normal, unforced endexspiration to provide a stable image uneffected by respiration.

The studies were recorded on a videotape for subsequent analysis. Echocardiograms of sufficient quality and at all subsequent stages were obtained in 52 patients, and the data of these patients will be presented in this paper.

The patients were divided into two groups, group A with an infarct time – onset of symptoms until reperfusion of less than 210 minutes – and group B more than 210 minutes.

Analysis

Echocardiographic studies were analyzed blindly. For each of the two apical views that were recorded the endocardial outline was traced with a felt pen on a

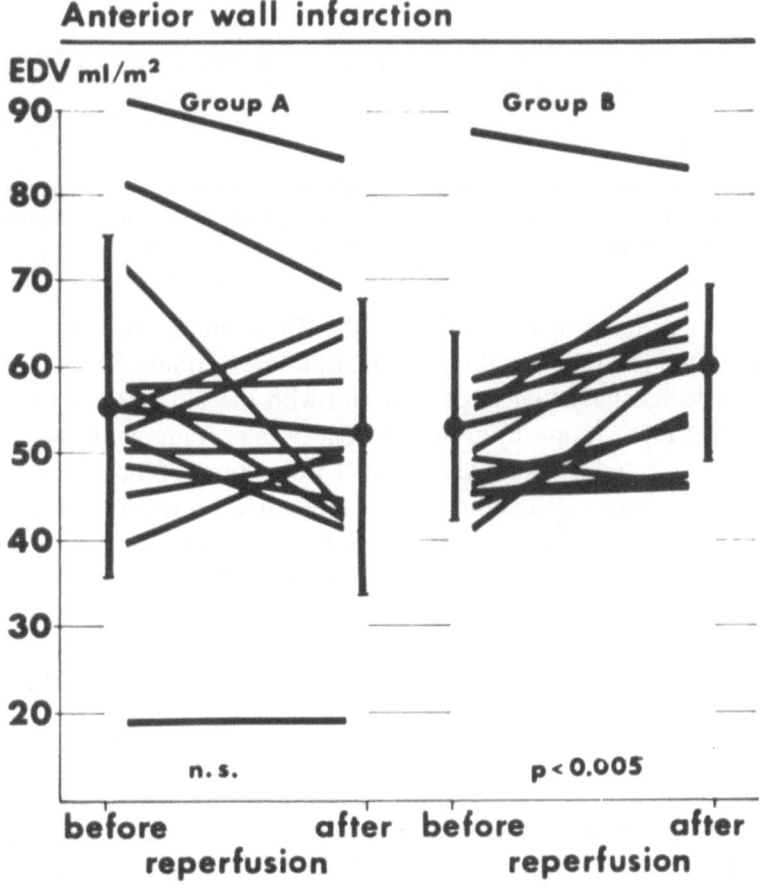

Figure 1. Enddiastolic volume index in both groups with anterior myocardial infarction before and immediately after reestablishment of perfusion. In group A (short infarct time) no change of EDV index; in group B (long infarct time) significant increase of EDV index.

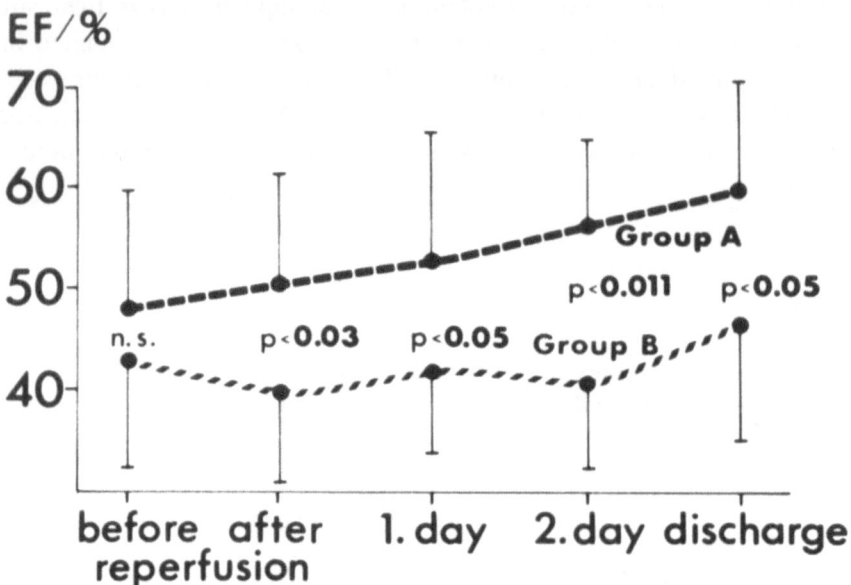

Figure 2. Endsystolic volume index in both groups with anterior myocardial infarction before and immediately after reestablishment of perfusion. In Group A (short infarct time) no change of ESV index; in group B (long infarct time) significant increase of EDV index.

transparent sheet fixed to the surface of the TV-monitor. The tape was first viewed in real time and slow motion, and finally frame by frame. The enddiastolic frame was selected by visual inspection and with the aid of the ECG-signal. Advancing the tape, frame by frame the endsystolic frame with the smallest silhouette was selected from the same beat. Three actions of the two views were evaluated. For volume calculations the disc method as previously described was used [5] and corrected for body surface area. From volume calculations ejection fraction was derived. Data were expressed as the mean ± SD. Statistical analysis was performed using paired and unpaired t-tests, whenever appropriate.

Results

Fifty-two patients were analyzed. None of those had a history of previous myocardial infarction. Of the 52 patients there were 27 with anterior myocardial infarction and 25 with posterior myocardial infarction, none of those had an elevation of CK before thrombolytic intervention was started.

All patients were divided into group A and group B. In the patients with anterior myocardial infarction mean infarct time was 179 ± 21 min in group A and

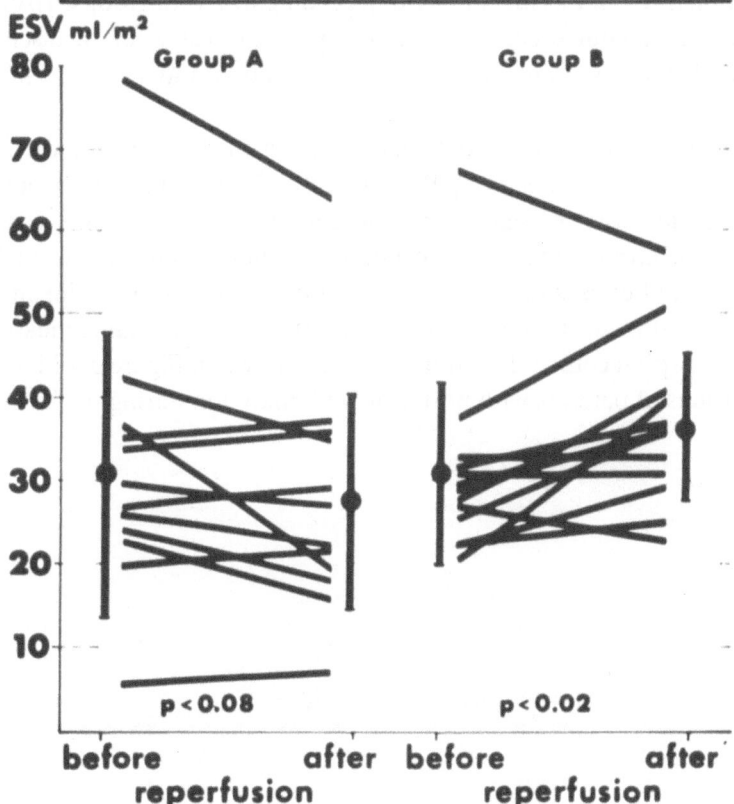

Figure 3. Ejection fractions in group A and group B with anterior myocardial infarctions. Significant increase of EF in group A – patients with short infarct time. No increase of EF in group B with long infarct time. Before recanalization no significant difference of EF between both groups.

273 ± 88 min in group B, and in patients with posterior myocardial infarction mean latency time was 163 ± 36 min in group A and 288 ± 45 min in group B.

Figure 1 and Figure 2 show changes of enddiastolic volume and endsystolic volume before and immediately after establishment of reperfusion in the two groups with anterior myocardial infarction. Enddiastolic volume changes were not found in group A, whereas in group B there was an increase of enddiastolic volume after reperfusion. Mean enddiastolic volume index increased from $53 \pm 11,5$ ml/m^2 (p0.05). In group A endsystolic volume index did not change immediately after reperfusion, in group B end-systolic volume index increased from 31 ± 11 ml/m^2 to 37 ± 10 ml/m^2 (p0.05). Ejection fractions obtained from the echocardiographic volume data during the hospital course in both groups of patients with anterior myocardial infarction are shown in Figure 3.

Before recanalization ejection fraction in group A was $48 \pm 10,5\%$ and in group B $43 \pm 11\%$; there was no significant difference in ejection fraction be-

108

tween both groups before the procedure. Already immediately after recanalization ejection fraction was higher in group A compared with group B (p 0,05). The more favourable course continued in group A till evaluation at discharge. At discharge ejection fraction was $59 \pm 11\%$ in group A and $46 \pm 12\%$ in group B (p 0.05).

In patients with posterior myocardial infarction ejection fraction was $56 \pm 12\%$ in group A and $55 \pm 11\%$ in group B before thrombolytic therapy. In both groups ejection fraction was not significantly altered after the procedure, a difference between both groups after the procedure was not found, either. In Figure 4 enddiastolic and endsystolic volumes of both groups with posterior myocardial infarction are shown; there was not significant change in volume measurements during the hospital course. Ejection fractions, shown in Figure 5, did not change in both groups of patients with posterior wall infarction during the hospital stay.

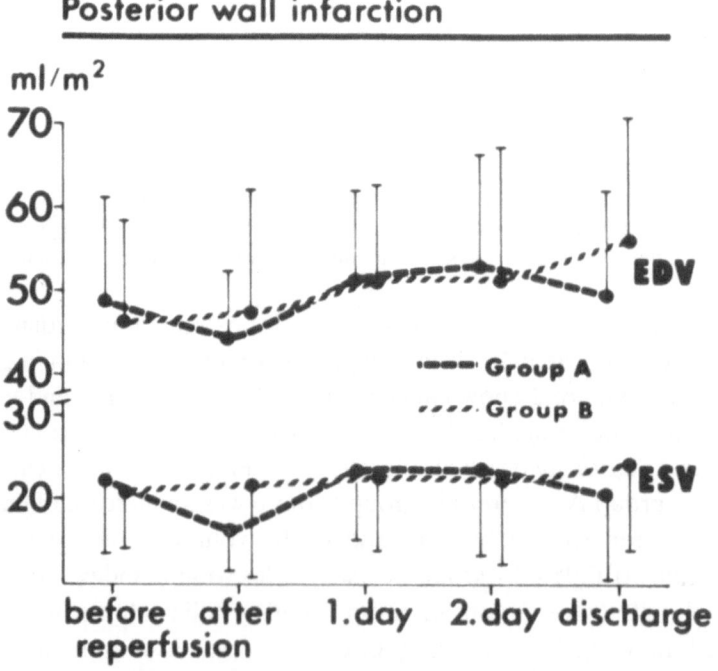

Figure 4. EDV index and ESV index in both groups of patients with posterior myocardial infarction. In both groups no change of volume indices before and after recanalization and during the hospital course, either. No difference between both groups.

Posterior wall infarction

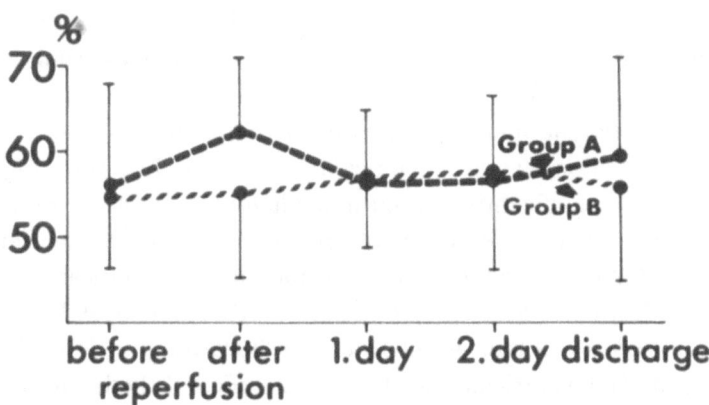

Figure 5. Ejection fractions of group A and group B with posterior myocardial infarction. No change of ejection fractions in both groups before and after recanalization and during the hospital course, either. No difference between both groups.

Discussion

Serial measurements of left ventricular function in the course of acute myocardial infarction have been performed by invasive methods [4] and by radionuclide methods [7].

Since two-dimensional echocardiography bears advantages of being noninvasive and repeatedly applicable, even in the critically ill patient, it appears attractive to assess left ventricular function in the course of acute myocardial infarction. Only recently serial echocardiographic assessments of left ventricular function during the course of myocardial infarction were published [8, 9].

Whether intracoronary thrombolysis is effective in improving left ventricular performance is a matter of debate in the current literature. Some studies demonstrate improvement of left ventricular performance after establishment of reperfusion in patients with acute myocardial infarction [9, 2, 3]. A recent report showed no improvement of LV-function despite effective reopening of the occluded coronary artery [4].

All patients who were analyzed in this study had a hospital course without complications such as infarct extension or reinfarction, defined as a new period of ischemic pain accompanied by CK elevation and ECG changes; and coronary angiography at the end of the hospital period showed patency of the occluded coronary artery reestablished and maintained over the study period.

Since infarct size and functional impairment is closely related to the time of coronary artery occlusion, as has been shown in experimental work [10], the lack of improvement in left ventricular function despite restoration of coronary blood flow may be related to the fact that coronary reperfusion was achieved at a time when the development of the infarct was complete. Therefore, in our study all patients were divided into two groups, one [1] with a short infarct time (less than 3,5 h between onset of symptoms and restoration of blood flow) and one (B) with an infarct time longer than 3,5 h.

Before thrombolytic therapy, ejection fraction of both groups with anterior myocardial infarction was not significantly different. In both groups ejection fraction was not significantly altered immediately after the procedure. But in group A on subsequent measurements ejection fraction rose and at discharge (3–4 weeks after recanalization) ejection fraction was significantly higher than before recanalization, whereas in group B an improvement of global left ventricular function was not found at subsequent echocardiographic evaluations. At discharge global left ventricular function was significantly higher in group A when compared with those of group B. These data are consistent with a recent publication [9]. Recovery of contractile function after coronary occlusion has been shown in experimental work to require several days [11]. In those patients with long occlusion time (B) the infarct size according to the perfusion area may be complete with irreversible ischemic injury and reperfusion did not salvage myocardium.

Volume measurements also disclosed the functional impairment of left ventricular myocardium in the group with long occlusion time and the more favourable course of those patients with short occlusion time.

In the group with posterior myocardial infarction the difference of both groups was not apparent in our data, possibly because infarct size of posterior myocardial infarction is too small for global functional impairment. Evaluation of regional contractile function also showed an improvement in those patients with short coronary occlusion time (unpublished data).

Our data show, as others have shown [9], that patients with acute myocardial infarction may benefit from early reperfusion.

References

1. Rentrop P, Blunke H, Karsch KR, Kaiser H, Kostering H, Leitz K (1981) Selective intracoronary thrombolysis in acute myocardial infarction and unstable angina pectoris. Circulation 63: 307–317
2. Mathey DG, Kuck KH, Tilsner V, Krebber JH, Bleifeld W (1981) Nonsurgical coronary artery recanalization in acute transmural myocardial infarction. Circulation 63: 489–497
3. Ganz W, Buchbinder N, Marcus H, Mondkar A, Maddahl J, Charuzi Y, O'Connor L, Fischbein M, Kass R, Myamoto A, Swan HJC (1981) Am Heart J 101: 4–13
4. Rentrop P, Feit F, Schneider R, Blanke H, Stecy P, Rey M, Horowitz S, Goldmann R (1984) Mt. Sinai – New York University randomized reperfusion trial: pilot phase. N Engl J Med 311: 1457–1463
5. Erbel R, Schweizer P, Lamberth H, Heun G, Meyer J, Krebs W, Effert S (1983) Echoventriculography. A simultaneous analysis of two dimensional echocardiography and cineventriculography. Circulation 67: 205–214

6. Erbel R, Pop T, Meinertz T, Kasper W, Rückel A, Schreiner G, Pfeiffer C, Meyer J (1983) Combined Mechanical and Medical Recanalization in acute myocardial infarction. Circulation 68, Suppl. III: III–326

7. Shal PK, Pichler M, Berman DS, Singh BN, Swan HJC (1980) Left ventricular ejection fraction determined by rationuclide ventriculography in early stages of first transmural infarction. Am J Cardiol 45: 542–546

8. Kan G, Visser CA, Lie KI, Darrer D (1984) Serial left ventricular ejection fraction in acute myocardial infarction by cross-sectional echocardiography: correlation of changing ejection fraction with clinical course. Europ Heart J 5: 470–476

9. Charuzi Y, Beeder C, Marshall L, Sasaki H, Pack N, Geft J, Ganz W (1984) Improvement in Regional and Global Left Ventricular Function after Intracoronary Thrombolysis: Assessment with Two-Dimensional Echocardiography. Am J Cardiol 53: 662–665

10. Gottmik M, Zimmer P, Wüsten B, Hofmann M, Winkler B, Schaper W (1981) Experimental myocardial infarction in a closed-chest canine model. Observations of temporal and spatial evolution over 24 hours. Basic Res Cardiol 76, 670–680

11. Pari PS (1975) Constructile and biochemical effects of coronary reperfusion after extended periods of coronary occlusions. Am J Cardiol 36: 244–251

Right ventricular infarction: Echocardiographic, hemodynamic feature

H.-J. RUPPRECHT, R. ERBEL, K.-H. SCHÖTER, G. SCHREINER,
K.-L. HENNRICHS and J. MEYER

Introduction

According to pathological and scintigraphic studies, right ventricular infarction (RVI) can be seen in more than 40% of patients with acute inferior myocardial infarction, but its clinical feature with an elevated systemic venous pressure, clear lungs, and arterial hypotension is often unapparent [1, 2, 3]. Early diagnosis of right ventricular infarction, however, is important with respect to therapeutic interventions, such as volume loading, in order to improve cardiac output and systolic arterial pressure. Two-dimensional echocardiography has been shown to be useful in detecting right ventricular abnormalities secondary to right ventricular infarction [4–7].

In the present study, we examined electrocardiographic, hemodynamic, echocardiographic and angiographic data in a series of 84 patients with acute inferior myocardial infarction, in particular with regard to echocardiographic evidence of right ventricular infarction.

Methods

Eighty-four consecutive patients with acute inferior myocardial infarction (AIMI) as diagnosed by electrocardiographic and enzyme changes were submitted within six hours after onset of chest-pain in our clinic. There were 71 men and 13 women with a mean age of $55 + 9$ respectively $65 + 10$ years. A standard 12 lead electrocardiogram and the right precordial leads from Vr3 to Vr6 were obtained in each patient. The latter were evaluated for the presence of at least 0.05 or 0.1 mV ST-segment elevation, measured 0.02 second after the J-point. All patients underwent coronary angiography and hemodynamic measurements including cardiac index, mean right atrial pressure and pulmonary artery enddiastolic pressure in the acute stage followed by a combined medical-mechanical recanalisation therapy, as previously described [8]. Echocardiographic evidence of right ventricular dilatation or wallmotion abnormality in the apical four-chamber-view led to the diagnosis of right ventricular involvement in 35/84 patients (42%, group A). In 49 patients (58%, group B) there were no echocardiographic signs of impaired right ventricular function. Quantitative evaluation of the shortening fraction of right ventricular area in the apical four-chamber-view was performed subsequently. In 66 patients repeated hemodynamic and angiographic data could be obtained after four weeks and 2-dimensional echocardiography was available up to a three months period. In 18 patients complete data could not be obtained due to missing of informed consent or death.

Results

Electrocardiogram

The electrocardiogram showed in at least one of the right precordial leads from Vr3 to Vr6 transient ST-segment -elevations of more than 0.05 mV in 89% of the patients in group A but also in 40% of the patients in group B. ST-segment elevations of more than 0.1 mV were seen in 50% of the patients with right ventricular involvement and in 16% of group B patients, so that increasing specifity was followed by decreasing sensitivity [9]. A typical ECG with signs of an acute inferior myocardial infarction and distinct elevation of the ST-segment in the right precordial leads is shown in Figure 1, demonstrating furthermore an ST-elevation in lead V1. We exhibited this particular finding, which was recently reported [10] to be caused by right ventricular infarction [11], in 5 patients of group A. (Figure 1)

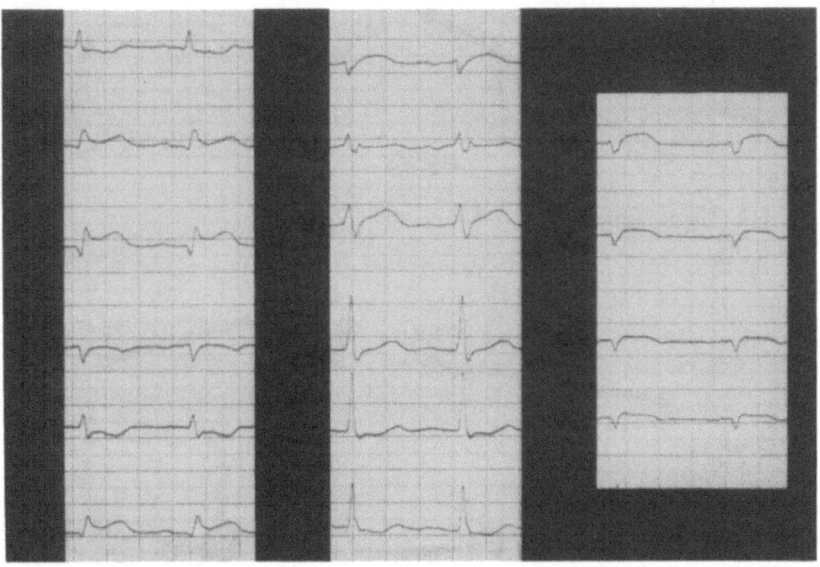

Figure 1. Electrocardiographic evidence of right ventricular involvement in a patient with acute inferior myocardial infarction.

Hemodynamics

Hemodynamic measurements in the acute stage confirmed former results of our Aachener working-group [12, 13]. So we found a significant lowered systolic blood pressure and elevated right atrial pressure, as well as slight depressed heart-rate in the group with right ventricular involvement. (Table 1) Hemo-

Table 1. Hemodynamics in acute inferior myocardial infarction.

	Group A	Group B	p-Value
SBP (mmHg)	99 + 30	122 + 29	0.01
HR (1/min.)	75 + 20	86 + 15	NS
MRAP (mmHg)	11.2 + 6.0	7.5 + 3.9	0.01
PAEDP (mmHg)	13.7 + 6.2	12.7 + 5.3	NS
CI (L/min*m²)	2.9 + 0.7	3.1 + 0.7	NS

SBP = systolic blood pressure; HR = heart rate; MRAP = mean right atrial pressure; PAEDP = pulmonary artery enddiastolic pressure; CI = cardiac index.

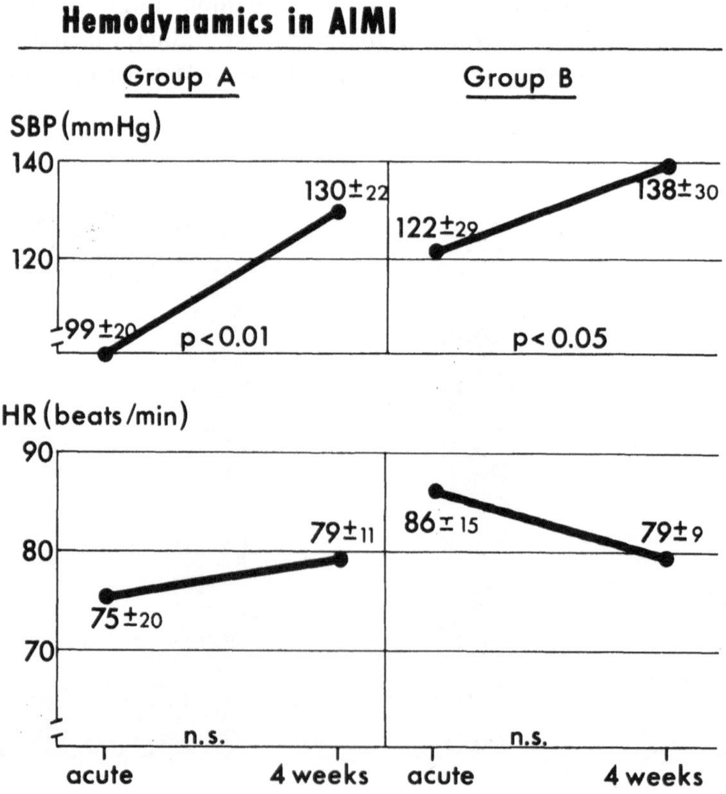

Figure 2. Hemodynamic changes within 4 weeks after inferior myocardial infarction with regard to right ventricular involvement.

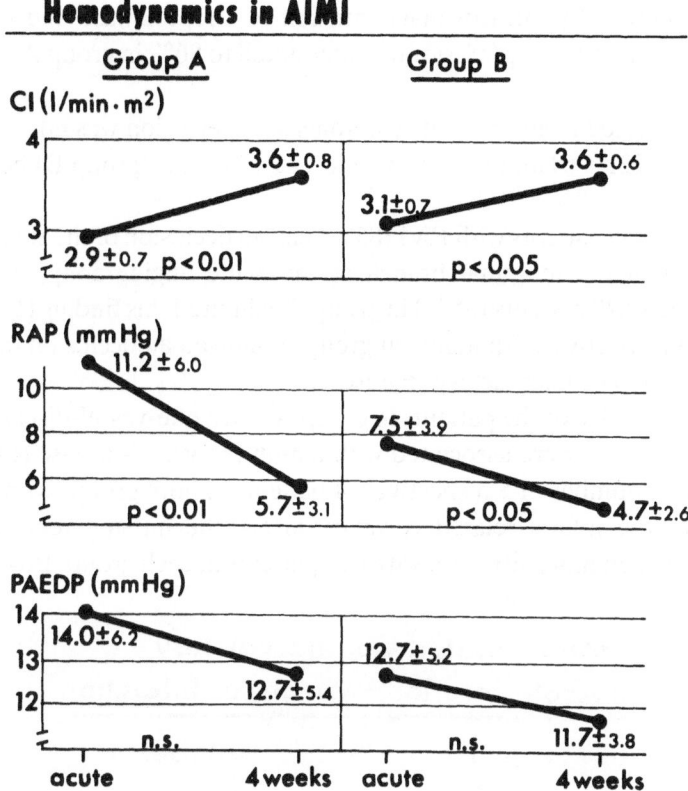

Figure 3. Hemodynamic changes within 4 weeks after inferior myocardial infarction with regard to right ventricular involvement.

dynamic measurements revealed at the 4-week-control significant improvement of cardiac output irrespective of right ventricular involvement. A noteworthy decrease of MRAP in both groups from 11.2 to 5.7 mmHg and also from 7.5 to 4.7 mmHg in group B were observed. Systolic blood pressure rose significantly from 99 to 130 mmHg in group A. Thus, we could not state any significant difference of hemodynamic data at the 4-week-control between the two groups. (Figures 2, 3)

Angiography

Combined medical-mechanical recanalisation therapy was performed in all patients. Four out of 35 patients (11%) in group A showed an open infarct-related coronary artery at the first angiography compared to seventeen out of 49 patients (35%) in group B.

In 5 patients of group A (15%) and in 4 patients in group B (8%) we did not succeed in reperfusion of the coronary artery. In all other patients reperfusion

116

could be achieved by intracoronary infusion of streptokinase and mechanical treatment, so that total reperfusionrate amounted to 86% in group A and 92% in group B.

The time elapsed from onset of symptoms to reperfusion was not significantly different with $221 + 69$ min (group A) and $225 + 78$ min. (group B) between the two groups.

Thirty out of 35 patients with RVI (85%) had an occlusion of the right coronary artery proximal the marginal branch at the acute angiography, wereas only seventeen out of 49 patients (35%) in group B exhibited this finding [14]. Accordingly only 3 respectively 2 patients in group A showed an occlusion of the distal part of the right coronary artery (Figure 4).

Beyond that, 60% of the patients in group A had a one-vessel-disease but 60% of group B patients were associated with a multiple-vessel-disease (Figure 5).

In the small number of 5 respectively 4 patients in both groups with persistent occlusion of the infarct-related coronary artery the missing reperfusion was followed by a high mortality rate, with two patients in each group. Beyond that in

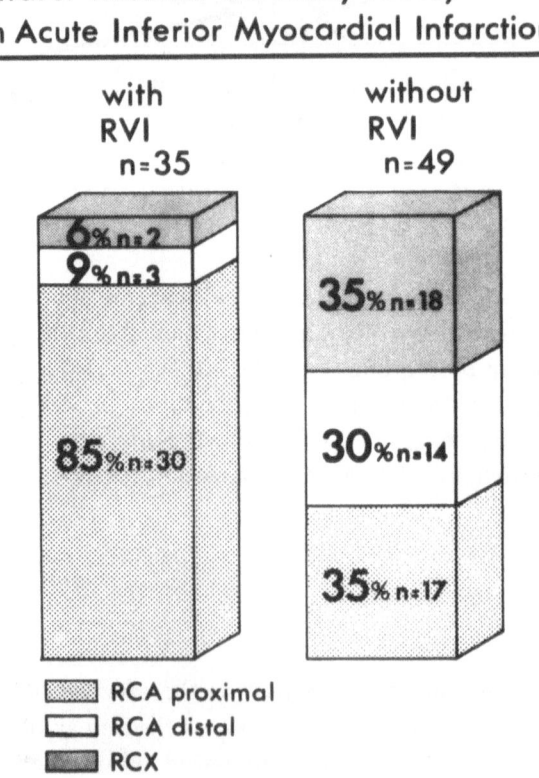

Figure 4. Infarct-related coronary artery in acute inferior myocardial infarction with regard to right ventricular involvement.

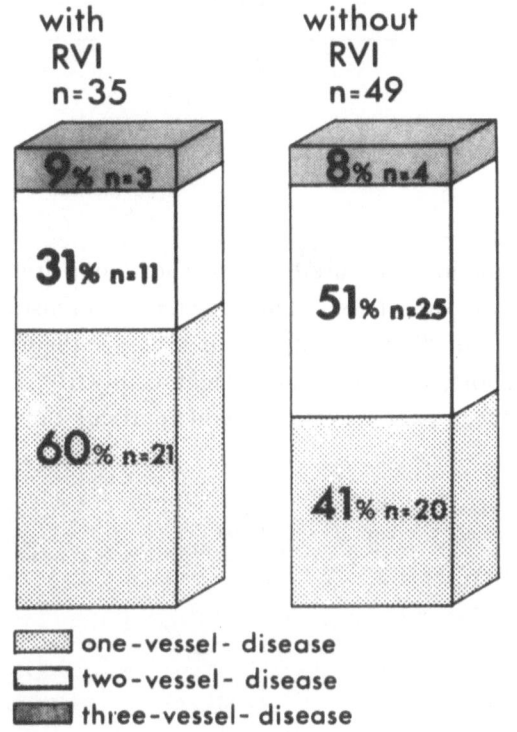

one - vessel - disease
two - vessel - disease
three - vessel - disease

Figure 5. One- or multiple-vessel-disease in acute inferior myocardial infarction with regard to right ventricular involvement.

three out of 4 patients in group B collateral blood flow was evident. On the other hand only one out of 5 patients in group A exhibited collateral vessels, but in this case we found an occlusion of the right coronary artery and the left circumflex artery. (Table 2)

In 28 patients of group A and 38 patients of group B repeated coronary angiography was performed 4 weeks after successful thrombolysis. Reocclusion of the infarct-related artery was found in six out of 28 patients (21%) in group A but only in four out of 38 patients (10%) in group B. (Table 3)

Table 2. Persistent occlusion in AIMI.

	Group A n = 5	Group B n = 4
Mortality	2	2
Collaterals	1	3

Table 3. Angiography 4 weeks after medical-mechanical treatment.

	Group A n = 28	Group B n = 38
Re-occlusion	6 (21%)	4 (10%)
Open coronary artery	22 (79%)	38 (90%)

Echocardiography

Right ventricular function measured by the shortening fraction of the right ventricular area in the apical four-chamber-view, demonstrated a depressed function in group A with 29% (tolerance limit 35%, see Figure 6). After thrombolysis-therapy the shortening fraction rose significantly from 29 to 38% in group A and from 37 to 44% in patients without right ventricular involvement. Within

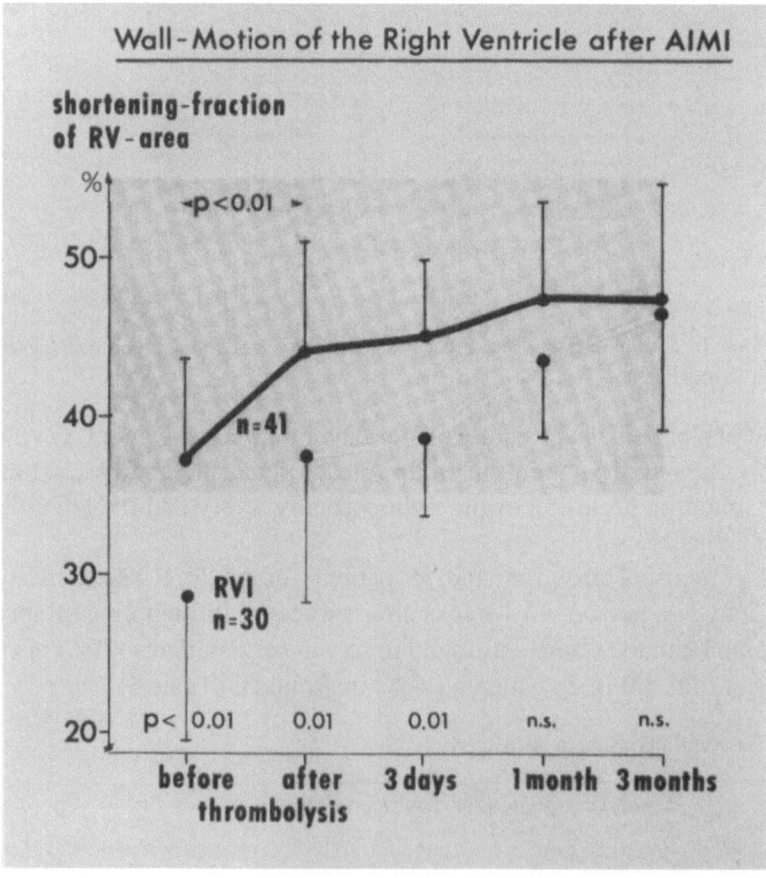

Figure 6. Shortening fraction of right ventricular area in acute inferior myocardial infarction with regard to right ventricular involvement.

three months both groups showed a further improvement to 47% and a similar course (Figure 6). Shortening fraction of the RV-area was examined with regard to the time elapsed from the onset of symptoms to successful reperfusion. We found a significant better shortening fraction (32%) when reperfusion resulted within the first 4 hours in comparison with 26% in patients with late recanalisation. Immediately after thrombolysis the difference persisted with gradual improvement at later controls and a similar quality of right ventricular function in both groups (Table 4).

Table 4. Right ventricular function and reperfusion – time.

| Shortening of RV – Area (%) | Reperfusion – time | | p – Value |
	<4 hours n = 18	>4 hours n = 13	
Before lysis	32 + 11	26 + 12	0.01
After lysis	41 + 5	35 + 9	0.01
3 days after lysis	40 + 9	39 + 8	NS
4 weeks after lysis	43 + 6	43 + 8	NS

Complications

The in-hospital course was complicated by high-degree-AV-conduction defects in eighteen out of 35 patients (51%) in group A, but only in six out of 49 patients (12%) without infarction of the right ventricle. Sinus-bradycardia and atrial fibrillation were also predominantly associated with the right ventricular infarction (Table 5).

Table 5. Complications in AIMI.

	Group a n = 35	Group b n = 49
AV-Block IIo/IIIo	18 (51%)	6 (12%)
Sinus-Bradycardia	4 (11%)	1 (2%)
Ventricular Asystoly	0	1 (2%)
Atrial fibrillation	4 (11%)	0
Ventricular fibrillation	3 (14%)	10 (20%)

Mortality

The mortality rate was not significantly different with 11% respectively 12% between the two groups, but all 4 deaths in group A were due to cardiogenic shock within 3 days in contrast to 1 patient in group B [15, 16]. (Table 6)

Table 6. Mortality, time, and cause of death in AIMI.

	Group A	Group B
Cardiogenic shock	4 (1.–3.d.)	1 (3.d.)
Ventricular asystoly	0	1 (1.d.)
Ventricular fibrillation	0	2 (4.d.; 6.w.)
Ventricular rupture	0	1 (3.d.)
Cerebrovascular Ins.	0	1 (6.w.)

Discussion

Right ventricular infarction has gained interest, when Cohn et al. [17] recognized its hemodynamic consequences in 1974. Since then several scintigraphic, pathological, hemodynamic and electrocardiographic studies [1–7, 9–15] have recognized that right ventricular infarction is a frequent companion of the infarction of the inferoposterior wall of the left ventricle.

Early recognition of this clinical entity is important in order to provide adequate therapy, in especially to avoid inappropriate treatment due to failure of the correct diagnosis.

Recent two-dimensional echocardiographic studies have shown this method to be useful in detecting right ventricular infarction [4–7].

In 42% of the patients with acute inferior myocardial infarction in our series right ventricular involvement was confirmed by 2-DE. This incidence was in accordance with previous reports cited above.

Electrocardiogram

A transient ST-segment elevation of more than 0.05 mV in at least one of the right-sided precordial leads from Vr3 to Vr6 was combined with a 89% sensitivity and a 60% specifity in identifying right ventricular infarction in this study. A threshold of 0.1 mV or greater was followed by a raise in specifity to 84% and a fall in sensitivity to 50%. These results indicate as several previous investigations [9, 10, 11, 18, 19] that early ECG changes may already refer to right ventricular involvement. With regard to either low specifity or low sensitivity this single parameter seems not to be reliable enough to identify right ventricular infarction.

Nonetheless, Croft et al. reported a 90% sensitivity and 91% specifity for this latter ECG-pattern. The first ECG in this study was obtained a mean of 17.2 + 13.6 hours after onset of symptoms (range 6 to 55). On the contrary our patients underwent electrocardiographic exploration within 6 hours after onset of chest-pain. These data might suggest, that repeated ECG-recordings, mainly at a later phase, are necessary, to detect right ventricular infarction. On the other side we noticed in accordance with other authors [18] that early ST-segment-elevations sometimes disappear within 2 hours after onset of chest-pain.

Thus one could assume, that a delay in ECG-recording of 6 to 55 hours is followed by a considerable decline in sensitivity. In addition there were only 19 patients with acute inferior myocardial infarction included in the forementioned study, clarifying that further prospective studies are necessary.

As recently shown by Geft et al. [10] ST-segment elevations from V1 to V5 can be related occasionally to right ventricular infarction, so far the amount of elevation is decreasing from V1 to V5. Correspondingly 5 patients in our group A exhibited this finding (see Figure 1), due to right coronary artery occlusion.

Hemodynamics

Initial measurements confirmed the well-known hemodynamic feature [12, 13, 16, 19, 20, 21] in patients with right ventricular infarction. Thus we found a significant elevated mean right atrial pressure and lowered systolic arterial blood pressure in group A, but no difference in left ventricular filling pressure (LVFP), measured as pulmonary artery enddiastolic pressure (PAEDP) between the two groups. Cardiac index, although slightly depressed, was within the same range, irrespective of right ventricular involvement.

Repeated hemodynamic investigations after 4 weeks revealed a significant fall of mean right atrial pressure and raise in systolic arterial blood pressure in group A. Beyond this a noteworthy improvement of cardiac output in both groups was recognized. Therefore, initial impairment of hemodynamics, mainly in patients with right ventricular infarction, was not detectable after 4 weeks.

It remains unclear, whether early reperfusion-treatment had influenced this favourable evolution or whether spontaneous changes determined the course, as reported by Legrand et al. [22].

Echocardiography

Patients in group A exhibited by definition initial echocardiographic evidence of right ventricular infarction as defined by akinesis, dyskinesis, hypokinesis or right ventricular dilatation [4–7, 12, 13, 21].

Subsequent quantitative evaluation of the shortening fraction of right ventricular area confirmed impaired right ventricular function in group A. After medical-mechanical recanalization therapy a significant improvement of shortening fraction in both groups could be achieved.

The initial shortening fraction was also dependent of the time elapsed between the onset of symptoms and reperfusion therapy. In contrast to other authors [4, 6] also patients with only hypokinetic right ventricular segments were thought to have a right ventricular infarction, since myocardial necrosis of the infero-posterior wall was established by typical ECG and enzyme changes.

Also hypokinesia is less specific for myocardial infarction than akinesia or dyskinesia, it seems to be highly sensitive, with a strong correlation to hemo-dynamic alterations [4, 6]. Thus, evaluation of wall-motion abnormalities by 2DE can lead to early detection of right ventricular involvement in patients with inferior myocardial infarction.

Angiographic findings

In accordance with previous reports [14, 21, 23] occlusion of the proximal part of the right coronary artery was a common finding in group A. In only 15% of these patients right ventricular infarction was related to the left circumflex artery. Nevertheless in about one third of the patients without echocardiographic evidence of right ventricular infarction a lesion of the proximal part of the right coronary artery was evident. In these patients only the infero-posterior wall of the left ventricle was affected, with preservation of the right ventricle.

This finding may be due to the relatively lower metabolic demand of the right ventricle [24]. As Wade [25] pointed out the low resistance of the right ventricle opposed to the systolic coronary blood flow, could also prevent the development of right ventricular infarction despite extensive necrosis of the left ventricle. Obviously the right ventricular myocardium in endowed with better ischemic tolerance than the left ventricle. Accordingly the patients in group B demonstrated frequently open coronary arteries at the first angiography.

Failure of reperfusion or reocclusion was more common in group A. Only one patient with persistent occlusion and right ventricular infarction exhibited collateral nutrition, but this patient had an occlusion of the right coronary artery and the left circumflex artery. On the other hand all 4 patients with unsuccessful reperfusion in group B demonstrated collateral vessels, which may have prevented them from right ventricular involvement. Beyond this the patients of group B suffered predominantly from multiple-vessel-disease, which is often followed by extensive development of collateral vessels. Thus a typical angiographic feature, causing prolonged ischemia, is often seen in patients with right ventricular infarction.

Complications and mortality

High degree AV-conduction defects were seen in 51% of our group A patients, compared to 12% in group B. Previous investigators found an incidence of 23–90% for this complication in patients with right ventricular involvement [17, 20, 21, 23].

The mortality rate was with 11% respectively 12% not significantly different between the two groups, but clearly lower than in previous reports [16, 20].

It is remarkable that 2 out of 5 patients in group A and 2 out of 4 patients in group B with failure of reperfusion died, elucidating the favourable effect of early reperfusion-therapy. All four deaths in group A were due to cardiogenic shock, as pointed out in previous reports [16, 20].

In conclusion two-dimensional echocardiography is a useful noninvasive method in order to detect as early as possible right ventricular involvement in patients with inferior myocardial infarction. Echocardiographic results were in accordance with hemodynamic, electrocardiographic and angiographic data. Prognosis is serious if recanalization-therapy fails, but becomes promising after successful reperfusion with corresponding improvement of hemodynamic and echocardiographic findings.

References

1. Erhard LR, Ring A (1974) Clinical and pathological observations in different types of acute myocardial infarction. Europ J Cardiol 4: 411–418
2. Sharpe DN, Botivinick EH, Shames DM, Schiller NB, Massie BM, Chatterjee K, Parmley WW (1978) The non invasive diagnosis of right ventricular infarction. Circulation 57: 483–490
3. Wackers FJT, Lie KJ, Busemann SE, Res J, van der Schoot JB, Durrer D (1978) Prevalence of right ventricular involvement in inferior wall infarction assessed myocardial imaging with Thallium – 201 and Technetium – 99 m pyrophosphate. Am J Cardiol 42: 358–362
4. D'Arcy B, Nanda NC (1982) Two-dimensional echocardiographic features of right ventricular infarction. Circulation 65: 176–173
5. Vannucci A, Cecchi F, Zuppiroli A, Marchionni N, Pini R, Di Bari M, Calamandrei M, Conti A, Ferrucci L, Greppi B, De Alfieri W (1983) Right ventricular infarction: Clinical, hemodynamic, mono- and two-dimensional echocardiographic features. Europ Heart J: 854–864
6. Lopez-Sendon J, Garcia-Fernandez MA, Coma-Canella J, Yangüela MM, Banuelos F, (1983) Segmental right ventricular function after acute myocardial infarction: Two-dimensional echocardiographic study in 63 patients. Am J Cardiol 51: 390–396
7. Jugdutt BJ, Sussex BA, Sivoram CA, Rossal RR (1984) Right ventricular infarction: Two-dimensional echocardiographic evaluation. Am Heart J 107(3): 505–518
8. Erbel R, Pop T, Henkel B, Schreiner G, Steuernagel C, Beck FJ, Henrichs KJ, Meyer J (1985) Medical-mechanical treatment of myocardial infarction. In: J. Meyer, R. Erbel (eds) Improvement of myocardial perfusion, M. Nijhoff, Dordrecht
9. Croft CH, Nicol P, Corbett JR, Lewis SE, Huxley R, Mukharji J, Willerson J, Rude R, (1982) Detection of acute right ventricular infarction by right precordial electrocardiography. Am Heart J 50: 421–427
10. Geft JL, Shah PK, Rodriguez L, Hulse S, Maddahi J, Berman DS, Ganz W, (1984) ST-elevations in leads V1 to V5 may be caused by right coronary artery occlusion and acute right ventricular infarction. Am Heart J 53(8): 991–996
11. Chou TC, Van der Bel-Kahn J, Allen J, Brockmeier L, Fowler NO, (1981) Electrocardiographic diagnosis of right ventricular infarction. Am J Med 70: 1175–1180
12. Meyer J, Merx W, v Essen R, Erbel R, Rupprecht H-J, Püllen C, Effert S, (1982) Rechtsherzinsuffizienz beim Infarkt der rechten Kammer. Prognose und Therapie. Dtsch Med Wschr 107: 615–619

13. Merx W, Meyer J, v Essen R, Erbel R, Schweizer P, Püllen C, Rupprecht H-J; Effert S (1982) Rechtsherzinsuffizienz beim Infarkt der rechten Kammer. Diagnose und Häufigkeit. Dtsch Med Wschr 107: 565–570

14. Rackley CE, Russel RO, Mantle JA, Rogers WJ, Papapietra SE, Schwartz KM, (1981) Right ventricular infarction and function. Am Heart J 100: 215–218

15. Tebbe U, Rahlf G, Sauer G, Kreuzer H, Neuhaus KL (1984) Verschluß der rechten Kranzarterie mit akutem Rechtsherzinfarkt und kardiogenem Schock. Z Kardiologie 73: 327–332

16. Gewirtz H, Gold H, Fallon J, Pasternak RC, Leinbach R, (1979) Role of right ventricular infarction in cardiogenic shock associated with inferior myocardial infarction. Br Heart J 42: 719–725

17. Cohn JN, Guiha NH, Broder MJ, Limas CJ, (1974) Right ventricular infarction. Clinical and hemodynamic features. Am J Cardiol 33: 209–214

18. Klein HO, Tordjman T, Ninio R, Sareli P, Oren V, Lang R, Gefen J, Pauzner C, Di Segni E, David D, Kaplinsky E, (1983) The early recognition of right ventricular infarction:Diagnostic accuracy of electrocardiographic V4r lead. Circulation 67(3): 558–565

19. Erhard LR, Sjögren A, Waldberg J, (1976) Single right sided precordial lead in the diagnosis of right ventricular involvement in inferior myocardial infarction. Am Heart J 91: 571–576

20. Coma-Canella J, Lopez-Sendon J, Gamallo C, (1979) Low output syndrom in right ventricular infarction. Am Heart J 98(5): 613–620

21. Isner JM, Roberts WC, (1978) Right ventricular infarction complicating left ventricular infarction secondary to coronary heart disease. Am J Cardiol 42: 885–894

22. Legrand V, Rigo P, Smeets JP, Demoulin JC, Collignon P, Kulbertus HE, (1983) Right ventricular myocardial infarction diagnosed by 99m Technetium pyrophosphate scintigraphy: Clinical course and follow-up. Europ Heart J 4: 9–19.

23. v Essen R, Merx W, Meyer J, Effert S (1980) Rechtsventrikulärer Infarkt – ohne Hämodynamik keine Diagnose und gezielte Therapie. Anaesth und Intensivmed 125: 379–385

24. Rotman M, Ratliff NB, Hawley J, (1974) Right ventricular infarction:hemodynamic diagnosis Br Heart J 36: 941–944

25. Wade WG (1959) The pathogenesis of infarction of the right ventricle. Br Heart J 21: 545–554

Limitation of myocardial necrosis by thrombolysis during acute myocardial infarction

ALLAN S. LEW and WILLIAM GANZ

Introduction

The introduction of coronary intensive care units in the 1960s facilitated the prevention and management of lethal arrhythmias and thereby fostered a progressive decline in mortality following acute myocardial infarction [1]. Since death following myocardial infarction was usually due to extensive myocardial necrosis, efforts were focused on the development of interventions that would limit the extent of necrosis and reduce infarction size. Although several of these interventions appeared to be effective in experimental studies, they proved to have little or no impact in clinical practice [2].

In the late 1970s it became apparent that a significant reduction in the extent of myocardial necrosis could be achieved by restoration of myocardial perfusion to the ischemic myocardium [3] and consequently, clinical interventions that can restore antegrade coronary perfusion were considered. Surgical bypass or mechanical dilation of the artery of infarction and more recently, lysis of the occlusive coronary thrombus with fibrinolytic drugs all proved effective methods of achieving reperfusion but thrombolysis is currently the most practical method of achieving early repefusion during an acute myocardial infarction.

Pathophysiological considerations

Following coronary artery ligation, regional contractile function usually ceases and the ischemic myocardium becomes dyskinetic [4]. Creatine kinase, adenosine triphosphate (ATP) and glycogen are depleted and there is an accumulation of lactate [5]. In the dog, myocardial necrosis begins near the endocardium within 15–20 minutes following occlusion and gradually progresses to the epicardium in a 'wavefront of cell death' [6]. Reperfusion prior to completion of necrosis will arrest its progression and salvage variable portions of the jeopardized, but still viable, myocardium. The reversibly ischemic myocardium recovers in structure and function, whereas irreversibly damaged myocardium undergoes accelerated contraction band necrosis [7]. Intramyocardial hemorrhage may occur in regions of advanced necrosis that involve not only the myocardium but also the intramyocardial vasculature [8]. This 'reperfusion hemorrhage' is always confined to the necrotic myocardium, has no deleterious effects on the viable myocardium and does not interfere with myocardial healing or scar formation [9].

Very early reperfusion, within a few minutes of the onset of infarction, may completely prevent myocardial necrosis but this can rarely be achieved in clinical practice. The extent of myocardial salvage achieved with later reperfusion will depend on the extent of 'jeopardized' myocardium supplied by the occluded coronary artery, the rate at which myocardial necrosis is progressing and the time that has elapsed from the onset of infarction.

The rate at which myocardial necrosis progresses is inversely related to the amount residual perfusion of the ischemic myocardium [10]. When infarction is due to subtotal coronary occlusion and there is some residual antegrade perfusion, the rate of necrosis is slower than when infarction is due to complete coronary occlusion and the ischemic myocardium is perfused only via undeveloped collateral vessels.

This relation between the rate of necrosis and the magnitude of collateral perfusion is illustrated by species differences in the rate of myocardial necrosis related to the level of collateral flow via congenitally present epicardial collateral vessels. For example, the rabbit and the sheep have virtually no coronary collateral circulation and following coronary occlusion, myocardial necrosis is complete within about 15 to 20 minutes. In contrast, the dog and the baboon have relatively well developed collateral circulations providing 10–15% residual perfusion in the distribution of an occluded coronary artery, such that completion of necrosis requires 4–6 hours of ischemia [6, 11].

The rate of necrosis following coronary occlusion may be accelerated by hemodynamic factors that decrease collateral flow such as a low systemic blood pressure, which reduces collateral perfusion pressure and tachycardia, which reduces the duration of diastole. Therefore, hypotension and tachycardia during an acute myocardial infarction tend to worsen myocardial ischemia and accelerate the rate of myocardial necrosis. These factors are especially important in patients with multiple vessel coronary artery disease because the artery supplying the collaterals may have a severe stenosis which reduces collateral perfusion pressure compared to systemic blood pressure. In these patients, small falls in systemic blood pressure may significantly reduce collateral perfusion to the ischemic myocardium.

Clinical considerations

The pattern and time sequence of myocardial necrosis following complete occlusion of the coronary artery in man appears to be similar to that in the canine model. This relatively narrow 'time window' available for limitation of the extent of myocardial necrosis probably explains why interventions performed more than 6 hours after the onset of acute infarction have usually had little impact on the extent of infarction in clinical trials [12].

In the 10–15% of patients with acute myocardial infarction in whom the coronary artery is not completely occluded and in patients with well developed collateral vessels present prior to infarction, the rate of myocardial necrosis is slower than in patients with complete coronary occlusion and no significant collaterals and therefore, significant myocardial salvage is possible even after more than 5 to 6 hours of ischemia [13].

Since thrombotic coronary artery occlusion is the usual pathogenetic mechanism of acute myocardial infarction in man [14], reperfusion may be achieved by administration of thrombolytic agents that can rapidly lyse occlusive intracoronary thrombus. In clinical practice, both selective intracoronary [15, 16] and systemic intravenous administration [17, 18] of thrombolytic agents have proven very effective at restoring antegrade coronary perfusion during acute myocardial infarction. Intravenous administration is more widely applicable and avoids the delay inherent in preliminary coronary angiography. Reperfusion may also be achieved by surgical bypass [19] or mechanical dilation of the artery of infarction [20].

The possible role of interventions capable of slowing the rate of myocardial necrosis following coronary occlusion warrants investigation. In experimental studies pretreatment with beta adrenoreceptor blocking drugs or calcium channel antagonists has enhanced myocardial salvage by reperfusion [21].

Assessment of myocardial salvage

Reperfusion is usually associated with resolution of ischemic ST segment changes and rapid evolution of the electrocardiogram (Figure 1) [22]. The rate of resolution of the ST segment changes may be related to the rate of restoration of

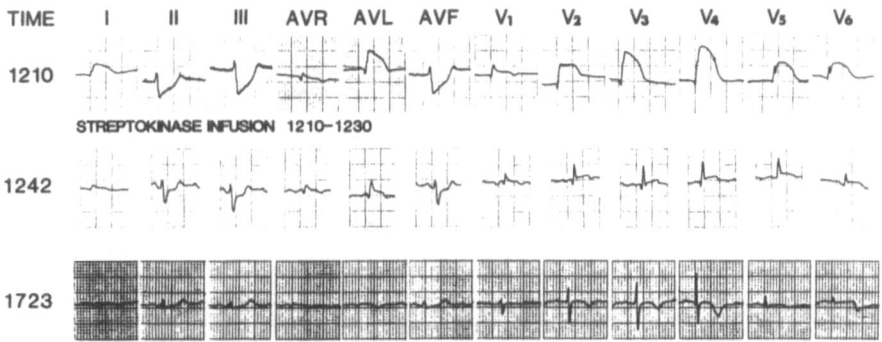

Figure 1. Serial 12 lead electrocardiograms demonstrating rapid resolution of marked anterior ST segment elevations following early reperfusion with intravenous streptokinase. In this instance pathological Q waves have not evolved. (From Lew AS, et al. Am J Cardiol 1984; 54: 450. Reproduced by permission).

myocardial perfusion whereby brisk restoration of coronary patency results in a rapid resolution of ST segment elevation and a gradual restoration of coronary flow results in a more gradual resolution of ST segment changes. In patients who have sustained no or minimal necrosis, there may be no development of pathological Q waves; however in clinical practice, reperfusion is rarely achieved early enough to completely prevent necrosis and Q waves evolution. Occasionally, abnormal Q waves are a transient electrocardiographic phenomenon [23].

In experimental studies, the extent of myocardial infarction can be accurately measured and expressed in grams or as either a percentage of the ischemic myocardium at risk or as a percentage of the total myocardial mass. An accurate clinical assessment of the extent of myocardial necrosis is not yet possible and therefore, the clinical assessment of myocardial salvage relies on indirect measurements of the extent of jeopardized myocardium and the extent of myocardial necrosis.

Thallium-201 exchanges with potassium and therefore its myocardial uptake is dependent on both myocardial perfusion and viability. When administered after occlusion of the coronary artery but prior to reperfusion, thallium-201 does not usually reach the non-perfused myocardium in a significant concentration and imaging reveals a perfusion defect corresponding to the extent of the non-

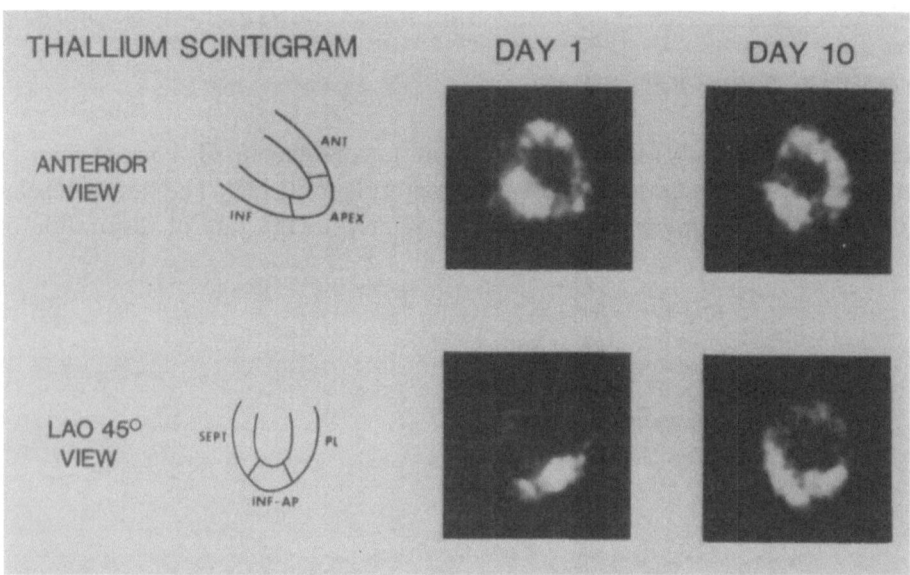

Figure 2. Thallium-201 scintigrams in the anterior and left anterior oblique (LAO) 45 degrees views performed on admission and 10 days after reperfusion with intravenous streptokinase. The day 1 image shows an extensive perfusion defect involving the anterior (ANT), apical (AP), septal (SEPT) and posterolateral (PL) walls of the left ventricle. The day 10 study reveals posterolateral and apical perfusion defects with marked improvement of anterior and septal isotope uptake. (From Lew AS, et al. Am J Cardiol 1984; 54: 450. Reproduced with permission).

perfused, or jeopardized myocardium. Following reperfusion, thallium-201 can reach the previously jeopardized myocardium and may be taken up by viable myocardium in that region but not by the necrotic myocardium and therefore, imaging following reperfusion will reveal a perfusion defect that represents the extent of infarcted myocardium in the jeopardized zone. The difference between these 2 perfusion defects (jeopardized myocardium – infarcted myocardium) represents the extent of jeopardized myocardium that may have been 'salvaged' (Figure 2).

Several clinical studies have used thallium-201 perfusion scintigraphy to assess the extent of myocardial salvage folowing reperfusion and have shown that the size of the perfusion defect decreases significantly following early reperfusion [24, 25]. Computer assisted quantification of thallium-201 uptake confirms a reduction in the severity of the perfusion defect following reperfusion [26] (Figure 3).

Technetium 99m pyrophosphate is a necrosis-avid radionuclide that binds to calcium ions. Myocardial uptake of technetium 99m pyrophosphate reflects the amount of intracellular calcium accumulation within the mitochondria and appears as a scintigraphic 'hot spot'. Following reperfusion, irreversibly damaged

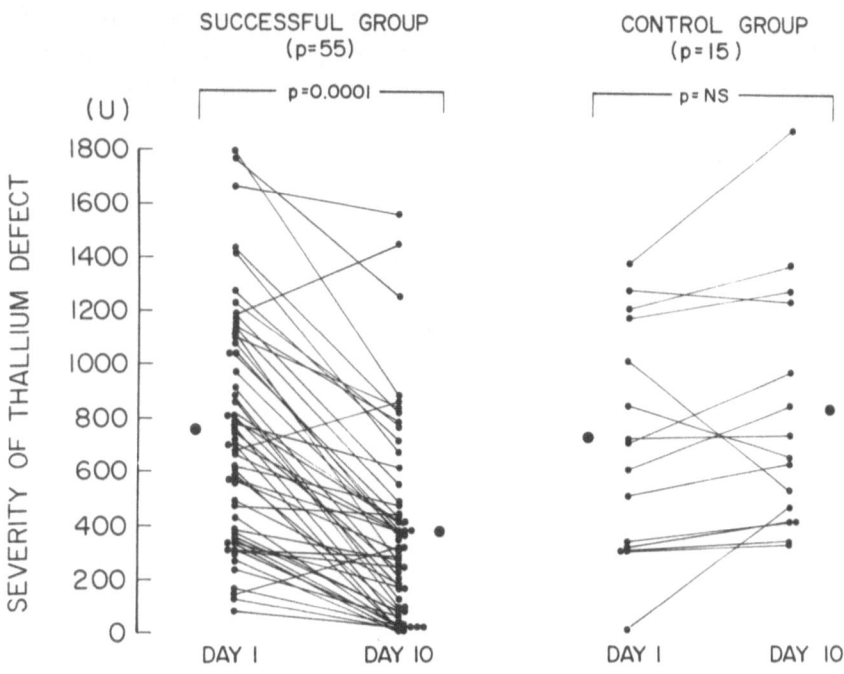

Figure 3. Graphic representation of the change in the severity of the thallium-201 perfusion defect from admission to day 10. In the Successful Group, reperfusion resulted in a significant decrease in the severity of the perfusion defect compared to a small increase in the Control Group. The severity of the perfusion defect was assessed by a computer assisted quantitative technique (45) and the for the day 1 study, thallium-201 was injected prior to administration of streptokinase.

and necrotic cells have a high affinity for technetium 99m pyrophosphate due to intracellular accumulation of calcium. By combining pre-reperfusion thallium-201 scintigraphy with post-reperfusion technetium 99m scintigraphy, myocardial salvage may be assessed by the difference in the size of the thallium-201 perfusion defect, representing the jeopardized myocardium, and the technetium 99m hot spot, representing the infarcted myocardium [27, 28].

Computerized tomography and positron emission tomography (PET) have also been used to assess myocardial salvage [29, 30]. The latter technique follows the fate of radiolabelled metabolic intermediaries such as sugars and free fatty acids. PET has shown that reperfusion effects a restoration of coronary flow to the jeopardized myocardium and that myocardial salvage is associated with a resumption of aerobic metabolism of free fatty acids and the recovery of high energy phosphate stores.

The release into the circulation of creatine kinase and the other cardiac enzymes is dramatically accelerated by reperfusion of the ischemic myocardium [31]. Following reperfusion, creatine kinase (CK) and CK MB are more completely and more rapidly 'washed out' and hence less inactivated [32]. Therefore, the total amount of CK and CK MB released into the circulation and their peak serum levels are 2–3 times higher than for an equivalent sized non-reperfused infarction (Figure 4). Due to this difference in the physiology of CK release from reperfused and non-reperfused infarctions, comparison of infarction size between reperfused and non-reperfused infarctions is not possible [33].

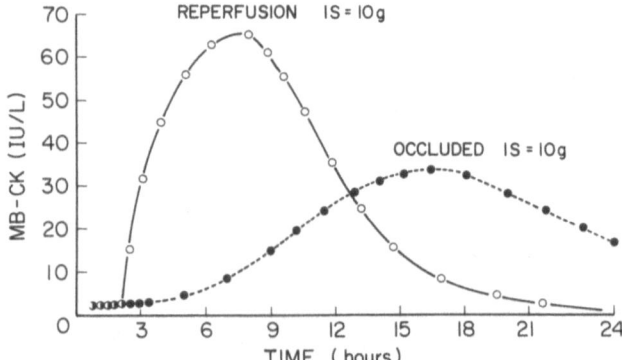

Figure 4. Creatine kinase MB release in 2 dogs with equivalent sized myocardial infarction. In the reperfused dog, the CK-MB time activity curve rises abruptly at the time of reperfusion and peaks early, within 9 hours of reperfusion. In the non-reperfused (Occluded) dog the CK-MB time activity curve rises slowly with a delayed peak. Even though both dogs have equivalent-sized infarctions, the peak level of CK-MB is about twice as high for the reperfused infarction compared with the non-reperfused infarction. (IS = infarction size).

Impact of myocardial salvage

1) Ventricular function

Following experimental reperfusion, the contractile function of the reperfused myocardium is initially depressed and gradually recovers over several days [34]. This so-called 'stunned' but viable myocardium is however, responsive to inotropic stimulation immediately after reperfusion [35] (Figure 5). This responsiveness has important clinical implications for the successful treatment of patients with severe cardiac failure or cardiogenic shock, in whom reperfusion plus inotropic therapy may markedly improve left ventricular function.

Clinical studies using either contrast left ventriculography, gated radionuclide ventriculography or 2-dimensional echocardiography have investigated recovery of ventricular function following reperfusion. Some studies have reported a significant improvement in left ventricular ejection fraction following reperfusion [13, 36–39] (Figure 6), while others have failed to show an improvement [40–43]. However, most studies have demonstrated significant improvement in regional function of the reperfused zone, even in patients without improvement of global function [38–41] (Figure 7).

The disparity between the results of global and regional function following reperfusion is probably due to the contribution of compensatory hyperfunction of the non-ischemic myocardium. In the early phase of acute infarction, the adverse

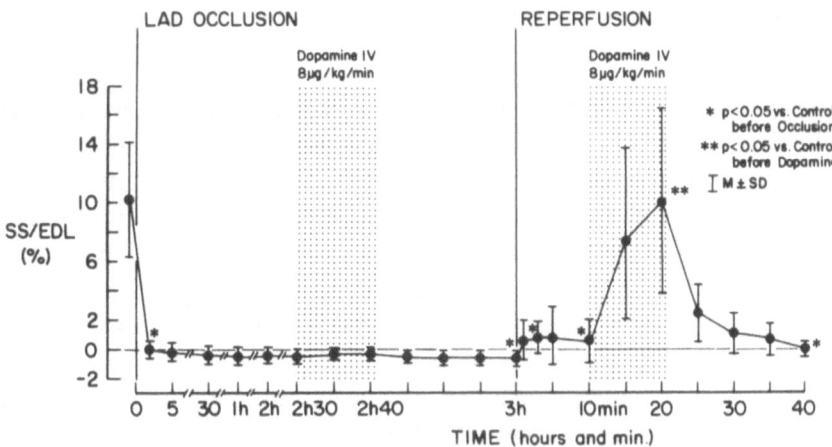

Figure 5. Graphic representation that apparently 'stunned' but viable myocardium is responsive to stimulation by catecholamine infusion, early after reperfusion. Regional anterior wall left ventricular function is represented on the abscissa by systolic shortening (SS) divided by end-diastolic length (EDL). Following left anterior descending artery (LAD) ligation, regional anterior wall function immediately deteriorated to dyskinesia and was not responsive to dopamine infusion. Following reperfusion, regional function improved slightly but, in contrast to pre-reperfusion, was markedly improved by infusion of dopamine.

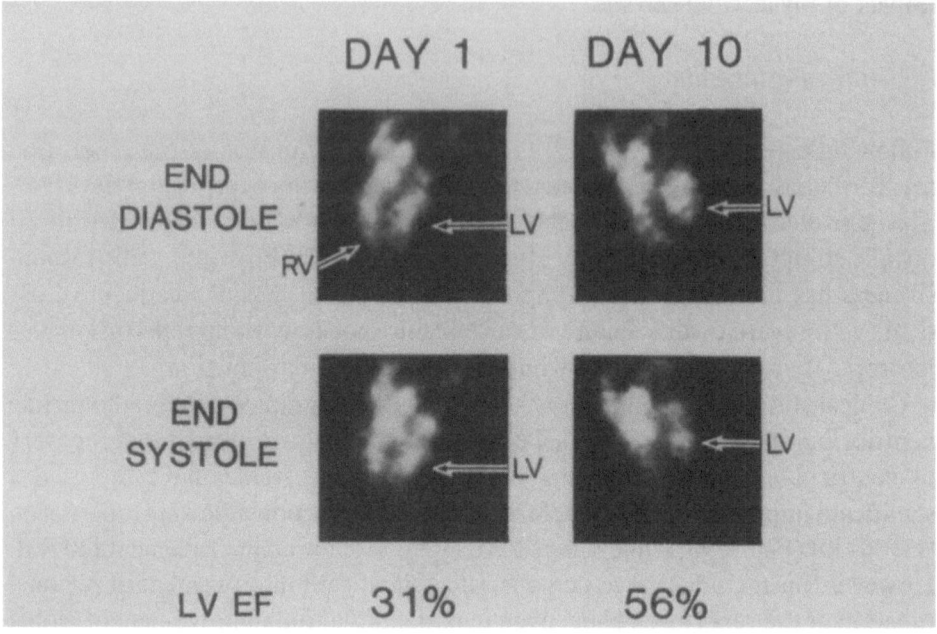

DAY 1   DAY 10

END
DIASTOLE   LV
              RV

END
SYSTOLE   LV

LV EF   31%   56%

Figure 6. Technetium 99m radionuclide wall motion studies in the left anterior oblique 45 degrees projection performed on admission and 10 days after reperfusion with intravenous streptokinase. The day 1 image shows a dilated and poorly functioning left ventricle with regional ventricular septal, inferoapical and posterolateral wall motion abnormalities. The day 10 study reveals significant improvement in both global and regional left ventricular function. (From Lew AS et al. Am J Cardiol 1984; 54: 450. Reproduced with permission).

effect on global function of the hypofunctioning ischemic region of myocardium is offset by compensatory hyperfunction of the non-ischemic myocardium. In the late phase of infarction, the favorable effect on global function of the improved regional function of the salvaged myocardium may, in turn, be offset by regression of compensatory hyperfunction of the non-ischemic myocardium [40].

The impact of these changes in regional function of both the ischemic and non-ischemic myocardium on global function depends on the relative extent of these two regions. When the ischemia is extensive, the impact of compensatory hyperfunction on early global function is relatively small and therefore, the impact of the regression of hyperfunction on late phase global function following reperfusion is also smaller. Therefore, when ischemia is extensive, late phase global function reflects functional changes in the ischemic, rather than the non-ischemic zone and myocardial salvage is likely to be reflected by improved global function. In contrast, when there is a relatively small extent of ischemia, early global function will be better preserved and there will be less late phase improvement in global function. This may be the reason that improvement in left ventricular function is usually more apparent in patients with extensive involvement and

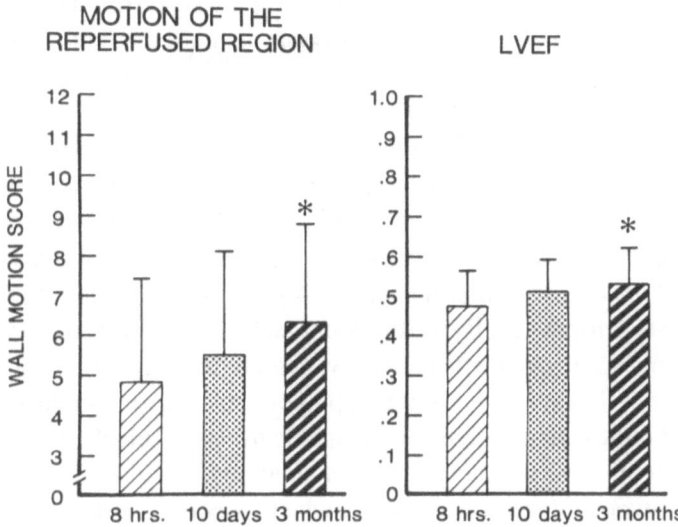

Figure 7. Graphic representation of the time course of recovery of ventricular function following reperfusion. There is significant early improvement in regional function of the reperfused zone with a modest improvement in global left ventricular function. At 3 months the improvement of both regional and global function is more apparent.

severe impairment of global function [44].

In patients with infarction and right ventricular dysfunction due to proximal right coronary occlusion, early reperfusion effects a rapid improvement of right ventricular function and may also improve survival [45].

Recently, it has been suggested that functional recovery of the reperfused and salvaged myocardium may be related to the level of perfusion achieved by reperfusion. Therefore, the degree of residual coronary stenosis may be an important determinant of functional recovery following reperfusion [46] and early coronary angioplasty or early coronary bypass surgery to the reperfused artery may improve perfusion and thereby improve function recovery of the reperfused zone.

Patients with incomplete coronary occlusion or extensive collateral supply to the infarcting myocardium, tend to show the most improvement in left ventricular function [47]. This may be consequent to the slower rate of myocardial necrosis and more extensive myocardial salvage.

2) Mortality

Several studies have reported an improved survival following reperfusion with streptokinase [13, 48, 49]. In a randomized study of intracoronary streptokinase by Kennedy et al. [48], the 30 day mortality was reduced from 11.2% to 3.7%. In our studies, in-hospital mortality was lower in patients who received either intracoronary or intravenous streptokinase than in a non-randomized group of conventionally treated patients [50].

The mechanisms by which coronary artery reperfusion improves survival are not yet identified. Theoretically, reperfusion may preserve a critical mass of functioning myocardium in patients with cardiogenic shock or severe cardiac failure. In other patients, reperfusion may salvage a subepicardial shell of myocardium and prevent transmural necrosis, a prerequisite for myocardial rupture and aneurysm formation. By terminating ischemia, reperfusion may prevent lethal ischemic ventricular arrhythmias which are the ultimate cause of death in many patients with extensive infarction [48] or may restore normal atrioventricular (A–V) conduction in patients with high degree A–V block block and thereby improve systemic and coronary hemodynamics and perfusion. Finally, reperfusion may prevent infarction extension which occurs in patients with subtotal occlusion when the thrombus progresses to total coronary occlusion.

Summary

Thrombolytic therapy is an effective means of achieving myocardial reperfusion during acute myocardial infarction. Consistent with experimental studies of the pathology of acute myocardial infarction, clinical reperfusion within 4 to 5 hours of the onset of infarction is likely to result in myocardial salvage, improved ventricular function and improved survival. In general, the earlier reperfusion is achieved, the greater is the extent of myocardial salvage. The clinical impact of reperfusion more than 6 hours after the onset of infarction and after completion of necrosis is unknown. Based on theoretical considerations late reperfusion may improve survival by mechanisms which are independent of myocardial salvage.

Acknowledgements

The authors are grateful to Jamshid Maddahi MD and Daniel S. Berman MD for their assisstance and expert advice during the preparation of this manuscript.

References

1. Kannel WB, Thom TJ (1984) Declining cardiovascular mortality. Circulation 70: 331–336
2. Rude RE, Muller JE, Braunwald E (1981) Efforts to limit the size of myocardial infarcts. Ann Intern Med 95: 736–761
3. Jennings RB, Reimer KA (1983) Factors involved in salvaging ischemic myocardium. Effect of reperfusion of arterial blood. Circulation 68: I-25–I-36

4. Tennant R, Wiggers CJ (1935) The effect of coronary occlusion on myocardial contraction. Am J Physiol 112: 351–361
5. Reimer KA, Jennings RB, Tatum AH (1983) Pathobiology of acute myocardial ischemia; metabolic, functional and ultrastructural studies. Am J Cardiol 52: 72A–81A
6. Reimer KA, Lowe JE, Rasmussen MM, Jennings RB (1977) The wave-front phenomenon of ischemic cell death. I. Myocardial infarct size vs duration of coronary occlusion in dogs. Circulation 56: 786–794
7. Schaper J, Schaper W (1983) Reperfusion of ischemic myocardium: ultrastructural and histochemical aspects. J Am Coll Cardiol 1: 1037–1046
8. Fishbein MC, Y-Rit J, Lando U, Kanmatsuse K, Mercier JC, Ganz W (1980) The relationship of vascular injury and myocardial hemorrhage to necrosis after reperfusion. Circulation 62: 1274–1279
9. Roberts CS, Schoen FJ, Kloner RA (1983) Effect of coronary reperfusion on myocardial hemorrhage and infarct healing. Am J Cardiol 52: 610–614
10. Schaper W, Pasyk S (1976) Influence of collateral flow on the ischemic tolerance of the heart following acute and subacute coronary occlusion. Circulation 53-I: I-57–62
11. Schaper W (1971) The collateral circulation of the heart. North-Holland Publishing Company, Amsterdam-New York
12. Swan HJC (1983) Thrombolysis in acute evolving myocardial infarction. A new potential for myocardial salvage. N Engl J Med 108: 1354–1358
13. Smalling RW, Fuentes F, Mathews MW, Freund GC, Hicks CH, Reduto LA, Walker WE, Sterling RP, Gould KL (1983) Sustained improvement in left ventricular function and mortality by intracoronary streptokinase administration during evolving myocardial infarction. Circulation 68: 131–138
14. DeWood MA, Spores J, Notske R, Mouser LT, Burroughs R, Golden MS, Lang HT (1981) Prevalence of total coronary occlusion during the early hours of transmural myocardial infarction. N Engl J Med 303: 897–902
15. Rentrop P, Blanke H, Karsch KR, Kaiser H, Kostering H, Leitz K (1981) Selective intracoronary thrombolysis in acute myocardial infarction and unstable angina pectoris. Circulation 63: 307–315
16. Ganz W, Buchbinder N, Marcus H, Mondkar A, Maddahi J, Charuzi Y, O'Conner L, Shell W, Fishbein MC, Kass R, Miyamoto A, Swan HJC (1981) Intracoronary thrombolysis in evolving myocardial infarction. Am Heart J 101: 4–13
17. Schroder R. Systemic versus intracoronary streptokinase infusion in the treatment of acute myocardial infarction (1983) J Am Coll Cardiol 1983 1: 1254–1261
18. Ganz W, Geft I, Shah PK, Lew AS, Rodriguez L, Weiss T, Maddahi J, Berman DS, Charuzi Y, Swan HJC (1984) Intravenous streptokinase in evolving myocardial infarction. Am J Cardiol 53: 1209–1216
19. Phillips SJ, Kongtahworn C, Skinner JR, Zeff RH (1983) Emergency coronary artery reperfusion: A choice therapy for evolving myocardial infarction. Results in 339 patients. J Thorac Cardiovasc Surg 86: 679–688
20. Hartzler GO, Rutherford BD, McConahay DR, Johnson WL, Ligon B. PTCA at initial coronary angiography – a safe and expeditious therapy (1984) Circulation 70-II: II-107
21. Hammerman H, Kloner RA, Briggs LL, Braunwald E (1984) Enhancement of salvage of reperfused myocardium by early beta-adrenergic blockade (Timolol). J Am Coll Cardiol 3: 1438–1443
22. Udall JA (1983) Noninvasive markers of intravenous streptokinase coronary thrombolysis. Clin Cardiol 6: 86–96
23. Bateman TM, Czer LSC, Gray RJ, Maddahi J, Raymond MJ, Geft IL, Ganz W, Shah PK, Berman DS (1983) Transient pathological Q waves during acute ischemic events: an electrocardiographic correlate of the stunned but viable myocardium. Am Heart J 106: 1421–1426
24. Markis JE, Malagold M, Parker A, Silverman KJ, Barry WH, Als AV, Paulin S, Grossman W, Braunwald E (1981) Myocardial salvage after intracoronary thrombolysis with streptokinase in

acute myocardial infarction. Assessment by intracoronary thallium-201. N Engl J Med 305: 777–782

25. Maddahi J, Ganz W, Ninomiya K, Hashida J, Fishbein MC, Mondkar A, Buchbinder N, Marcus H, Geft I, Shah PK, Rozanski A, Swan HJC, Berman DS (1981) Myocardial salvage by intracoronary thrombolysis in evolving acute myocardial infarction: Evaluation using intracoronary injection of thallium-201. Am Heart J 102: 664–674

26. Maddahi J, Weiss I, Geft I, Shah PK, Berman D, Swan HJC, Ganz W (1983) Coronary thrombolysis with intravenous streptokinase salvages jeopardized myocardium in evolving myocardial infarction: Assessment by quantitative Tl-201 imaging. Circulation 68-III: III-120

27. Maddahi J, Geft I, Berman D, Swan HJC, Ganz W (1982) Intracoronary technetium-99m pyrophosphate immediately demonstrates necrosis in reperfused myocardium and complements post-reperfusion intracoronary thallium-201 imaging. Circulation 66: II-86

28. Schofer J, Mathey DG, Montz R, Bleifeld W, Stritzke P (1983) Use of dual intracoronary scintigraphy with thallium-201 and technetium-99m pyrophosphate to predict improvement in left ventricular wall motion immediately after intracoronary thrombolysis in acute myocardial infarction. J Am Coll Cardiol 2: 737–744

29. Mancini GBJ, Peck WW, Slutsky RA, Ross J, Higgins CB (1984) Use of computerized tomography to assess myocardial infarct size and ventricular function in dogs during acute coronary occlusion and reperfusion. Am J Cardiol 53: 282–289

30. Bergmann SR, Lerch RA, Fox KA, Ludbrook PA, Welch MJ, Ter-Pogossian MM, Sobel BE (1982) Temporal dependence of beneficial effects of coronary thrombolysis characterized by positron tomography. Am J Med 73: 573–581

31. Shell W, Mickle DK, Swan HJC (1983) Effects of nonsurgical myocardial reperfusion of plasma creatine kinase kinetics in man. Am Heart J 106: 665–669

32. Sato Y, Degawa T, Isojima K, Y-Rit J, Fishbein MC, Karshmer DL, Shell WE, Ganz W (1984) Following early reperfusion, all the creatine kinase depleted from the necrotic myocardium appears in the blood. J Am Coll Cardiol 3: 22

33. Roberts R, Ishikawa Y (1983) Enzymatic estimation of infarct size during reperfusion. Circulation 68: I-83–I-89

34. Ellis SG, Henschke CI, Sandor T, Wynne J, Braunwald E, Kloner RA (1983) Time course of functional and biochemical recovery of myocardium salvaged by reperfusion. J Am Coll Cardiol 1: 1047–1055

35. Mercier JC, Lando U, Kanmatsuse K, Ninomya K, Meerbaum S, Fishbein MC, Swan HJC, Ganz W (1982) Divergent effects of ionotropic stimulation on the ischemic and severely depressed reperfused myocardium. Circulation 66: 397–400

36. Reduto LA, Smalling RW, Freund GC, Gould KL (1981) Intracoronary infusion of streptokinase in patients with acute myocardial infarction: effects of reperfusion on left ventricular performance. Am J Cardiol 48: 403–409

37. Anderson JL, Marshall HW, Bray BE, Lutz JR, Frederick PR, Yanowitz FG, Datz FL, Klausner SC, Hagan AD (1983) A randomized trial of intracoronary streptokinase in the treatment of acute myocardial infarction. N Engl J Med 308: 1312–1318

38. Anderson JL, Marshall HW, Askins JC, Lutz JR, Sorensen SG, Menlove RL, Yanowitz FG, Hagan AD (1984) A randomized trial of intravenous and intracoronary streptokinase in patients with acute myocardial infarction. Circulation 70: 606–618

39. Charuzi Y, Beder C, Marshall LA, Sasaki H, Pack NB, Geft I, Ganz W (1984) Improvement in regional and global left ventricular function after intracoronary thrombolysis: assessment with two-dimensional echocardiography. Am J Cardiol 53: 662–665

40. Sheehan FH, Mathey DG, Schofer J, Krebber HJ, Dodge HT (1983) Effect of interventions in salvaging left ventricular function in acute myocardial infarction: A study of intracoronary streptokinase. Am J Cardiol 52: 431–438

41. Stack RS, Phillips HR III, Grierson DS, Behar VS, Kong Y, Peter RH, Swain JL (1983)

Functional improvement of jeopardized myocardium following intracoronary streptokinase infusion in acute myocardial infarction. J Clin Invest 72: 84–95

42. Khaja F, Walton JA, Brymer JF, Lo E, Osterberger L, O,Neill WW, Colfer HT, Weiss R, Lee T, Kurian T, Goldberg AD, Pitt B, Goldstein S (1983) Intracoronary fibrinolytic therapy in acute myocardial infarction. Report of a prospective randomized trial. N Engl J Med 308: 1305–1311

43. Ritchie JL, Davis KB, Williams DL, Caldwell J, Kennedy JW (1984) Global and regional left ventricular function and tomographic radionuclide perfusion: The Western Washington intracoronary streptokinase in myocardial infarction trial. Circulation 70: 867–875

44. Rentrop P, Smith H, Painter L, Holt J (1983) Changes in left ventricular ejection fraction after intracoronary thrombolytic therapy. Results of the Registry of the European Society of Cardiology. Circulation 68-I: I-55–60

45. Schuler G, Hofmann M, Schwarz F, Mehmel H, Manthey J, Tillmanns H, Hartmann S, Kubler W (1984) Effect of successful thrombolytic therapy on right ventricular function in acute inferior wall myocardial infarction. Am J Cardiol 54: 951–957

46. Sheehan FH, Brown BG, Mathey DG, Dodge HT (1984) Effect of severe residual stenosis on recovery of function after streptokinase. J Am Coll Cardiol 3: 526

47. Rogers WJ, Hood WP Jr, Mantle JA, Baxley WA, Kirklin JK, Zorn GL, Nath HP (1984) Return of left ventricular function after reperfusion in patients with myocardial infarction: Importance of subtotal stenoses or intact collaterals. Circulation 69: 338–349

48. Kennedy JW, Ritchie JL, Davis KB, Fritz JK (1983) Western Washington randomized trial of intracoronary streptokinase in acute myocardial infarction. N Engl J Med 309: 1477–1482

49. Ferguson DW, White CW, Schwartz JL, Brayden GP, Kelly KJ, Kioschos JM, Kirchner PT, Marcus ML (1984) Influence of baseline ejection fraction and success of thrombolysis on mortality and ventricular function after acute myocardial infarction. Am J Cardiol 54: 705–711

50. Lew AS, Geft IL, Shah PK, Rodriguez L, Ganz W (1984) Intracoronary and intravenous streptokinase in acute myocardial infarction – a comparative report. Eur Heart J

Pathophysiology of transluminal angioplasty

WILFREDO CASTANEDA-ZUNIGA

Introduction

In their original description of the technique, Dotter and Judkins attributed the effectiveness of angioplasty to a redistribution and compression of the atheromatous intima [1]. Recent research, however, has shown that both complex morphologic and physiologic alterations are produced in the vessel wall by angioplasty. In this paper, we review the arterial pathophysiology of angioplasty in order to better understand the basis for its success and failure.

Morphologic changes produced by angioplasty

The most obvious changes produced in the arterial wall by the dilating balloon are morphologic. Acute morphologic changes produced by dilation consist of intimal splitting, medial stretching (often with intimal-medical dehiscence) and medial necrosis. Recent studies have demonstrated that the atherosclerotic intima is relatively incompressible (Figure 1) [2]. Therefore, when a balloon is inflated with sufficient pressure across an atherosclerotic stenoses, one of the first events which occurs is fracturing, or splitting, of the plaque (Figure 2). With only moderate dilation, this may be all that occurs. Frequently this is sufficient to obtain a significant increase in the arterial luminal diameter.

If larger balloons, longer inflation times and greater pressures are used during angioplasty, more significant morphologic changes are produced in the vessel wall. Following fracture of the plaque, actual separation of the atherosclerotic intima and surrounding media may occur. Separation of the intima and media, so-called intima-medial dehiscence, may actually be a common occurrence in clinical angioplasty. We have observed this phenomenon, both experimentally and clinically in arteries which have come to pathologic examination.

Histologic examination of dilated atherosclerotic vessels often reveals clefts which extend between the intima and media. The origin of these clefts appears to be most often located at the junction of a focal plaque and the more normal adjacent vessel lumen [3]. Complete separation of the intima and media with distal embolization of the plaque has been reported but this appears to be a very rare occurrence. Microembolization of atherosclerotic debris has also been investigated experimentally but has not been shown to be clinically significant [4, 5].

The radiographic picture of intimal-medial dehiscence is familiar to all experienced angiographers (Figure 3). On post-dilation angiograms, a linear extraluminal collection of contrast material is seen at the site of dilation. This, of course, represents the accumulation of contrast material under the dehisced intima. In most cases, the vessel appears to heal quickly without clinical sequelae.

Since the intimal cleft created by dilation may be a major mechanism by which lumen size is increased after angioplasty, it is reasonable to speculate the healing of this cleft may be one mechanism of restenosis. Some investigators, however, feel that remodeling of the fractured plaque occurs during the healing phase which results in a permanent increase in the luminal diameter [6]. It is also possible that when the more normal arterial media is separated from the encasing atherosclerotic intima, it can more easily increase its diameter in response to blood flow demands. These effects may be important means by which angioplasty produced its effect. It is apparent, however, that actual stretching of the media occurs during balloon inflation which results in an immediate mechanical increase in vessel diameter.

Angioplasty's effect has been described as a 'controlled vessel injury'. The 'injury' is especially apparent in the media of the dilated artery. Within 24 hours of dilation, the normal medial architecture begins to degenerate. Fusiform shaped smooth muscle cells lose their shape and disintegrate. Invading macrophages clear away medial debris and fibroblastic proliferation results in repair of the damaged artery. A large part of this process appears to occur. Within the first few days of dilation, however, complete repair of the vessel may require 4 to 6 weeks.

One other morphologic sequela of the dilating process remains to be discussed. With almost any vascular trauma, including angioplasty, denudation of the endothelial surface occurs. This exposes a relatively thrombogenic surface which results in platelet and fibrin deposition. One rationale for the use of aspirin after angioplasty therefore is to decrease the aggregation of platelets at the site of dilation. Acute occlusion of the dilated vessel may be due in certain cases to thrombosis. Some investigators, however, feel that aspirin may also decrease the amount of intimal proliferation which occurs after angioplasty [7]. Neointima formation is important after endothelial denudation in order to provide new northrombogenic flow surface. Intimal proliferation, or overgrowth, however may be one mechanism of restenosis following angioplasty. Certain physiologic alterations which may mediate this phenomenon will be discussed next.

Physiologic changes produced by angioplasty

Any mechanical trauma which alters a tissue morphologically, also produces physiologic changes. As expected then, angioplasty also effects vessel wall physiology to a significant extent. The artery's nutrient supply, contractility and metabolism are all affected by dilation. Many physiologic alterations may be a direct result of altered vessel wall morphology after angioplasty; i.e. disruption of the media may also decrease the vessel's contractile ability. Less well understood, however, is the concept that physiology changes induced by arterial trauma may also determine the long term morphologic outcome of the procedure; e.g. release of arachidonate metabolites from platelets or the vessel wall may be responsible for intimal proliferation. We have recently studied several aspects of vessel physiology after angioplasty.

The vasa vasorum nourish the walls of most larger systemic arteries. Interruption of the vasa vasorum has been implicated in both aneurysm formation an accelerated atherogenesis. Therefore, we investigated the effect of angioplasty on the vasa vasorum [8]. Although the vasa vasorum do not appear to be interrupted or altered morphologically by angioplasty, it is clear that they respond dramatically to the apparent trauma of dilation. Using sequential injections of differently labeled radioactive microspheres, we were able to show that angioplasty results in a dramatic increase in blood flow through the vasa vasorum of the dilated artery. This vessel wall hyperemia is persistent and is not unexpected in view of the previously demonstrated vessel injury which is produced by angioplasty. Interestingly, however, the hyperemia can be significantly alternated by administration of aspirin (10 mg/kg, IV) before the procedure [9]. This suggests that aspirin, which is an inhibitor of prostaglandin synthesis, may decrease the production and release of vasodilating prostaglandins after angioplasty. Prostacyclin, a well known vasodilating prostaglandin, produced in vessel endothelium, has now been shown to be released acutely after angioplasty. Vessel wall hyperemia then is a manifestation of altered physiology after angioplasty. Whether aspirin should be used to inhibit this phenomenon requires further study.

A second physiology manifestation of altered vessel wall morphology after angioplasty is an acute decrease in the contractility of the vessel wall [10]. The isometric tension which a dilated vessel generates in the presence of norepinephrine is significantly less than the normal vessel. With damage to the media this is expected. By administering indomethocin, however, which acts similar to aspirin, the contractile ability of the vessel is significantly enhanced suggesting again that the balance of vasoconstriction and vasodilation is altered by angioplasty. These findings may be important in selecting the type and dose of antithrombotic medication used following angioplasty.

Finally, using radiochromatography we have measured the production of various prostaglandin metabolites in the dilated arterial wall [11]. An unexpected an potentially important finding is that the production of newly discovered prostaglandin derivatives, the hydroperoxy-acids, is significantly augmented by angioplasty. The hydroperoxy-acids have been linked to vessel spasm, atherogenesis and inflammation. Aspirin and other aspirin-like drugs may be effective in decreasing the degree of restenosis following angioplasty. Prostaglandins and their metabolites may play a role, therefore, in such phenomena as vessel spasm and intimal proliferation which occur after angioplasty. Intimal proliferation and accelerated atherogenesis may be morphologic manifestations of altered vessel wall physiology which can and should be modified pharmacologically. The best type of intervention as well as the larger question of differential plately and prostaglandin inhibition requires additional study.

In summary, angioplasty is known to produce its effect primarily by mechanical deformation of the arterial wall. Significant changes are produced acutely including intimal splitting, intimal-medial dehiscence and medial necrosis. Repair of the vessel is generally complete with enlargement of the vessel lumen due in part to permanent stretching of the arterial media. Less well understood, though perhaps equally important, are the physiologic changes which are produced in the vessel wall by angioplasty. Disruption of the vessel's nutrient supply and prostaglandin metabolism may affect the long term morphologic outcome of the procedure. Aspirin may produce long term benefits by inhibiting local vessel wall prostaglandin metabolism.

References

1. Dotter CT, Judkins MP (1964) Transluminal treatment of arteriosclerotic obstruction: Description of a new technique and a preliminary report of its application. Circulation 30: 654–670
2. Castaneda-Zuniga WR, Formanek A, Tadavarthy M (1980) The mechanism of angioplasty. Radiology 135: 565–571
3. Laerum F, Castaneda-Zuniga WR, Rysavy J, Moore B, Amplatz K (1982) The site of wall rupture in transluminal angioplasty: An experimental study. Radiology 144: 769–770
4. Saffitz JE, Totty WG, McClennan BL, Gilula LA (1981) Percutaneous transluminal angioplasty. Radiological-pathological correlation. Radiology 141: 651–654
5. Sanborn TA, Faxon DP, Waugh D, Small DM, Haudenschild C, Gottsman SB, Ryan TJ (1982) Transluminal angioplasty in experimental atherosclerosis. Analysis for embolization using an in vivo perfusion system. Circulation 66: 917–922
6. Block PC (1980) Percutaneous transluminal coronary angioplasty. AJR 135: 955–959
7. Hagen P, Wang Z, Mikat EM, Hackel DB (1981) Antiplatelet therapy reduces aortic intimal hyperplasia distal to small diameter vascular prosthese (PTFE) in non-human primates. Ann Surg 195: 328–339
8. Cragg AH, Einzig S, Rysavy JA, Castaneda-Zuniga WR, Borgwardt B, Amplatz K (1983) The vaso vasorum and angioplasty. Radiology 148: 75–80
9. Cragg A, Einzig S, Rysavy J, Castaneda-Zuniga W, Borgwardt B, Amplatz K (1983) Effect of angioplasty on angioplasty-induced vessel wall hyperemia. AJR 140: 1233–1238
10. Zollikofer CL, Cragg AH, Einzig S (1984) Prostaglandins and angioplasty: An experimental study in canine arteries. Radiology
11. Cragg A, Einzig S, Castaneda-Zuniga W, Amplast K, White JG, Rao GR (1983) Vessel wall arachidonate metabolism after angioplasty: Possible mediators of postangioplasty vasospasm. Am J Cardiol 51: 1441–1445

Does angioplasty improve or accelerate atherosclerosis?

PETER C. BLOCK

Though the pathophysiological changes that occur immediately after transluminal angioplasty are now known, exactly how these changes effect the atherosclerotic process is less well understood. It was first thought that transluminal
angioplasty (using a dilating balloon) produces compression of the atherosclerotic plaque against the arterial wall. This has been difficult to document experimentally though some investigations indicate that compression may play a slight
role [1]. Instead, most studies have shown focal injury to the atherosclerotic
plaque with splitting or the intima and media. Angioplasty performed in the
coronary arteries of autopsied human hearts showed that the coronary atherosclerotic plaques were frequently split to the internal elastic membrane [2].
This raised questions as to the frequency with which angioplasty might be
associated with arterial dissection or perforation. Since dissection and perforation did not occur commonly, the issue of whether human autopsy material
reacted identically to living tissue *in vivo* caused doubts as to the reliability of
these data.

Experimental models have also been used to evaluate the changes that occur
after angioplasty. Angioplasty performed in canine coronary arteries produces
desquamation of endothelial cells and deposition of platelets in the area of
denuded subendothelial connective tissue matrix [3] (Figure 1). Platelets are
deposited despite the use of platelet inhibitors such as aspirin and dipyridamole,
or anticoagulant agents such as heparin. The same changes are seen in studies
using an atherosclerotic rabbit model. In arteries where the size of the inflated
balloon and the artery are almost the same, endothelium is injured and platelets
are deposited immediately. In areas where the size of the expanded angioplasty
balloon is larger than that of the stenosed arterial lumen, the atherosclerotic
plaque splits at its weakest portion [4, 5] (Figure 2). This is similar to the clinical
situation in man. The split frequently extends to the internal elastic membrane
and usually extends circumferentially around the arterial wall.

A similar picture of splitting of the plaque has also been seen in pathological
sections of peripheral and coronary arteries studied after successful angioplasty in
man [6].

After the intima and inner media are split and as the angioplasty balloon is fully

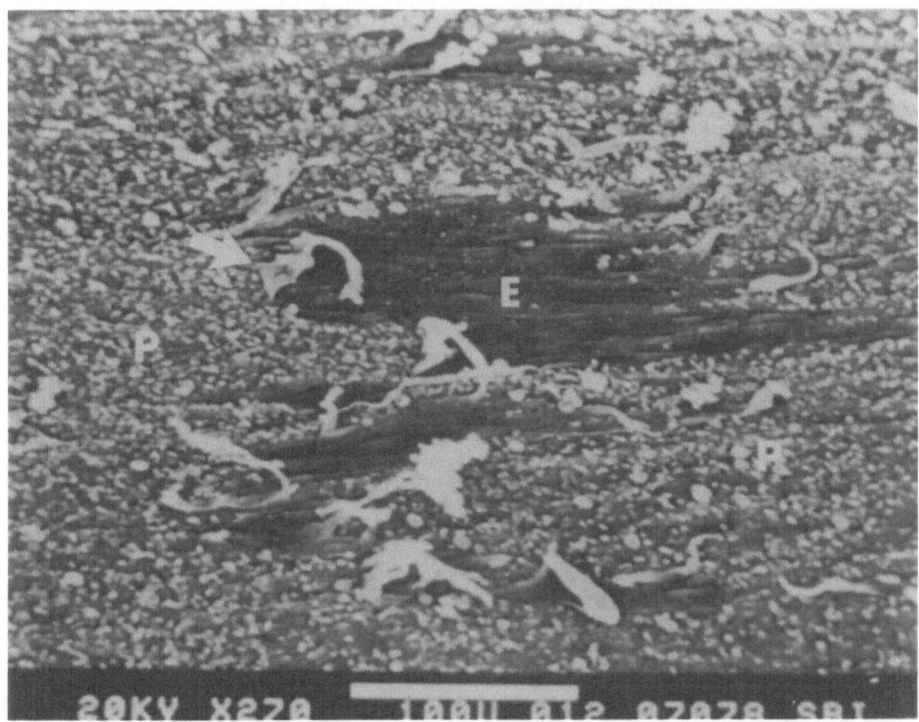

Figure 1. Electron micrograph of a normal canine coronary artery immediately after transluminal angioplasty. Small areas of intact endothelium (E) are present. Most of the endothelium has been injured. Partially adherent endothelial cells (arrow) and large numbers of platelets (P) are seen.

inflated, the outer media and adventitia stretch over the expanded angioplasty balloon. Multiple inflations of the balloon damage medial muscle cells. This may aid in expanding the adventitia and media due to loss of elasticity of these layers as medial cells and elastic tissue are injured. Electron and light microscopic studies of arteries after angioplasty in dogs have shown medial myocytes with a 'cork screw' appearance of their nuclei related to nuclear injury [7, 8].

In summary, the morphologic changes that occur after angioplasty are the following (Figure 3):

1. The dilating balloon begins to inflate within the stenosed atherosclerotic segment and the atherosclerotic plaque resists stretching. There may be some extrusion of liquid from the plaque and possibly some compression of plaque (Figure 3B).

2. Pressure mounts within the angioplasty balloon and the dilating force exceeds the tensil strength of the plaque at its weakest (usually thinnest) portion. The plaque splits, and the balloon then continues to inflate to its full diameter.

3. Full inflation occurs and the split in the atherosclerotic plaque widens circumferentially. The outer media and adventitia are stretched over the expanded

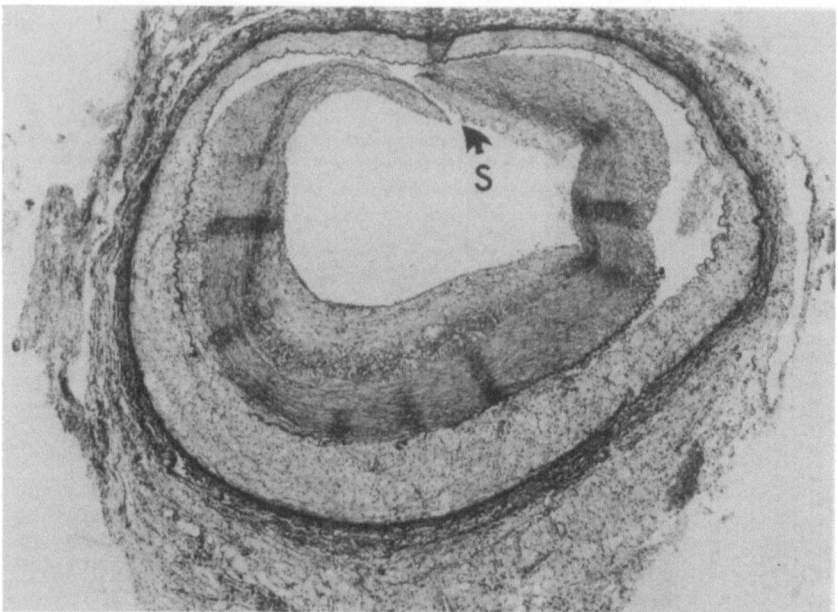

Figure 2. Microscopic section of a rabbit atherosclerotic iliac artery immediately after angioplasty. The atherosclerotic plaque has been split (S) at its weakest point. The split extends to the internal elastic membrane and extends circumferentially.

dilating balloon (Figure 3C). Microscopically myocytes are injured as stretching occurs, elastic fibers lose their characteristic undulated morphology, and there may be fragmentation of elastic fibers as well.

4. The balloon is deflated. The atherosclerotic plaque remains split and the outer layers of the artery remain fixed in a dilated position (Figure 3D).

Hemodynamic data support this concept of the changes that occur with angioplasty. The first inflation of a dilating balloon often does not abolish the pressure gradient across the arterial stenosis. More than one dilation may be necessary to diminish the gradient or abolish it (Figure 4). Thus, the outer layers of the artery must be progressively stretched after the atheromatous plaque is split. Multiple dilations of the artery cause progressive injury to medial myocytes and stretching of elastic tissue. Elastic recoil is then gradually lost. Finally, the artery remains fixed in a dilated position. Occasionally, the pressure gradient across the stenosis recurs in the first few minutes after angioplasty (Figure 5). To account for this, the outer layers of the artery must re-establish muscular tone and elastic recoil. This diminishes the circumference of the outer layers of the artery to less than the circumference of the fully expanded angioplasty balloon and the trans-stenotic pressure gradient returns. Multiple balloon inflations damage the outer layers of the artery further and leave them in a permanently fixed, dilated position.

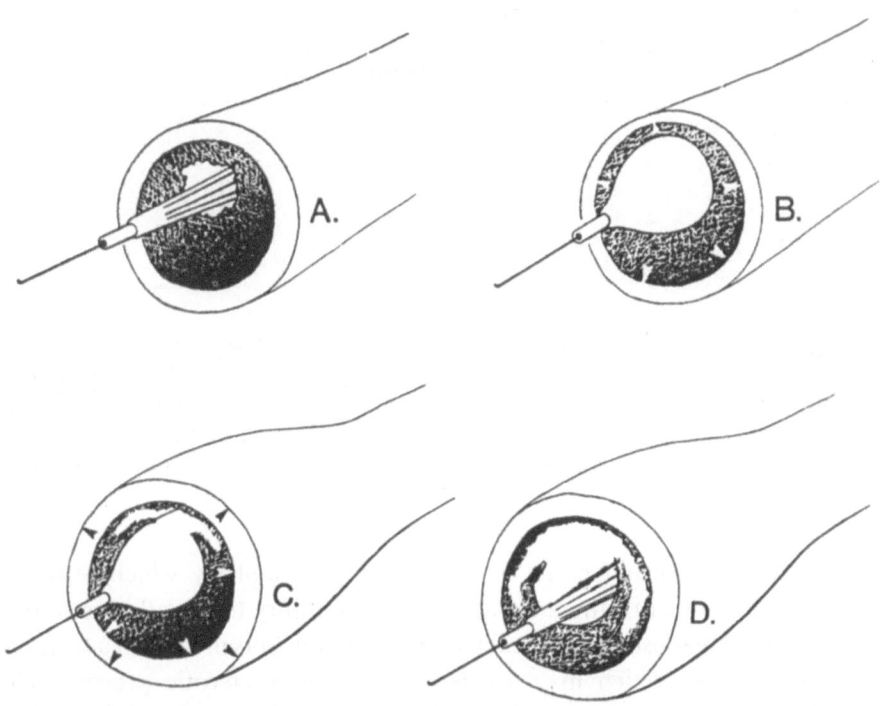

Figure 3. Diagram of the morphologic changes that occur after angioplasty. A. Dilating balloon in position within the atherosclerotic plaque. B. The dilating balloon begins to inflate within the atherosclerotic segment. The atherosclerotic plaque resists stretching. C. As the balloon is fully inflated, the atherosclerotic plaque splits at its weakest portion. The split widens circumferentially and the outer media and adventitia are stretched over the expanded balloon. D. The balloon is deflated and the artery remains fixed in a dilated position. The atherosclerotic plaque is split.

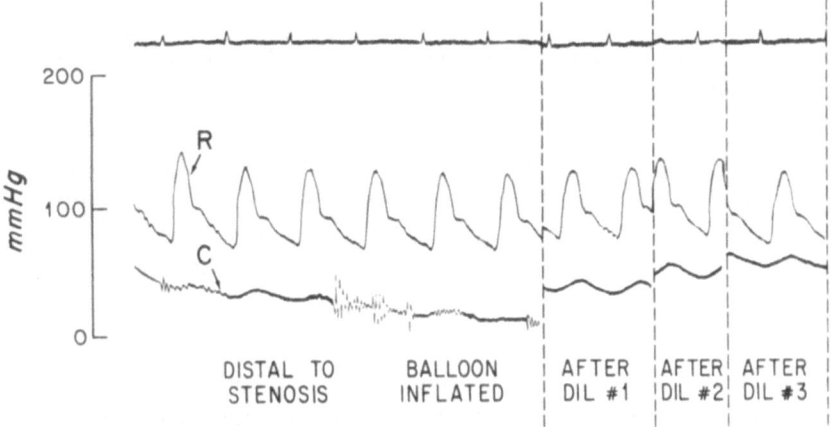

Figure 4. Hemodynamic measurements before and immediately after angioplasty. Initial pressure gradient across the stenosis is approximately 50 mm Hg. After the first dilation, the pressure gradient is diminished only slightly (DIL #1). After 3 dilations (DIL #3), the pressure gradient has been diminished to approximately 15 mm Hg. (R; radial artery pressure; C; coronary artery pressure measured from the coronary artery distal to the stenosis).

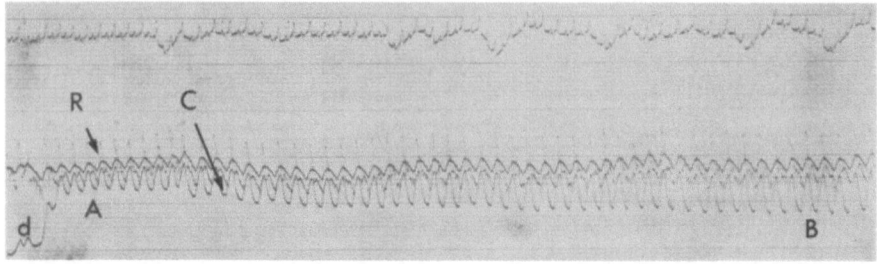

Figure 5. Hemodynamic measurements during coronary angioplasty showing immediate return of elastic recoil of the outer artery with increase in the pressure gradient. Immediately after balloon deflation (d), the gradient across the coronary stenosis is approximately 20 mm Hg (A). The pressure gradient across the coronary stenosis, however, increases as elastic recoil of the outer layers of the coronary artery occurs (B). (R; radial artery pressure). (C; coronary artery pressure measured distal to the coronary stenosis).

Thus, it is mechanical factors associated with angioplasty which result in immediate enlargement of the arterial lumen. The injury to the atherosclerotic plaque produced by these mechanical factors, however, sets in motion a series of physiological factors which may accelerate the atherosclerotic process. The re-stenosis rate after successful angioplasty ranges from 25% to 35% [9]. Possible mechanisms for reversal of the beneficial effects of angioplasty may be due to a loss of the initial mechanical effects or may be due to an acceleration of the atherosclerotic process.

Loss of Mechanical Effects

1. *Loss of adventitial 'stretch'.* Re-stenosis may occur because of return of elasticity of the outer arterial wall. As medial myocytes regenerate and regain vasoactive function and the outer elastic elements are repaired, vascular tone returns. The volume of the atherosclerotic plaque is unchanged after angioplasty. Therefore, any diminution in the amount of stretching of the outer layers of the artery reduces lumen size back toward the size of the lumen before angioplasty. The amount of re-stenosis depends upon the amount of recoil of the outer layers of the vessel.

2. *Platelet thrombus formation.* Immediately after angioplasty platelets become firmly attached to exposed collagen fibers in subendothelial layers. Platelets spread over the damaged area, pseudopod formation occurs, and intracellular granules discharge (Figure 6). There are three types of platelet granules:
a. Alpha granules which contain platelet derived growth factor (PDGF), beta-thromboglobulin, platelet factor IV, fibrinogen, and coagulation factors VIII and V.

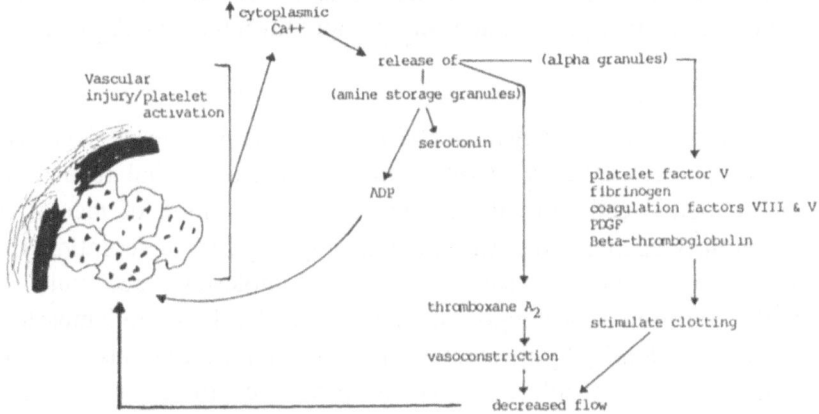

Figure 6. Diagram of the physiologic factors that occur after angioplasty which may promote re-stenosis. Vascular injury produces platelet aggregation and an increase in platelet cytoplasmic calcium. Platelet granules are released and the arachidonic acid pathway is stimulated with production of thromboxane A_2. These factors tend to diminish vascular flow and promote further platelet activation.

b. Amine storage granules which contain serotonin and ADP.

c. Lysosomal vesicles.

As the platelet mass builds due to platelet aggregation, there is an increase in cytoplasmic calcium [10] which leads to the release of platelet granule constituents – especially ADP. The arachidonic acid pathway is activated with production of thromboxane A_2. ADP and thromboxane A_2 further stimulate platelet aggregation. This increases the release of ADP and perpetuates the process. In addition, the platelet thrombi themselves may partially occlude the lumen after angioplasty and diminish blood flow. Since blood flow is inversely related to platelet deposition, as flow diminishes more platelets are deposited and blood flow is increasingly diminished. This sets up a vicious cycle: platelet thrombi cause a decrease in blood flow, which causes a further increase in platelet deposition, which causes a further decrease in blood flow, etc.

The clotting mechanism itself may be activated during platelet adhesion and thrombin may be generated at the site of injury. Alterations in the platelet membrane result in release of phospholipoprotein platelet factor III, which enhances the action of coagulation factors II and XII and generates thrombin by means of the intrinsic coagulation pathway. The degree of injury is important. If damage to the endothelium is minor, small platelet thrombi form and then break off. If there is more extensive injury large segments of subendothelial connective tissue are exposed. If blood flow is not increased, thrombus may form.

3. *Effect of thromboxane A_2.* Thromboxane A_2, a potent vasoconstrictor, is released by platelets. If medial muscle cells in the area of angioplasty are not badly damaged and are able to respond to the effect of thromboxane A_2, vas-

oconstriction may occur in the area of angioplasty. This diminishes blood flow and may enhance further platelet deposition, more thromboxane A_2 release, etc. (Figure 6).

4. *Acceleration of the underlying atherosclerotic process*. Platelet derived growth factor (PDGF) is released by platelets and accelerates medial regeneration, migration of medial cells into the intima, and proliferation of medial cells. Platelets that have aggregated at the site of angioplasty form a neointima that is permeable to lipids and cholesterol. Lipids and cholesterol accumulate and stimulate the secretion of proteoglycans and collagen by the smooth muscle cells in the media. Low density lipoproteins, which carry cholesterol, also can stimulate smooth muscle cell proliferation. As this process continues, smooth muscle cells proliferate, collagen and proteoglycans are continually secreted, and cholesterol accumulates – resulting in a mature atherosclerotic plaque. This may account for late re-stenosis over 3 to 6 months in many patients after successful angioplasty.

In summary, the ultimate fate of the angioplasty area depends on a balance of mechanical and physiological factors. Depending on which predominates, the vessel may remain patent or there may be progression of atherosclerosis.

Factors favoring maintainence of a patent lumen

1. Change in flow characteristics of the dilated area cause remodeling and reabsorption of atherosclerotic material in the area of angioplasty. This accounts for a smooth lumen and larger lumen size seen in follow-up angiograms six months or more after angioplasty.

2. An increase in blood flow minimizes platelet deposition. Therefore, less thromboxane A_2 and PDGF are released and there is less effect of these agents on the arterial wall. Damage to medial cells diminishes the responsiveness of the arterial media to thromboxane A_2 and may diminish the effect of PDGF on the media later.

3. If the adventitia and outer layers of the media remain fixed in the dilated position after angioplasty, some atherosclerosis may recur, but the impact of the volume of the atherosclerotic plaque may be small and not affect blood flow appreciably.

Factors promoting re-stenosis and the atherosclerotic process

1. Platelets, deposited in the area of angioplasty because of focal injury, release thromboxane A_2. This causes local vasoconstriction, diminishes local blood flow, and promotes further platelet deposition in the area.

2. Thrombus formation in the area of angioplasty may organize and ingrowth of fibrocellular tissue may diminish lumen size.

3. The release of PDGF stimulates medial cells, which have escaped injury, to migrate proliferate. Medial cells migrate to the intima and re-establish the atherosclerotic process.

How these various factors interact has not been established. Whether or not the use of platelet inhibitor therapy, vasodilating agents, and dietary factors affect the complex physiology which occurs after successful angioplasty is unknown. A clearer understanding of the interplay of these factors will help us to better understand and avoid re-stenosis after angioplasty.

References

1. Kaltenbach M, Beyer J, Klepzig H, Schmidts L, Hubner K (1982) Effect of 5 kg/cm^2 pressure on atherosclerotic vessel wall segments. In: Transluminal Coronary Angioplasty and Intracoronary Thrombolysis. Springer-Verlag Berlin Heidelberg: 189–193
2. Baughman KL, Pasternak RC, Fallon JT, Block PC (1978) Coronary transluminal angioplasty in autopsied human hearts. Circ. 80 (Suppl II): 57–58
3. O'Gara PT, Guerrero JL, Feldman B, Fallon JT, Block PC (1984) Effect of dextran and aspirin on platelet adherence following transluminal angioplasty of normal canine coronary arteries. Am J Cardiol 53: 1695–1698
4. Block PC (1980) Angioplasty: Lessons from the laboratory. Amer J Radiol 135: 907–912
5. Schmidt-Moritz AD, Schneider M, Kunkel B, Kaltenbach M (1982) Histological changes following transluminal angioplasty of experimentally induced atherosclerosis in miniature pigs. In: Transluminal Coronary Angioplasty and Intracoronary Thrombolysis. Springer-Verlag Berlin Heidelberg: 176–182
6. Block PC, Myler RK, Stertzer SS, Fallon JT (1981) The pathophysiological mechanism of transluminal angioplasty in humans. New Engl J Med 305: 382–385
7. Block PC (1984) Mechanism of transluminal angioplasty. Am J Cardiol 53: 69–71
8. Castenida-Zuniga WR, Sibley R, Amplatz K (1984) The pathologic basis of angioplasty. Angiology 35: 195–205
9. Holmes DR, Vlietstra RE, Smith HC, Vetrovec GW, Kent KM, Cowley MJ, Faxon DP, Gruntzig AR, Kelsey SF, Detre KM, Van Raden MJ, Mock MB (1984) Restenosis after percutaneous transluminal coronary angioplasty (PTCA): A report from the PTCA Registry of the National Heart, Lung and Blood Institute. Am J Cardiol 53: 77–81
10. Frishman WH (1982) Antiplatelet therapy in coronary heart disease. Hospital Practice 73–86

Elective PCTA of totally occluded coronary arteries not associated with acute myocardial infarction: short and long term results

PATRICK W. SERRUYS, VICTOR ULMANS, GUY R. HEYNDRICKX, MARCEL v.d. BRAND, PIM J. DE FEYTER, WILLIAM WIJNS, BRIAN JASKI and PAUL G. HUGENHOLTZ

Abstract

Of 652 consecutive patients referred for coronary angioplasty between September 1980 and March 1984, 49 patients presented with total or functional 'occlusion' of the involved vessel. Total vessel occlusion was defined as absent antegrade filling beyond the lesion. Functional occlusion was defined as faint, late antegrade opacification of the distal segment in the absence of a discernible luminal continuity. In 39 patients, the total or functional occlusion represented a progression, without acute myocardial infarction, of a previously diagnosed stenotic lesion.

The maximal potential duration of occlusion was estimated to be 4 weeks or less in 21 patients, more than 4 to 8 weeks in 12, and more than 8 weeks in 16. Dilation of the occluded artery was attempted in the left anterior descending coronary artery in 30 patients, in the right coronary artery in 8, in the circumflex coronary in 7 and in 4 jumpgrafts. For the whole group, angioplasty was successful in 28 patients (57%). The primary success rate with the functionally occluded vessel (81%) was significantly higher than with the total occlusion (45%). In 33 patients with an occlusion estimated to be of 8 weeks or less, angioplasty was successful in 65%. In the 16 patients with an occlusion estimated to be of more than 8 weeks duration, dilation was successful in 44%. Of the 21 patients in whom angioplasty was an unsuccessful attempt, 11 required surgery (1 urgent with persistent pain and ST elevation and 10 elective). Ten patients were maintained on medical treatment. Of the 28 patients in whom angioplasty was successful, 10 patients had recurrence of symptoms during follow-up (1–42 months). Four were kept on medical therapy, three required bypass surgery and three underwent repeat PTCA.

After primary success, late angiographic studies obtained in 20 out of 28 patients showed reocclusion in 8.

In conclusion, elective PTCA of totally occluded coronary arteries is feasible but the primary success rate is lower (57%) than that associated with conventional lesions. The longterm clinical results following successful angioplasty are satisfactory (64%), but the incidence of reocclusion is higher (40%).

Introduction

Coronary angioplasty was introduced in 1978 by Grüntzig et al. [1] as a non operative technique for treatment of single, discrete and proximal coronary artery stenosis in patients with symptomatic ischemic heart disease.

Today, after six years of experience with PTCA, these indications have been extended to include distal stenotic lesions in up to three vessels requiring multiple dilations [2]. Patients with unstable angina [3] and impaired ventricular function [4] have been included. Furthermore, PTCA is performed in stenotic bypass grafts [5] and for residual stenosis after fibrinolytic recanalization [6] during acute or impending myocardial infarction.

In 1982, we reported [7] that a fixed guide wire angioplasty catheter could be used to dilate totally occluded coronary arteries and in the same year, Savage et al. [8] reported 39 patients who had progressed to total or functional total occlusion between their diagnostic angiogram and scheduled dilatation and in whom angioplasty was attempted despite arterial occlusion.

Recently, Dervan et al. [9] emphasized the advantages of a movable guide wire system for performing coronary angioplasty of functionally occluded vessels and Holmes et al. [10] demonstrated that the duration of occlusion is an important factor determining the primary success rate. This study describes our experience in 49 patients with attention to the short and long term clinical results.

Methods

Study population

Of 652 consecutive patients referred for coronary angioplasty at the Thoraxcenter and at the University Hospital of Gent between September 1980 and March 1984, 49 patients presented with total or functional 'occlusion' of the involved vessel. According to the criteria proposed by Dervan et al. [9], total vessel occlusion was defined as absent antegrade filling beyond the lesion whereas functional occlusion was defined as faint, late antegrade opacification of the distal segment in the absence of a discernible luminal continuity.

The study population consisted of 44 males and 5 females. The mean age was 54 ± 11 years. Eight patients had a previously documented transmural myocardial infarction in the region of distribution of the occluded vessel.

At the time of the attempted angioplasty no patient had a documented evolving transmural infarction and none of them had received fibrinolytic therapy. All patients had prior recurrent angina pectoris (mean duration 21 m; range; 0.5–156 m) unresponsive to drug therapy. Sixteen were in New York Heart Association functional class IV, 22 were in class III and 11 were in class II. A retrospective review of the clinical records in the study group showed that all but 4 patients had experienced recent exacerbation of their anginal symptoms. In the 39 patients with recent coronary occlusion, as evidenced by sequential angiograms, no patient had overt clinical or electrocardiographic signs of recently sustained acute myocardial infarction. One patient with right coronary artery involvement was suspected of having developed a silent myocardial infarction, since a new Q wave appeared in the inferior leads of his electrocardiogram.

Angiographic findings prior to PTCA

Ten patients had a total occlusion at the time of the initial diagnostic studies which were performed a mean of 52 days (range 7–240) before attempted angioplasty (Figure 1).

Thirty two patients had a non occluded discrete stenotic lesion at the time of the diagnotic angiography that was thought to be technically suitable for angioplasty. In these patients, the time interval between diagnostic angiography and angioplasty was 67 days (range 1–293). Nine of these 32 patients progressed from severe stenosis to functional occlusion over this time interval, while 23 of these patients progressed to total occlusion.

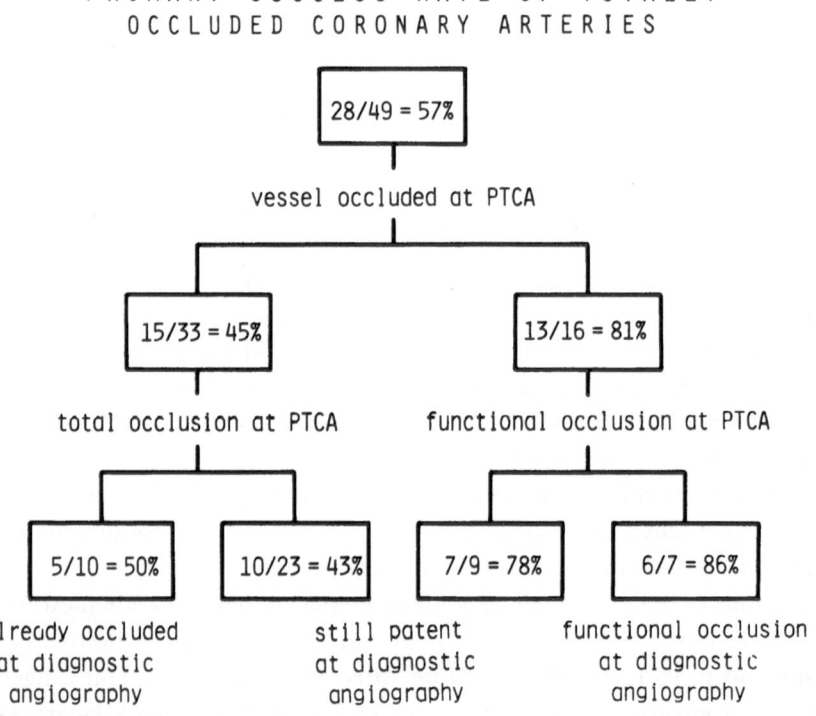

Figure 1. Primary success rate of angioplasty according to the angiographic finding at the time of the diagnostic angiography.

The remaining 7 patients had a functional occlusion at the time of diagnostic angiography.

The occluded vessel was the left anterior descending coronary artery in 30 patients, the right coronary artery in 8, the circumflex coronary artery in 7, and a coronary artery bypass graft in 4 (Figure 2).

At the time of the diagnostic angigraphy, collateral vessels were seen in 8 of the 10 patients with total occlusion, in 5 of the 7 patients with functional occlusion and in 11 of the 32 patients with a patent vessel.

At the time of angioplasty, collateral vessels provided some degree of opacification in 37 of the 49 patients; the collateral filling was provided by the

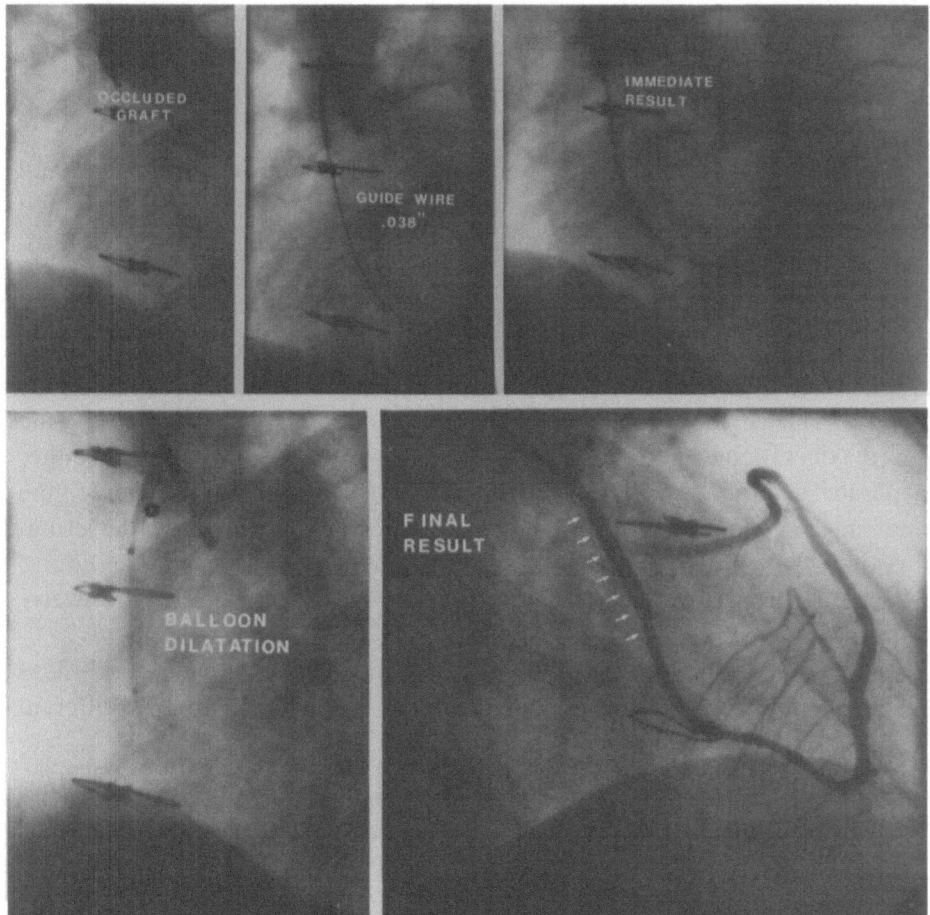

Figure 2. Example of successful dilatation of occluded coronary artery bypass graft. A. Pre-PTCA angiogram demonstrating total occlusion of graft. B. Successful perforation with .38″ guide wire. C. Angiogram following recanalization with guide wire. D. Dilatation with 3.7 mm balloon. E. Post-PTCA angiogram of successfully dilated bypass graft. Arrows indicate area of minor vessel dissection.

contralateral coronary artery alone in 21, from the ipsilateral coronary artery alone in 9, and from both coronary arteries in 7.

Duration of occlusion

In 32 patients the maximal possible duration of occlusion was defined as the time interval elapsed between diagnostic angiography and the time of attempted dilation. This time interval averaged 65 days (range 1–293 days).

In the remaining 17 patients with functional or total occlusion at diagnostic angiography, the minimal established duration of occlusion was on the average 49 days (range 7 to 240 days).

Angioplasty technique

After puncturing the femoral vein and artery, one hundred mg of heparin and 250 mg acetosalicylic acid were administered intravenously. Before attempted recanalization and angioplasty and following baseline angiography, 3 mg of iso-sorbide dinitrate and 0.2 mg nifedipine was injected into the involved vessel to exclude coronary spasm and to improve collateral filling of the distal vessel so that the course of the post-occlusion vesssel could be assessed. Since our early experience in 1980, the technique of recanalization has varied considerably (Table 1). Thirteen occlusions were crossed with the soft guide wire affixed to the tip of the dilatation catheter, while 10 occlusions required initial passage of either a separate stiffer guide wire (.032, .035, .038 inch) or a thin 3F catheter. In the remaining 26 patients, a movable guide wire system was used to cross the lesion. After that, the balloon catheter was advanced into the stenosis, a series of three to 10 balloon inflations were carried out at pressures varying from four to twelve atmospheres.

The total occlusion time varied from 10 up to 750 seconds. Individual occlusions ranged from 10 to 70 seconds. Stenotic areas were filmed in two different

Table 1. Left ventricular volume or ejection fraction derived from pre- and post-PTCA ventriculo-grams.

	pre-PTCA (n = 9)		Late follow up (n = 9)
EDV ml/m^2	83 ± 35	ns	70 ± 14
ESV ml/m^2	26 ± 10	ns	25 ± 9
EF %	68 ± 9	ns	64 ± 6

Abbreviations: EDV: end diastolic volume; ESV: end systolic volume; EF: ejection fraction; ns: non significant.

projections in procedures on the right (RCA) and circumflex (LCX) coronary arteries and in at least three projections including one cranio-caudal in stenoses of the left anterior descending artery (LAD).

After the dilatation procedure the sheath was left in place for the next 24 hours and nifedipine 10 mg every two hours was given during the first 24 hours. From the second day following angioplasty, all patients received 500 mg aceto salicylic acid and nifedipine, 60 mg a day. This regimen was continued during the next six months.

A dilatation was considered successful when the remaining stenosis was less than 50% and the mean pressure gradient (mmHg) across the stenosis, normalized for mean aortic pressure, was less than 0.2 Quantitative analysis of selected coronary segments was carried out with the Coronary Angiographic Analysis System (CAAS) [11, 12], which measures lumen diameters in absolute values (mm). From these measurements the relative obstruction of a vessel after the PTCA procedure can be defined [13].

Analysis of global and regional LV function

Global and regional left ventricular function was studied from the 30° right anterior oblique left ventricular cine-angiogram with an automated hardwired endocardial contour detector linked to a mini-computer [14]. Left ventricular volume was computed according Simpson's rule. Systolic regional wall displacement is determined along a system of 20 coordinates based on the pattern of actual endocardial wall motion in normal individuals [15] and generalized as a mathematical expression amenable to automatic data processing [16]. For each segment, segmental volume is computed from the local radius (R) and the height of each segment (1/10 of left ventricular long axis length (L) according the formula: $1/20 \, \P \, R^2 L$. When normalized for end-diastolic volume, the systolic segmental volume change can be considered as a parameter of regional pump function (Figure 3). During systole this parameter expresses quantitatively the contribution of a particular segment to global ejection fraction, termed regional contribution to global ejection fraction of CREF [16].

The sum of the values for all segments equals the global ejection fraction.

Statistical analysis

Data are expressed as mean ± SD; a paired or unpaired t test of Student was applied to the hemodynamic data, as appropriate; differences in baseline characteristics between groups were tested by the Fischer's exact test.

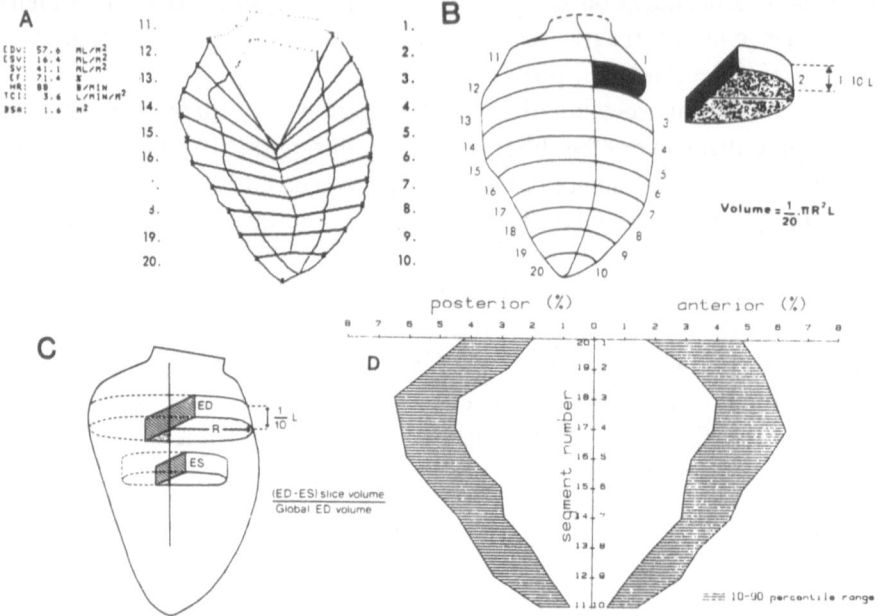

Figure 3. A. Example of the computer output showing the enddiastolic and endsystolic contours of the 30° RAO left ventriculogram and the system of coordinates along which left ventricular segmental wall displacement is determined. The corresponding volume data, ejection fraction and other parameters are shown in the upper right corner. B. The left ventricular enddiastolic cavity is divided into twenty half slices. The volume of each half slice is computed according to the given formula, R is radius and L is left ventricular long axis length. C. The regional contribution to global ejection fraction (CREF) is determined from the systolic decrease of volume of the half slice which corresponds to a particular wall segment. The systolic volume change is mainly a consequence of the decrease of radius (R) of the half slice, which is expressed by the X-component (x) of the displacement vector (d). D. The shaded zones represent the 10th–90th percentiles area of CREF values in normal individuals. On the X-axis the CREF values of the anterior and infero-posterior wall areas are displayed (%), while on the Y-axis the segment numbers of the anterior wall (1–10) and of the infero-posterior wall (11–20) are depicted.

Results

Outcome of dilatation procedure

The occlusion was successfully recanalized in 43 patients (88%), but the stenotic lesion could be crossed with the balloon catheter in only 38 patients (78%). A successful dilatation according to the criteria mentioned above obtained in 28 patients (57%): 19 (63%) of the 30 patients with a left anterior descending coronary occlusion, 5 (63%) of the 8 with a right coronary artery occlusion, 3 of the 7 (43%) with a circumflex coronary artery occlusion, and 1 of the 4 (25%) with a jumpgraft occlusion. The residual percentage diameter stenosis in the 28 patients whose arteries were successfully dilated was $34.6 \pm 10.5\%$ while the mean pressure gradient normalized for mean aortic pressure decreased from 0.51 ± 0.15 to 0.18 ± 0.11. The success rate was significantly higher in patients with functional occlusion (13/16, 81%) than in those with total occlusion (15/33, 45%, p = 0,04).

In these 33 patients with total occlusion at the time of angioplasty, the success rate was similar between those who had a total occlusion at the time of diagnostic angiography (5/10, 50%) and those who previously had a stenotic lesion (10/23, 43%).

Occlusion duration and outcome of dilation procedure

The outcome of the dilatation procedure was evaluated by taking into account the duration (estimated or established) of occlusion and the functional or total nature of the occlusion. The success rate for the patients in whom the occlusion was estimated to be less than 4 weeks was 62% (13/21) and for those in whom the occlusion was more than 4 weeks but less than 8 weeks, it was 67% (8/12).

Of the patients in whom the duration of occlusion was estimated to be more than 8 weeks the success rate was only 44% (7/16). The primary success rates in patients with functional or total occlusion versus the time elapsed since diagnostic angiography are shown in Figure 4.

Hospital course

Ten of 21 patients with unsuccessful PTCA underwent elective coronary artery

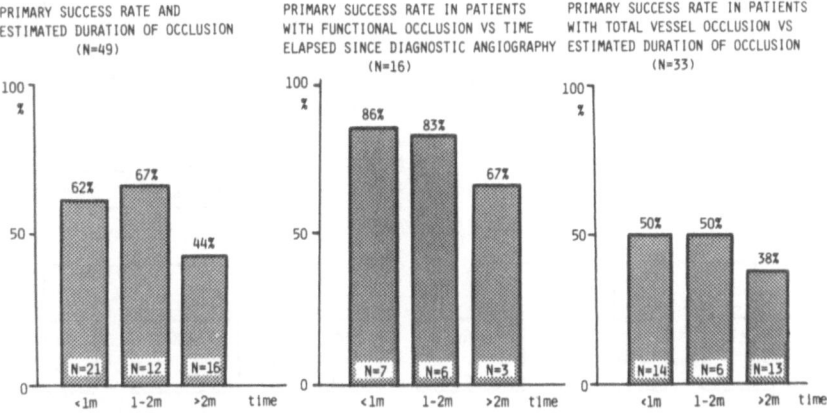

Figure 4. Primary success rates in patients with total and/or functional occlusion versus the time elapsed since diagnostic angiography.

bypass surgery, while one had emergency surgery because of persisting chest pain following attempted recanalization. The remaining 10 patients were kept on medical therapy.

Of the 28 patients with primary success, 8 had an elevation of serum creatine phosphokinase (61–190 U), but without appearance of a new Q waves or loss of R wave.

One patient had a subarachnoid hemorrhage several hours following the procedure which necessitated a trepanation – the neurological deficit initially observed subsided completely following the neurosurgical intervention.

Longterm angiographic and clinical follow-up

Of the 28 patients with successful dilatation, 10 patients had recurrence of anginal symptoms at a mean follow-up of 7 months (range 1–42 months). Nine of these ten patients underwent follow-up angiography which showed reocclusion in six (Figures 5 and 6). Three patients required coronary artery bypass graft surgery, three had repeat dilatation for re-stenosis (n = 2) or reocclusion (n = 1) while four were maintained on medical therapy. Eighteen patients were asymptomatic. Late angiographic follow-up was available in 11 of the asymptomatic patients. Cineangiogram disclosed two reocclusions, 5 partial restenoses (an increase of 20% in luminal diameter stenosis) and four persistent successful dilatations (Figure 5).

The 9 patients with either partial restenosis or persistent successful dilatation underwent follow-up left ventriculography. All had LAD lesions. No significant

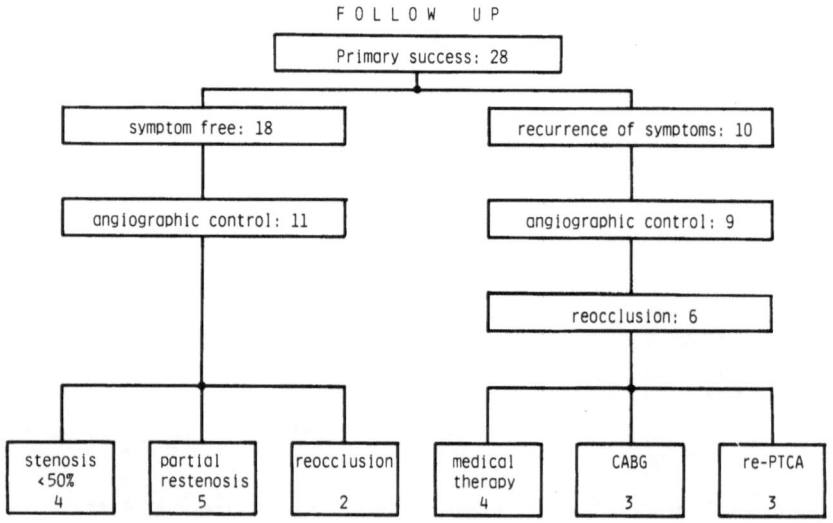

Figure 5. Long term angiographic and clinical follow-up of 28 patients who underwent a successful angioplasty.

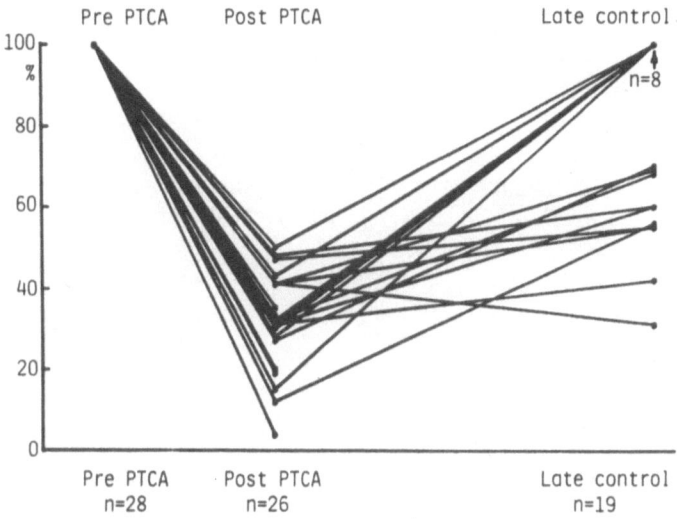

Figure 6. Percentage diameter stenosis following successful angioplasty and during late angiographic follow up. In 8 patients, reocclusion was observed.

Table 2. Technique of recanalization and dilatation.

	Pts	Recanalization	Dilatation	Primary success
Guide wire .032/.035/.038	6	4	4	1
3F perfusion catheter	4	4	1	1
Guide wire affixed to the tip of the dilatation catheter	13	10	10	9
Movable guide wire angioplasty system	26	25	23	17
	100%	88%	78%	57%

changes in left ventricular volume or ejection fraction were found when comparing the pre and post PTCA left ventriculograms (Table 2). The regional contributions to the global ejection fraction were also not affected by the intercurrent episode of coronary occlusion (Figure 7).

Discussion

Progression to complete occlusion

Unexpected progression to complete obstruction (total or functional) was observed in 6% of all PTCA candidates. Although it has been demonstrated that

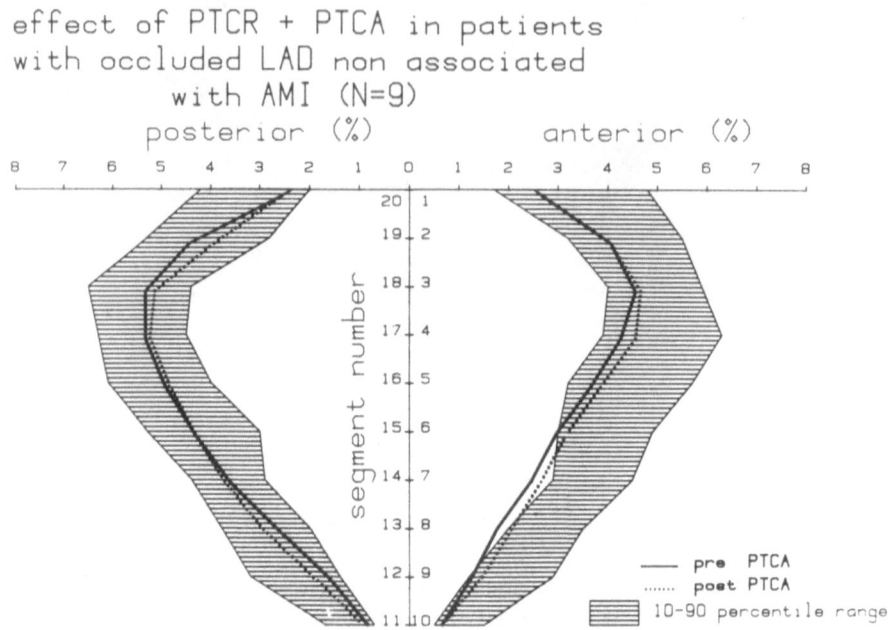

Figure 7. Regional contribution to the global ejection fraction in 9 patients with intercurrent occlusion of the left anterior descending artery (LAD). Solid line: wall motion at the time of the diagnostic angiography, when the LAD was still patent. Dotted line: wall motion during late angiographic follow up.

certain risk factors may predispose to rapid progression to total occlusion [18], we were previously unable, to predict this progression. When compared to other patients at the time of diagnostic angiography, this subgroup showed no difference in the severity of the coronary lesions, quantitatively analyzed [19]. Specifically, the severity of the coronary stenosis on the diagnostic angiogram was not predictive of progression to complete occlusion.

In the present study, no patients with functional occlusion progressed to total occlusion. Thus it was similarly difficult to predict which patients would progress to a total occlusion based on the severity of their stenosis at the time of diagnostic study.

One may speculate that occlusion of the PTCA-related vessel in these patients is not related to rapidly progressive atherosclerosis but is due to a thrombotic process. Evolving coronary thrombosis has been reported in unstable angina [20] and a review of the clinical records in our patients shows that progression to complete obstruction was clearly associated with worsening and unstability of the anginal symptoms, but without occurrence of myocardial necrosis probably prevented by the development of collaterals.

Collaterals and myocardial viability

Controversy exists over the role of the collateral circulation in preserving myocardial function [21–24], although it has become increasingly evident that certain collateral vessels provide sufficient blood flow to maintain myocardial viability.

This fact is substantiated by the studies of Baroldi [25], Levin [26] and Hamby [23] who found no evidence of myocardial infarction in respectively 44%, 30% and 28% percent of patients with a totally occluded coronary artery and it is also supported by several case reports [27, 28] of patients with complete obstruction of the left main coronary artery and preserved left ventricular function.

Part of this controversy stems from the fact that the mere angiographic presence of collateral vessel does not provide complete information concerning the physiologic significance of the vessel. It is well established that coronary cineangiography for evaluation of collateral vessels underestimates the fine collateral network that is detected by post mortem angiography [29] and correlates poorly with normal resting myocardial blood flow distribution through these vessels [30].

Therefore, it is not surprising to see that some of our patients, despite preserved regional wall function, did not exhibit discrete visualization of collateral filling of the post occlusive coronary segment. In our opinion, the visualization of distal occlusive luminal anatomy is not an absolute requirement for attempted dilatation. We assume that collateral filling, even when not angiographically demonstrable, is potentially sufficient to preserve good wall motion. Kolibash et al. [30] demonstrated that the prevalence of wall motion abnormalities was significantly less in the 'distribution' areas of totally occluded native vessels with normal perfusion at rest assessed from radio-isotopic studies even in the absence of demonstrable angiographic collaterals. The purpose of this study was not to evaluate the contribution of the coronary collateral circulation to the perservation of myocardial function; however, our wall motion analysis clearly indicates that collaterals may serve an important protective function since no deterioration in wall motion occurred despite prolonged periods of coronary occlusion in our patients with persistent longterm lesion patency.

Outcome of the dilatation procedure

The primary success rate of transluminal angioplasty of occluded coronary arteries reported in the literature varied between 54% and 67%. To interpret this report with those percentages, the distinction between functional and total occlusion is meaningful since the success rates with these two types of occlusion differ considerably (81% vs 45%). On the other hand, our results partially corroborate recent suggestions [10, 31] that either functional or total occlusions present for periods greater that 2 months are associated with lower primary success rates. In these patients the high percentage of failure may be related to progressive organization and fibrosis in the occluded area.

The success rate with the movable guide wire angioplasty system was higher (65%, 17/26) than with the previous techniques, (48%, 11/23) which required the initial use of either a separate stiff guide wire, catheter or guide wire affixed to the tip of a dilatation catheter.

Finally, although we have had no angiographic evidence of peripheral embolization, 8 patients had a slight elevation of myocardial enzymes and 2 of them experienced prolonged chest pain.

Long term follow-up

In patients with an initially successful result, follow-up angiography was available in 20. In 12 of these patients, left ventriculography was of sufficient quality to permit comparison to the left ventriculogram obtained at the time of diagnostic angiography.

Although several studies have demonstrated the physiologic capabilities of collateral vessels to maintain a normal resting LV function in the distribution of a totally occluded native vessel, it has also been clearly established that collaterals may be unable to provide adequate myocardial perfusion during exercise [30, 32]. Hence, it is not surprising to see that virtually all our patients had still severe exertional angina unresponsive to medical treatment at the time of angioplasty.

The early results were extremely promising since only one patient remained symptomatic. With long term follow-up, however, the rate of recurrence of symptoms in these patients (36%) did not differ significantly from the rate usually reported in patients with dilatation of conventional stenoses [33].

Among the asymptomatic patients who underwent an angiographic follow-up study, two showed a reocclusion of their dilated lesion; both had a normal exercise stress test and one of them had even a normal myocardial perfusion scintigraphy during exercise. In contrast to the rate of recurrence of symptoms, the incidence of reocclusion in these patients was alarmingly high (8 of 20 angiographic studies) when compared to either angioplasty of conventional 60 to 95% stenoses or even angioplasty following fibrinolytic recanalization [6].

Two reasons may account for the high incidence of reocclusion in patients following successful dilatation of a recently occluded coronary lesion.

First, this group may represent a subset of the total PTCA population with a demonstrated intrinsic vascular or hematologic propensity to acute occlusion of existing atherosclerotic lesions.

Second, if the morphologic character of the recent occlusion is thrombus, then one would anticipate the presence of a progressively organizing dense fibrocellular tissue [34]. Instrumental recanalization and dilatation of this lesion must produce histologic disruption through the longitudinal and radial shearing of the

atherosclerotic and fibrocellular material. This could initiate a non-specific pro-
liferative process that could contribute to reocclusion of the vessel [35–37]. In
addition, this disrupted material could provide a substrate prone to rethrombosis
[38, 39].

Accordingly, there is a theoretical reason for adopting special antiplatelet or
even antiinflammatory measures after angioplasty of an occluded coronary artery
[40–43].

In summary, elective angioplasty of occluded coronary arteries is feasible,
although the overall primary success rate (57%) is lower than that associated with
conventional lesions. However, it is evident that the primary success rate is
significantly higher in patients with functional occlusion (81%) than in patients
with total occlusion (45%).

The likelihood of successful recanalization is inversely related to the duration
of the occlusion. Despite a long duration of occlusion, no significant deterioration
of wall motion or regional myocardial function may be present. The time between
diagnostic angiography and angioplasty should be kept to a minium to prevent the
progression of a significant stenosis to an occlusion.

Finally, the long term clinical results following successful recanalization were
satisfactory in 64% of our patients. The incidence of restenosis or reocclusion has
tended to be higher, though, than that seen in patients undergoing dilatation of
conventional stenosis.

References

1. Grüntzig A (1978) Transluminal dilatation of coronary artery stenosis. (letter to the editor) Lancet
   1: 263
2. Vlietstra RE, Holmes DR, Reeder GS, Mock MB, Bove AA (1984) Balloon angioplasty in
   multivessel coronary disease: importance of anatomic subtyping. JACC 3: 469
3. de Feyter PJ, van den Brand M, Serruys PW (1984) Emergency PTCA in patients with impending
   infarction, unresponsive to medical treatment. Eur H J 5: 93
4. Hartzler G, Rutherford B, Mc Conahay DR (1984) Multiple lesion coronary angioplasty in 'high
   risk' patients sub-groups. JACC 3: 469
5. Dorros G, Johnson DW, Tector AJ, Schmahl T, Kalush SL, Janke L (1984) Percutaneous
   Transluminal coronary angioplasty in patients with prior coronary artery bypass grafting. In:
   Thorac cardiovasc Surg 87: 17–26
6. Serruys PW, Wijns W, van den Brand M, Ribeiro V, Fioretti P, Simoons ML, Kooijman CJ,
   Reiber JHC, Hugenholtz PG (1983) Is transluminal coronary angioplasty mandatory after successful thrombolysis? Br Heart J 50: 257–65
7. Heyndrickx GR, Serruys PW, van den Brand M, Vandormael M, Reiber JHC (1982) Transluminal angioplasty after mechanical recanalisation in patients with chronic occlusion of coronary
   artery. Circulation 66 (suppl II) II-5
8. Savage R, Hollman J, Grüntzig A, King S, Douglas J, Tankersley R (1982) Can percutaneous
   transluminal coronary angioplasty be performed in patients with total occlusions. Circulation 66
   (suppl II) II-330
9. Dervan JP, Baim DS, Cherniles J, Grossman W (1983) Transluminal angioplasty of occluded
   coronary arteries: use of a movable guide wire system. Circulation 68: 776–784

164

10. Holmes DR, Vlietstra RE, Reeder GS, Bresnahan JF, Smith HC, Bove AA, Schaff HV (1984) Angioplasty in total coronary artery occlusion. JACC 3: 845–9

11. Reiber JHC, Gerbrands JJ, Kooijman CJ, Schuurbiers JCH, Slager CJ, den Boer A, Serruys PW (1984) Quantitative coronary angiography with automated contour detection and densitometry: technical aspects. In: Just H, Heintzen PH (eds) Angiocardiography, Current status and future developments. Heidelberg: Springer-Verlag (in press)

12. Kooijman CJ, Reiber JHC, Gerbrands JJ, Schuurbiers JCH, Slager CJ, den Boer A, Serruys PW (1982) Computer-aided quantitation of the severity of coronary obstruction from single view cineangiograms. International symposium on medical imaging and image interpretation. IEEE catalog no 82 CH 1804–4, 59–64

13. Serruys PW, Reiber JHC, Wijns W, Kooijman CJ, van den Brand M, ten Katen HJ, Hugenholtz PG. Assessment of percutaneous transluminal coronary angioplasty by quantitative coronary angiography: diameter vs densitometric area measurements. Am J Card, in press

14. Slager CJ, Reiber JHC, Schuurbiers JCH, Meester GT (1978) Contouromat- a hardwired left ventricular angio processing system. Design and application. Comp Biomed Res 11: 491–502

15. Slager CJ, Hooghoudt TEH, Reiber JCH, Booman F, Meester GT (1980) Left ventricular contour segmentation from anatomical landmark trajectories and its application to wall motion analysis. In Computers in Cardiology. Los Angeles, 1980, IEEE Computer Society, pp 347–350

16. Hooghoudt TEH, Slager CJ, Reiber JHC, Serruys PW, Schuurbiers JCH, Meester GT, Hugenholtz PG (1980) 'Regional contribution to global ejection fraction' used to assess the applicability of a new wall motion model to the detection of regional wall motion in patients with asynergy. In Computers in Cardiology. Los Angeles, IEEE Computer Society, pp 253–256

17. Serruys PW, Wijns W, van den Brand M, Meij S, Slager CJ, Schuurbiers JCH, Hugenholtz PG, Brower RW (1984) Left ventricular performance, regional blood flow, wall motion and lactate metabolism during transluminal angioplasty. Circulation 70: 25–36

18. Shub C, Vlietstra RE, Smith HC, Fulton RE, Elveback LR (1981) The unpredictable progression of symptomatic coronary artery disease. A serial clinical-angiographic analysis. Mayo Clin Proc 56: 155–160

19. Wijns W, Serruys PW, van den Brand M, Suryapranata H, Kooijman CJ, Reiber JHC, Hugenholtz PG (1983) Progression to complete coronary obstruction without myocardial infarction in patients who are candidates for percutaneous transluminal angioplasty. A 90-day angiographic follow-up. In: Roskam H (ed) Prognosis of coronary heart disease. Progression of coronary arteriosclerosis. Springer-Verlag, Berlin-Heidelberg-New York-Tokyo, pp 190–195

20. Rentrop P, Blanke H, Karsch KR, Kaiser H, Kostering H, Leitz (1981) Selective intracoronary thrombolysis in acute myocardial infarction and unstable angina pectoris. Circulation 63: 307–317

21. Helfant RH, Kemp HG, Gorlin R (1970) Coronary atherosclerosis, coronary collaterals and their relation to cardiac function. Ann Intern Med 189: 189–98

22. Carroll RJ, Verani MS, Falsetti HL (1974) The effect of collateral circulation on segmental left ventricular contraction. Circulation 50: 709–13

23. Hamby RI, Aintablin A, Schwartz A (1976) Reappraisal of the functional significance of the coronary collateral circulation. Am J Cardiol 38: 304–9

24. Schwartz F, Flameng W, Ensslen R, Sesto M, Thormann J (1978) Effect of coronary collaterals on left ventricular function at rest and during stress. Am Heart J 95: 570–7

25. Baroldi G (1973) Coronary heart disease: significance of the morphologic lesions. Am Heart J 85: 1–5

26. Levin DC (1974) Pathways and functional significance of the coronary collateral circulation. Circulation 50: 831–7

27. Frick MH, Valle M, Korhola O, Rukimaki E, Wiljasalo M (1976) Analysis of coronary collaterals in ischemic heart disease by angiography during pacing induced ischemia. Br Heart J 38: 186–96

28. Frye RL, Gura GM, Chesebro JH, Ritman EL (1977) Complete occlusion of the left main coronary artery and the importace of coronary collateral circulation. Mayo Clin Proc 52: 742–5

29. Fulton WFM (1965) The coronary arteries. Springfield, IL: Charles C Thomas 213
30. Kolibash AJ, Bush CA, Wepsic RA, Schroeder DP, Tetalman MR, Lewis RP (1982) Coronary collateral vessels: Spectrum of physiologic capabilities with respect to providing rest and stress myocardial perfusion, maintainance of left ventricular function and protection against infarction. Am J Cardiol 50: 230–238
31. Giorgi LV, Hartzler GO, Rutherford BD, Mc Conahay DR (1983) Angina following total coronary occlusion: definitive treatment with percutaneous coronary angioplasty. JACC 1: 656
32. Eng C, Patterson RE, Horowitz SF, Halgash DA, Pichard A, Midwall J, Verman MV, Gorlin R (1982) Coronary collateral function during exercise. Circulation 66: 309–316
33. Kent KM, Bentivoglio LG, Block PC, Bourassa MG, Cowley MJ, Dorros G, Detre KM, Gosselin AJ, Grüntzig AR, Kelsey SF, Mock MB, Mullin ZM, Passamani ER, Myler RK, Simpson J, Stertzler SH, Van Raden MJ, Williams DO (1984) Long term efficacy of percutaneous transluminal coronary angioplasty (PTCA): Report from the National heart, lung and blood institute PTCA registry. Am J Cardiol 53: 27–31
34. Abela GS, Conti R, Norman S, Feldman RL, Pepine CJ (1984) A new model for investigation of transluminal recanalization: human atherosclerotic coronary artery xenografts. Am J Cardiol 54: 200–205
35. Waller BF, McManns BM, Gorfinkel HJ, Kishel JC, Schmidt CH, Kent KM, Roberts WC (1983) Status of the major epicardial coronary arteries 80–150 days after percutaneous transluminal coronary angioplasty. Am J Cardiol 51: 81–84
36. Hollman J, Austin GE, Gruentzig AR, Douglas JS, King SB (1983) Coronary artery spasm at the site of angioplasty in the first two months after successful percutaneous transluminal coronary angioplasty. JACC 2: 1039–1045
37. Essed CE, Van den Brand M, Becker AE (1983) Transluminal angioplasty and early restenosis. Fibrocellular occlusion after wall laceration. Br Heart J 49: 393–396
38. Steele PM, Chesebro JH, Lamb HB, Stanson AW, Badimon L, Fuster V (1983) Natural history of balloon angioplasty in pigs: wall injury, platelet-thrombus deposition and intimal hyperplasio. Circulation 68, Supp III 264
39. Enzekowitz MD, Pope CF, Smith EO, Glickman M, Rapoport S, Zaret BL (1983) Indium-III Platelet deposition at sites of percutaneous transluminal peripheral angioplasty. Circulation 68, suppl III, p 144
40. Steele PM, Chesebro JH, Lamb HB, Stanson AW, Holmes DR, Dewanjee MK, Badimon L, Fuster V (1983) Balloon angioplasty in pigs: effect of platelet-inhibitor drugs. Circulation 68, suppl III, 264
41. Kaltenbach M, Scherer D, Vallbracht C, Kober G (1984) Longterm result of coronary angioplasty. Eur Heart J 5: 75
42. Sanborn TA, Faxon DP, Haudenschild C, Gottsman SB, Ryan TJ (1983) Sulfintyrazone inhibition of restenosis after experimental angioplasty. JACC 2: 644
43. Thornton MA, Gruentzig AR, Hollman J, King SB, Douglas JS (1984) Coumadin and aspirine in prevention of recurrence after transluminal coronary angioplasty, a randomized study. Circulation 69: 721–7

Acute changes of myocardial function by PTCA. Evaluation by two-dimensional echocardiography

BERND HENKEL, RAIMUND ERBEL, WERNER CLAS, GERHARD SCHREINER, HELMUT KOPP, TIBERIUS POP and JÜRGEN MEYER

Introduction

Two-dimensional echocardiography allows a detailed analysis of global and regional left ventricular function [1]. The aim of our study was to analyse continuously the left ventricular function during percutaneous transluminal coronary angioplasty (PTCA) by two-dimensional echocardiography.

Methods

We examined 10 patients (9 male and 1 female, mean age: 52 ± 8 years). 8 patients had left-anterior-descending-stenoses (LAD), 1 a left-circumflex stenosis, and 1 patient had a stenosis of the right coronary artery. Luminal narrowness measured more than 80% in all stenoses. PTCA was performed with a Grüntzig – balloon – catheter in the usual technique [2, 3]. The average balloon inflation time was 41 ± 22 seconds. PTCA was stopped, when angina pectoris occurred [4]. ECG and aortic and coronary perfusion pressure were recorded simultaneously. Two-dimensional echocardiographic studies were performed with a commercially available Diasonics CV 3400 R Ultrasonograph equipped with a 2.25 MHz phased-array transducer. Apical echocardiograms of the left ventricle in the right anterior oblique equivalent view were recorded continuously before, during, and after PTCA on a 1/2- or 3/4 inch videocasette recorder for subsequent analysis. The end-diastolic and end-systolic contours of the left ventricle were digitized by a computer system (Kontron, Kardia 80) in intervals of 10 seconds. The end-diastolic and end-systolic volumes of the left ventricle and left ventricular ejection fraction were calculated using a disc method [5, 6, 7]. The regional abnormalities of contraction were analysed with a radiant method, which was developed in our laboratory [8]. Statistically significant differences were determined with the t-test for dependent means.

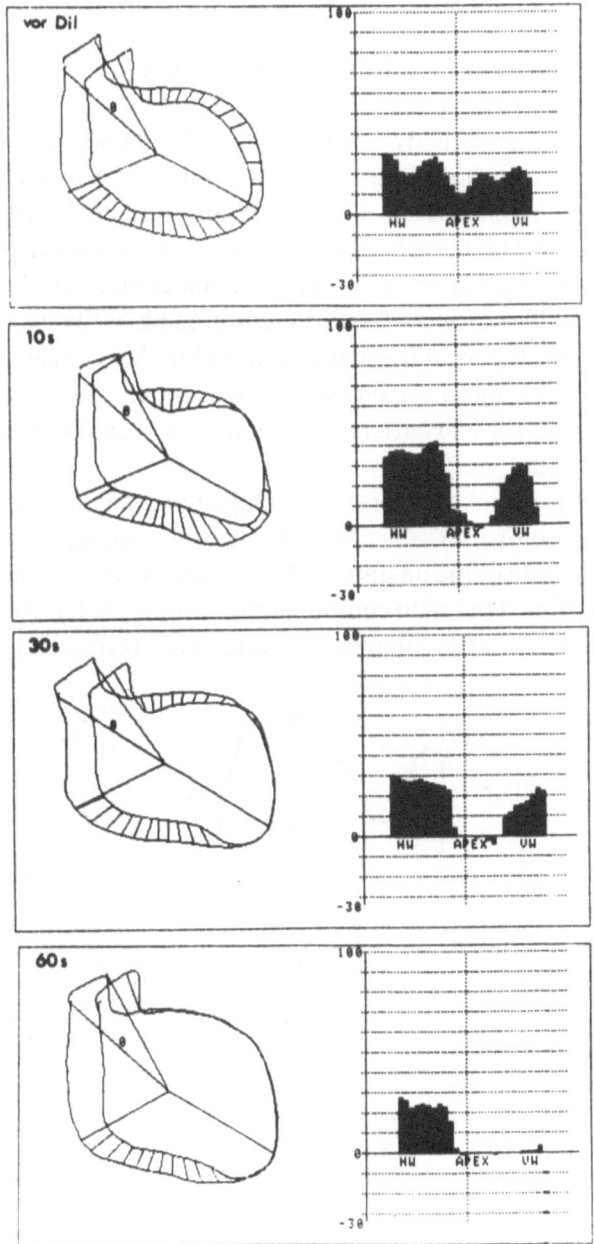

Figure 1. LAD PTCA. Enddiastolic and endsystolic outlines of the left ventricle before PTCA and after 10, 30, and 60 seconds of PTCA – duration on the left side. Shown on the right side the fractional shortening of 28 radiants. The stepwise developement of an akinesia of the anterior wall is demonstrated.

Results

Regional dysfunction of the left ventricle during PTCA

The first sign of left ventricle dysfunction during PTCA was characterized by a regional hypokinesis in the supply area of the concerned coronary artery. We observed this local hypokinesis 14 + 8 seconds after the beginning of the dilatation. Regional abnormalities of contraction occurred earlier than ST segment changes, which appeared after 24 + 7 seconds, and earlier than angina pectoris, which was noticed 39 + 22 seconds after the beginning of the dilatation. During the LAD-dilatations the local hypokinesis started in the supraapical area of the anterior wall and the apical region of the left ventricle and in the case of the dilatation of the right coronary artery the hypokinesis began in the basal segments of the posterior wall.

Subsequently the initial hypokinesis developed into an akinesia in 6 of the 10 patients. In the case of LAD-dilatation the akinesia extended to the complete anterior wall at the end of the dilatation. An example is demonstrated in Figure 1. During the dilatation of the right coronary artery and of the left circumflex artery the akinesia extended to the complete posterior wall, respectively the complete

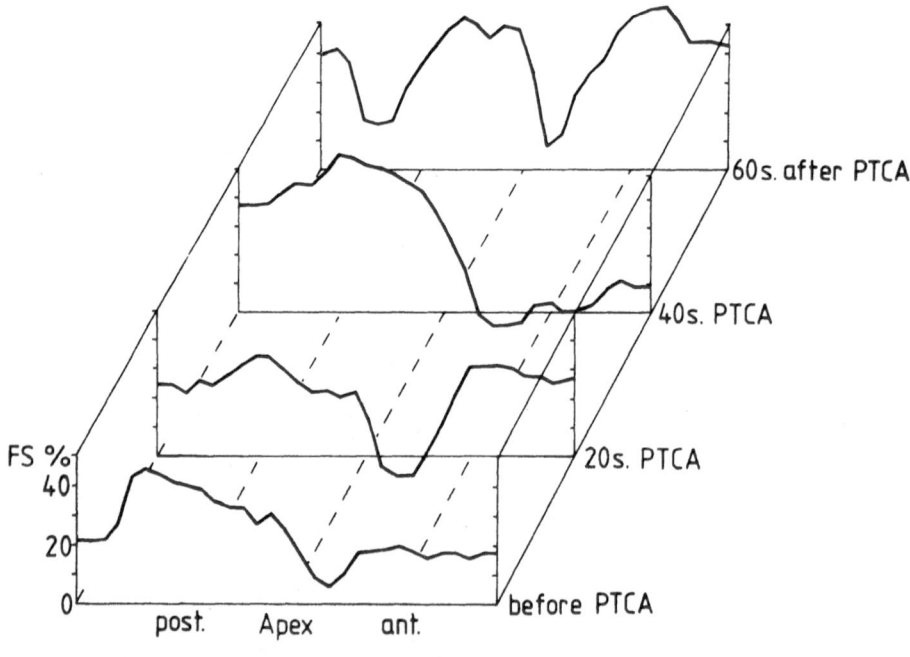

Dyskinesia with contralat. hyperkinesia

Figure 2. 3 – dimensional display of the regional fractional shortening of the 28 radiants in relation to time during LAD – PTCA. The developement of an anterior dyskinesia with contralateral compensatory hyperkinesis during PTCA is shown.

posterior – lateral wall of the left ventricle.

In 4 of the 10 patients the initial hypokinesis developed into a dyskinesia with an akinesia in the adjacent area, as it is demonstrated in Figure 2. In this example the circumscript dyskinesia of the apical anterior wall started already 20 seconds after balloon inflation, 20 seconds later the akinesia of the adjacent anterior wall was observed.

The majority of the patients developed a compensatory hyperkinesia of the contralateral wall during PTCA. In the group with an akinesia a compensatory hyperkinesia was observed in 5 of 6 patients and in the group with dyskinesia in 2 of 4 patients. Figure 2 shows the developement of a compensatory hyperkinesia of the posterior wall during LAD – PTCA of 40 seconds duration. The maximal hyperkinesia of the posterior wall was observed 40 seconds after balloon infla-tion. At this time we saw the dyskinesia with the adjacent akinesia of the anterior wall. Figure 3 demonstrates the developement of a dyskinesia of the anterior wall without a compensatory hyperkinesia of the posterior wall during the dilatation of the left anterior descending artery. The absence of the compensatory hyper-kinesia during PTCA can be explained by another lesion of the contralateral wall. This indicates, that the developement of regional dysfunction and contralateral compensatory function are closely related to coronary morphology.

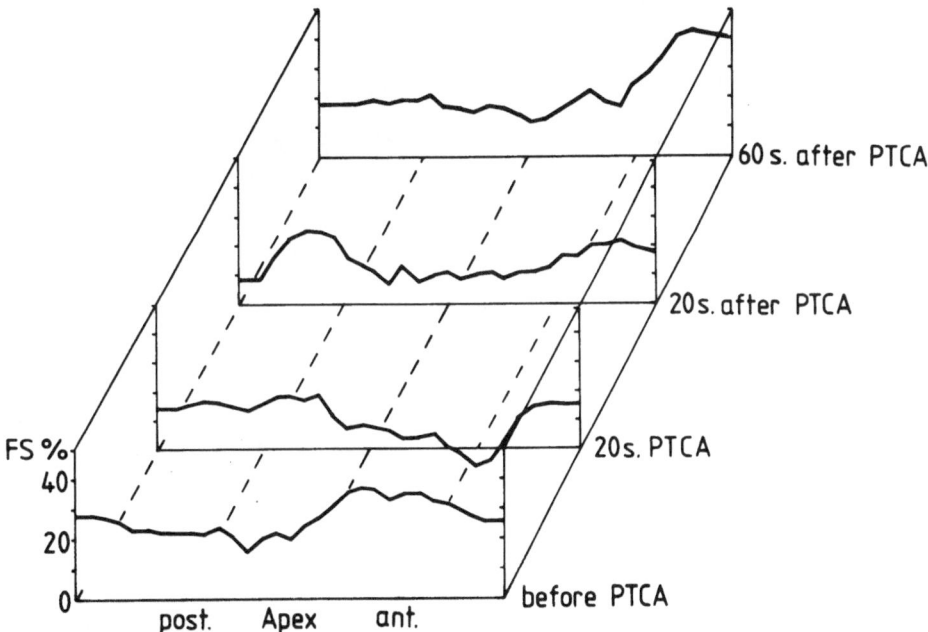

Dyskinesia without contralat. hyperkinesia

Figure 3. 3 – dimensional display of the regional fractional shortening of the 28 radiants in relation to time during LAD – PTCA. The developement of an anterior dyskinesia without contralateral compensatory hyperkinesia during PTCA is shown.

170

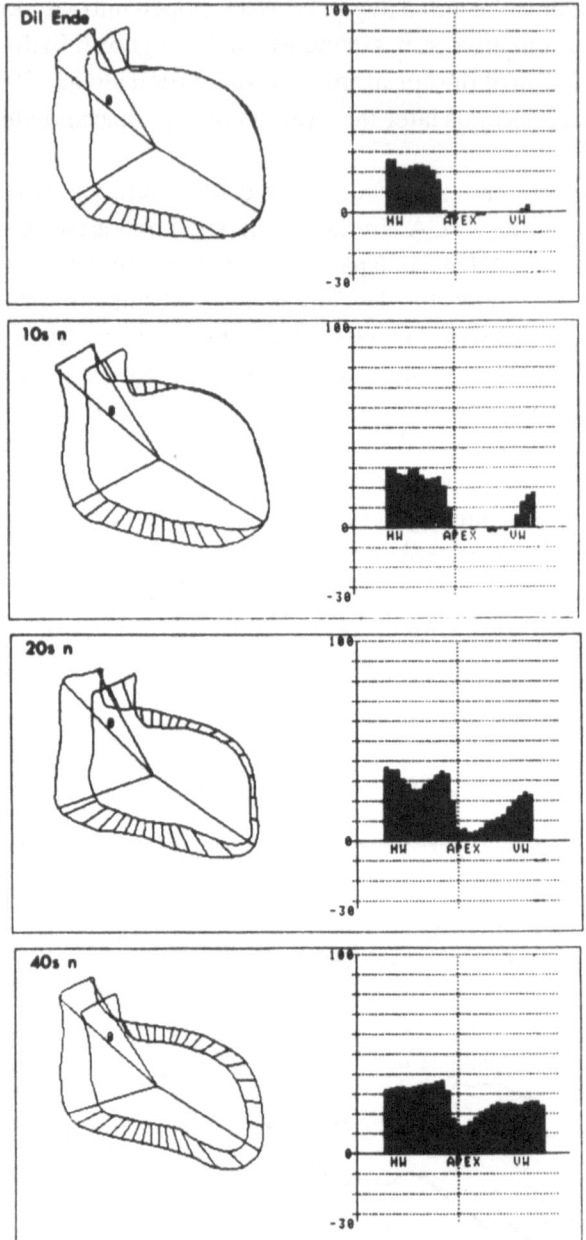

Figure 4. Recovery period after LAD – PTCA. Enddiastolic and endsystolic outlines of the left ventricle at the end of the dilatation and after 10, 20, and 40 seconds on the left side. Shown on the right side the fractional shortening of the 28 radiants. The stepwise normalization of the left ventricular function is demonstrated.

During the recovery period a stepwise normalization of the regional left ventricular dysfunction was observed. But 40 seconds after dilatation the starting point was not reached in all patients. Figure 4 displays the recovery period after a dilatation of the left anterior descending artery. The normalization started in the basal segments of the anterior wall 10 seconds after the balloon deflation. Subsequently the other parts of the anterior wall recovered and finally wall motion normalized in the apical and supraapical area, where the regional dysfunction started. This pattern of recovery was observed in all patients.

Global dysfunction of the left ventricle during PTCA

The regional abnormalities of contraction caused the global left ventricular dysfunction, which we observed during PTCA.

In our 10 cases we observed only a slight increase of the end – diastolic left ventricular volume during the coronary angioplasty. The mean end – diastolic left ventricular volume index increased from 80 ± 13 ml/m^2 to 84 ± 15 ml/m^2. This increase of the end – diastolic volume index was not significant. Figure 5 shows the developement of the mean end – diastolic volume index during PTCA.

In contrast to the end – diastolic volumes the left ventricular end – systolic volume indices increased significantly from 35 ± 9 ml/m^2 to 57 ± 9 ml/m^2, as it is shown in Figure 6. This progressive increase of the end – systolic volume index started before ST segment changes or angina pectoris occurred.

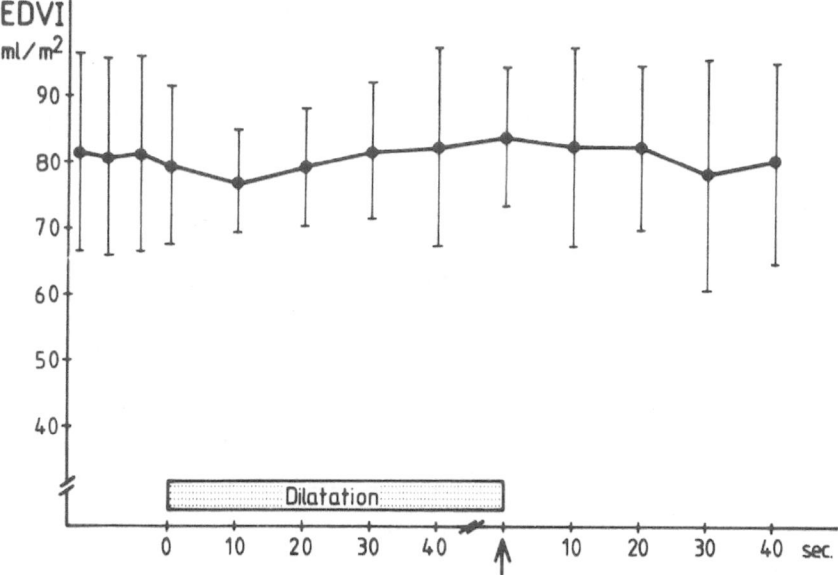

Figure 5. Changes of the mean left ventricular enddiastolic volume index (EDVI) and standard deviation during PTCA and in the recovery period. n = 10.

172

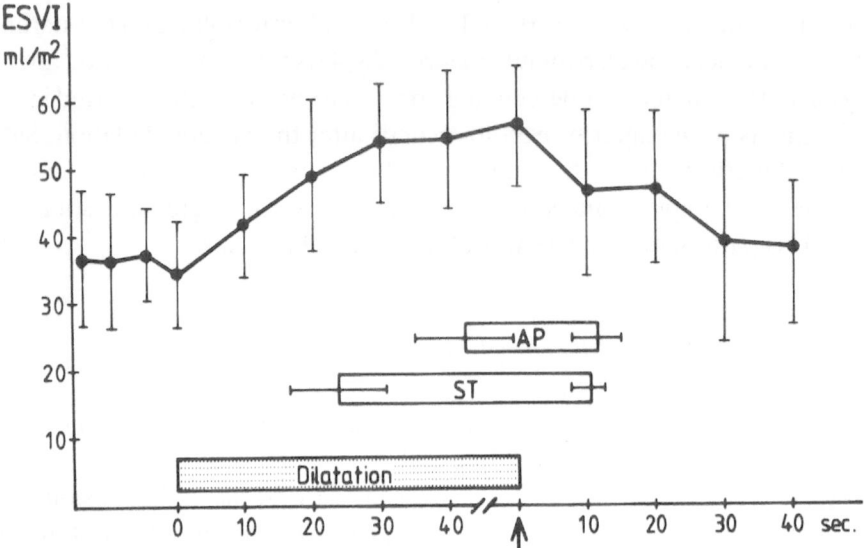

Figure 6. Increase in the mean left ventricular endsystolic volume index (ESVI) and standard deviation during PTCA and in the recovery period. ST: ST segment changes in the ECG. AP: angina pectoris. n = 10.

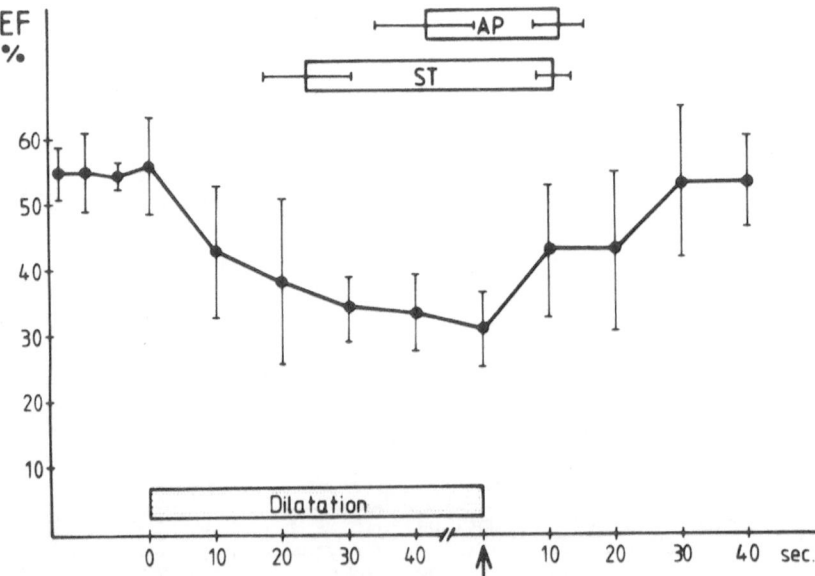

Figure 7. Decrease and recovery of the mean left ventricular ejection fraction (EF) and standard deviation during PTCA respectively in the recovery period. ST: ST segment changes in the ECG. AP: angina pectoris. n = 10.

ST segment changes were observed after 24 ± 7 seconds, and angina pectoris after 39 ± 22 seconds. Normalization of ventricular size occurred within 40 seconds after the end of the dilatation. The observed abnormalities of contraction persisted clearly longer than ST segment changes or angina pectoris. Resultant from these changes of the end – diastolic and end – systolic left ventricular volumes the stroke volume decreased progressively during the coronary angioplasty.

Accordingly the ejection fraction decreased rapidly during the dilatation from $55 \pm 3\%$ to $31 \pm 6\%$. This pronounced decrease in ejection fraction began already 10 seconds after the start of the PTCA. As shown in figure 7, the decrease in ejection fraction started earlier and persisted longer than ECG – changes and angina pectoris.

Summary

During PTCA we observed:
- only a small increase in the end-diastolic left ventricular volume,
- a significant increase in the end-systolic left ventricular volume,
- and thus a significant decrease of stroke volume and left ventricular ejection fraction.

During PTCA regional and global left ventricular dysfunction occur earlier than ST segment changes and angina pectoris and persist longer than electrocardiographic changes and angina pectoris.

References

1. Erbel R, Schweizer P, Pyhel N, Hadre U, Meyer J, Krebs W, Effert S (1980) Quantitative Analyse regionaler Kontraktionsstörungen des linken Ventrikels im zweidimensionalen Echokardiogramm. Z Kardiol 69: 562–572
2. Grüntzig A (1978) Transluminal dilatation of coronary artery stenosis. Lancet. I, p 263
3. Grüntzig A, Senning A, Siegenthaler WE (1979) Nonoperative dilatation of coronary artery stenosis. Percutaneous transluminal coronary angioplasty. New Engl J Med 301, p 61
4. Aueron F, Grüntzig A, Meier B (1984) Significance of chest pain during percutaneous transluminal coronary angioplasty. Amer Heart J 107: 578–580
5. Erbel R, Schweizer P, Henn G, Meyer J, Effert S (1982) Apikale zweidimensionale Echokardiographie. Normalwerte für die monoplane und biplane Bestimmung der Volumina und der Ejektionsfraktion des linken Ventrikels. Dtsch Med Wschr 107: 1872–1877
6. Erbel R, Schweizer P, Meyer J, Krebs W, Effert S (1983) Quantifizierung der Funktion des linken Ventrikels mittels zweidimensionaler Echokardiographie. Ultraschall 4: 228–236
7. Erbel R (1983) Funktionsdiagnostik des linken Ventrikels mittels zweidimensionaler Echokardiographie. Steinkopff Verlag, Darmstadt
8. Clas W, Henkel B, Erbel R, Schreiner G, Kopp H, Brennecke R, Meyer J (1984) Computergestützte Analyse regionaler Wandbewegungsstörungen bei transluminaler Angioplastie. Biomed Tech 29, Ergänzungsband, p 276

Coronary sinus potassium and pH during percutaneous transluminal angioplasty: Temporal relation to contractility and action potential duration

P.A. POOLE-WILSON and S.C. WEBB

Introduction

Arrythmias are common during the initial ten minutes following the onset of acute myocardial ischaemia. Early changes in electrolyte concentrations in the ischemic heart muscle and in the plasma perfusing adjacent normal muscle may be important to the genesis of arrhythmias and a prime cause of sudden death. Ionic alterations in ischaemic tissue may also be a contributory factor to arrhythmias occurring later (say after three hours) during the progression of a myocardial infarct.

The introduction of percutaneous transluminal angioplasty (PTCA) [1] gave rise to some concern about the potential risk of arrhythmias during this procedure since short periods of ischaemia followed by reperfusion are known to be arrythmogenic in animals. Fortunately such arrhythmias seem to be rare in clinical practice and PTCA has become an established form of treatment for patients with angina pectoris.

PTCA also provides an opportunity to study the early ionic changes during myocardial ischaemia in man and thus allow a comparison with results previously obtained in animals. In patients, ischaemia commonly occurs in the presence of preexisting severe coronary artery disease, often with extensive collateral formation. In animals ischaemia is usually studied by acute occlusion of a single artery. In some species such as the guinea pig and, to a lesser extent, some breeds of dog there is an extensive collateral network [2]. In other species such as rabbit and possibly the rat there is almost no collateral network. Hence results obtained in animals need to be confirmed in man whenever possible. PTCA provides such an opportunity.

Intracellular ions early in ischaemia

Little is known about intracellular ion concentrations during myocardial ischaemia. In part this is because only recently have techniques become available for the measurement of ion concentrations in the cell cytosol. Cytosolic calcium concentration has been studied under hypoxic conditions and in the presence of metabolic inhibitors but the results are inconsistent [3]. Intracellular sodium has recently been measured and shown to be unchanged over the initial fifteen minutes of ischaemia [4].

Most interest in the past has been concerned with intracellular pH, because acidosis may be a major determinant of the loss of myocardial contractility, and with the extracellular accummulation of potassium, because this is a major factor determining the observed changes in the action potential early in ischaemia.

Potassium ions

Several groups have reported that potassium is lost from myocardial cells within seconds of the onset of ischaemia and accumulates in the extracellular space [5, 6, 7, 8, 9]. Extracellular potassium concentration rises rapidly and can double within the first three minutes (Figure 1). The initial loss of potassium is associated with reversible ischaemia [10]. After a plateau, extracellular potassium rises again and can exceed $30 \, mmol.l^{-1}$ after sixty minutes. This secondary rise is not reversible and has been linked to the necrosis of myocardial cells.

The increase of extracellular potassium concentration is due to an increased efflux of potassium and not a reduced influx [10]. Evidence strongly suggests that

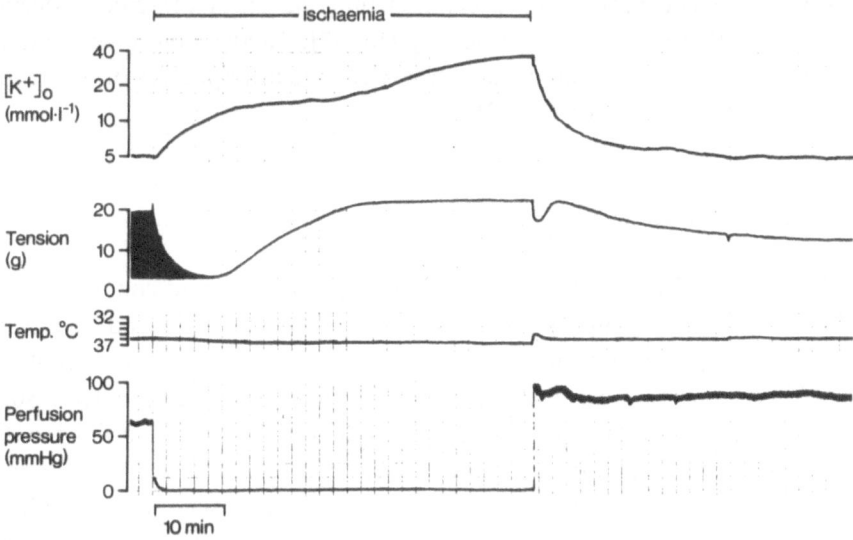

Figure 1. The accumulation of potassium ions in the extracellular space during total and global ischaemia in a Langendorff perfused rabbit heart. The potassium concentration was measured with a small ion selective electrode. Note the rapid initial rise of the potassium concentration, the existence of a plateau after ten minutes and the secondary rise of the potassium concentration. On reperfusion the concentration returns to the control value over a period of fifteen minutes [8].

the Na-K pump is not inhibited [4, 10] and the intracellular sodium does not increase [4]. Possible mechanisms for potassium efflux include increased permeability to this ion as a direct effect of ischaemia, a rise of intracellular calcium increasing potassium conductance, lack of ATP to phosphorylate channels in the membrane which remain open [11, 12], or transport of K^+ out of the cell accompanied by phosphate or lactate [13]. An increase of membrane permeability to potassium alone would not cause an increase efflux of potassium in diastole since the membrane potential is so close to the equilibrium potential for potassium. During systole and phase 2 of the action potential some potassium loss could result from an alteration of inward rectification. Most of the potassium loss is probably linked to the movement of an anion or a cation moving the opposite direction.

Hydrogen ions

It was suggested many years ago that acidosis during ischaemia was a major cause of the early loss of myocardial contractility [14]. Ample evidence exists to demonstrate that a substantial acidosis does develop during ischaemia and biochemical explanations have been proffered. Dispute has arisen partly because the mechanism by which acidosis affects myocardial contraction is uncertain and partly because of difficulties in quantifying the severity and rate of onset of acidosis in ischaemia [15]. Some authors have claimed that the onset of acidosis occurs concurrently with the fall of contractility [16, 17]. In the dog a washout of hydrogen ions into the coronary sinus can be detected after periods of ischaemia as short as twenty seconds (Figure 2).

Action potential duration

During myocardial ischaemia the action potential shortens and conduction velocity is reduced. In isolated muscle similar changes can be induced by raising perfusate potassium concentration, though a more accurate reproduction of the effects of ischaemia requires the additional presence of an acidosis [18]. Such experiments show only that these changes are a sufficient explanation for the known alteration of the action potential, not that the ionic changes are the only explanation. Later in myocardial ischaemia other factors such as intracellular lipid accumulation will undoubtedly have significant effects. Certainly the electrophysiological alterations provide a substrate for the genesis of arrhythmias.

In dogs in vivo it has been more difficult to reproduce the early changes in the action potential during ischaemia by elevation of the plasma potassium concentration [19, 20]. This is largely because it has not been possible to show that elevation of the plasma potassium, in vivo, brings about the same change in the

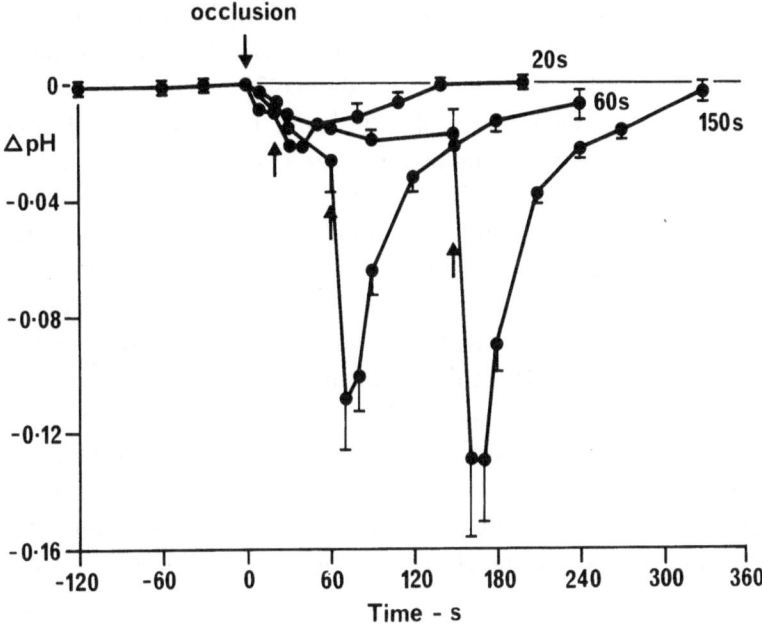

Figure 2. A pH ion selective electrode was placed in the great cardiac vein of the dog. During short occlusions of the left anterior descending coronary artery there were only small changes of pH. On release of the occlusion a rapid and transient change of pH was observed. The size of the pH change increased with the duration of the occlusion and was evident after an occlusion of only twenty seconds [17].

extracellular potassium concentration in the myocardium as occurs in the myocardium during ischaemia.

Man

In man the loss of potassium from the ischaemic myocardium and the development of acidosis has been confirmed by obtaining samples of blood from the coronary sinus during angina induced by atrial pacing [21].

The use of ion-selective electrodes has allowed the continuous recording of ionic concentrations in the coronary sinus during an atrial pacing test and during PTCA. Acidosis develops during an atrial pacing test and on cessation of pacing there is a washout of hydrogen ions [22] similar to that found in experiments in which the coronary artery has been transiently occluded in the dog [17]. An important consequence of this observation is that the timing of sampling from the coronary sinus during atrial pacing is crucial, particularly if it is the intention to draw conclusions about the metabolic state of the myocardium. Results will differ if samples are obtained before the end of the pacing, immediately on cessation of pacing or thirty seconds later.

The continous measurement of potassium in the coronary sinus has confirmed previously reported results. Increasing the heart rate by atrial pacing causes a transient loss of potassium from the myocardium [23]. Only if ischaemia develops is there a further secondary loss of potassium. On cessation of pacing the myocardium regains the loss of potassium over a period of minutes.

During PTCA the potassium concentration in the coronary sinus alters little [24]. This is because there is insufficient blood flow through the ischaemic region distal to the coronary occlusion to convey potassium to the recording electrode in the great cardiac vein. On deflation of the balloon a bolus of potassium rich blood is washed out of the ischaemic muscle and sensed in the great cardiac vein (Figure 3). The effect is repeatable. By reducing the time of balloon inflation it is possible to show that a potassium loss occurs even after occlusions of less than twenty seconds. The release of potassium detected by this method occurs before changes are observed on the surface electrocardiogram and considerably before the onset of chest pain. The administration of a bolus of potassium into a coronary artery causes the same changes on the electrocardiogram as are observed early during ischaemia [25].

Other recent studies have reported on the measurement of ventricular function [26, 27] and the monophasic action potential [28] during angioplasty. Alterations of contractility can be detected about the twentieth beat. The monophasic action potential can alter in duration in less than ten beats. The exact time of these changes may vary from patient to patient depending in particular on the extent of collateral flow. If collateral flow is high and the distal pressure does not fall to a low value as the coronary artery is occluded with the angioplasty balloon, then a considerable residual blood flow exists. Ischaemia is less severe and the consequences of ischaemia will be slower in onset.

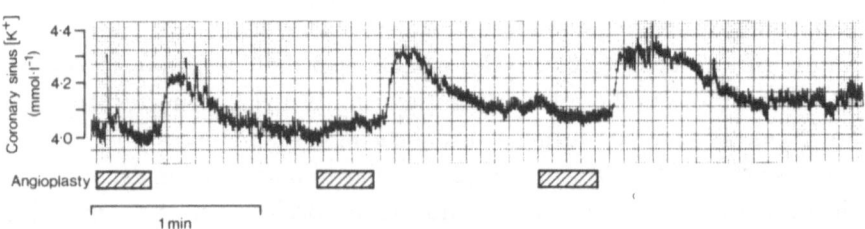

Figure 3. A potassium ion selective electrode was placed in the great coronary vein in a patient undergoing angioplasty. During inflation of the balloon there was almost no change in the potassium concentration but on deflation of the balloon a bolus of potassium passed into the vein. The effect was reproducible [23].

Conclusion

Information obtained during angioplasty demonstrated that most of the early changes during myocardial ischaemia in man are the same as those previously reported from experiments on animals. As in animals the severity of ischaemia depends on the extent of collateralisation. On abrupt occlusion the heart continues to function normally for up to four beats. Sufficient oxygen exists in the blood and myoglobin to provide the energy requirement for these beats. Subsequently creatine phosphate and adenosine triphosphate are used as energy sources. Anaerobic metabolism is stimulated. Between the fifth and twentieth heart beat contractility is reduced, the action potential shortened and potassium lost from the intracellular space. It is a plausible hypothesis that a large part of the decline of contractility is due to intracellular acidosis and that the action potential changes are the result of the combination of an accumulation of extracellular potassium and an intracellular acidosis.

References

1. Gruntzig AR, Senning A, Seigenthaler WE (1979) Non-operative dilatation of coronary-artery stenosis; percutaneous transluminal coronary angioplasty, N Eng J Med 301: 61–68
2. Schaper W, Experimental infarcts and the microcirculation. In: Hearse DJ, Yellon DM (eds) Therapeutic approaches to myocardial infarct size limitation. Raven Press, New York, pp 79–90
3. Poole-Wilson PA (1984) What causes cell death? In: Hearse DJ, Yellon DM (eds) Therapeutic approaches to myocardial infarct size limitation. Raven Press, New York, pp 43–60
4. Kleber AG (1983) Resting membrane potential, extracellular potassium activity and intracellular sodium activity during acute global ischaemia in isolated perfused guinea pig hearts. Circ Res 52: 442:450
5. Hirche HJ, Franz C, Bos L, Bissig R, Lang R, Schramm M (1980) Myocardial extracellular K^+ and H^+ increase and noradrenaline release as possible cause of early arrhythmias following acute coronary artery occlusion in pigs. J Mol Cell Cardiol 12: 579–594
6. Hill JL, Gettes LS (1980) Effect of acute coronary artery occlusion on local myocardial extracellular K^+ activity in swine. Circulation 61: 768–778
7. Wiegand V, Guggi M, Meesmann W, Kessler M, Greitschus F (1979) Extracellular potassium activity changes in the canine myocardium after acute coronary occlusion and the influence of B-blockade. Cardiovasc Res 13: 297–302
8. Webb SC, Fleetwood GG, Montgomery RAP, Poole-Wilson PA (1984) Absence of a relationship between extracellular potassium accummulation and contractile failure in the ischaemic or hypoxic rabbit heart. In: Dhalla and Rona (eds) Advances in myocardiology Vol. 6.
9. Weiss J, Shine KI (1982) Extracellular K^+ accumulation during myocardial ischaemia in isolated rabbit heart. Amer J Physiol 242: 619–628
10. Rau EE, Shine KI, Langer GA (1977) Potassium exchange and mechanical performance in anoxic mammalian myocardium. Am J Physiol 232: 85–94
11. Noma A (1983) ATP-regulated K^+ channels in cardiac muscle. Nature 305: 147–148
12. Bechem M, Pott L (1983) K-channels activated by loss of intracellular ATP in guinea-pig atrial cardioballs. J Physiol 348: 50P
13. Kleber AG (1984) Extracellular potassium accumulation in acute myocardial ischemia. J Mol Cell Cardiol 16(5): 389–394

14. Tennant R, Wiggers CJ (1935) The effect of coronary occlusion on myocardial contraction. Am J Physiol 112: 351–361
15. Jacobus WE, Pores IH, Lucas SK, Clayton HK, Weisfeldt, ML, Flaherty TJ. The role of intracellular pH in the control of normal and ischaemic myocardial contractility: a ^{31}P nuclear magnetic resonance and mass spectrometry study. In: Nuccitelli R, Deamer DW (eds). Intracellular pH: its function, regulation and utilization in cellular functions. Alan Liss, New York. pp 537–565
16. Cobbe SM, Poole-Wilson PA (1980) The time of onset and severity of acidosis in myocardial ischaemia. J Mol Cell Cardiol 12: 745–760
17. Cobbe SM, Parker DJ Poole-Wilson PA (1982) Tissue and coronary venous pH in ischaemic canine myocardium. Clin Cardiol 5: 153–156
18. Weiss J, Shine KI (1981) Extracellular potassium accumulation during myocardial ischemia: implications for arrhythmogenesis. J Mol Cell Cardiol 13(7): 699–704
19. Donaldson RM, Nashat FS, Noble D, Taggart P (1984) Differential effects of ischaemia and hyperkalaemia on myocardial repolarization and conduction tissues in the dog. J Physiol 353: 393–403
20. Morena H, Janse MJ, Fiolet JWT, Krieger WJG, Crijns H, Durrer H (1980) Comparison of the effects of regional ischaemia, hypoxia, hyperkalaemia and acidosis on intracellular and extracellular potentials and metabolism in the isolated porcine heart. Circ Res 46: 634–646
21. Parker JO, Chiong MA, West RO, Case RB (1970) The effects of ischaemia and alterations of heart rate on myocardial potassium balance in man. Circulation 42: 205–217
22. Cobbe SM, Poole-Wilson PA (1982) Continuous coronary sinus and arterial pH monitoring during pacing induced ischaemia in coronary artery disease Brit. H J 47: 369–374
23. Webb SC, Rickards AF, Poole-Wilson PA (1983) Coronary sinus potassium concentration recorded during coronary angiopasty. Brit H J 50: 146–148
24. Webb S, Canepa-Anson R, Fox K, Rickards AF, Poole-Wilson PA (1983) Evidence that myocardial potassium loss during ischaemia in man precedes electrocardiographic changes and chest pain. Clin Sci 65: 24P
25. Webb SC, Canepa-Anson R, Rickards AF, Poole-Wilson PA (1983) High potassium concentration in a parenteral preparation of glyceryl trinitrate. Need for caution if givenby intracoronary injection. Brit H J 50: 395–396
26. Brower RW, Meij S, Serruys PW (1983) A model of asynchronous left ventricular relaxation predicting the bi-expirential pressure decay. Cardiovasc. Res 17: 482–488
27. Serruys PW, Wijns W, Van den Brand M, Meij S, Slager C, Schuurbiers JCH, Hugenholtz PG, Brower RW (1984) Left ventricular performance, regional blood flow, wall motion and lactate metabolism during transluminal angioplasty. Circulation 70: 25–36
28. Donaldson RM, Taggart P, Bennett JG, Rickards AF (1984) Study of electrophysiological ischemic events during coronary angioplasty. Texas H Inst J 11: 24–30

Validity of myocardial scintigraphy, measurement of pulmonary artery pressure and intravenous digital subtraction angiocardiography in the evaluation of the effect of PTCA

P. SPILLER, E. SCHWAMMENTHAL, J. JEHLE, A. LAUBER, B. LÖSSE and F. LOOGEN

Introduction

Primary success of PTCA can easily be proved by coronary angiography. Since clinical symptoms and exercise electrocardiograms can only give limited information, quantitative evaluation of long term success implies repeated invasive diagnostic procedures.

The purpose of the study was to determine the value of myocardial scintigraphy, intravenous digital subtraction angiocardiography and measurement of pulmonary artery pressure to assess the effect of PTCA.

Methods

PTCA was performed in 36 patients (LAD 30; LCX 1; RCA 5). The dilatation was successful in 33 cases (LAD 27; LCX 1; RCA 5), unsuccessful in 3 cases (LAD 3). Before and after PTCA thallium-201-imaging (34 patients), digital subtraction angiocardiography (19 patients) and measurement of pulmonary artery pressure (28 patients) were performed at rest and during exercise.

Results

Thallium-201-imaging

After successful PTCA perfusion of the respective myocardial region during exercise improved in 94% (32/34), 44% (15/34) belonged to the subgroup 'marked change' [2] and normalization [3].

In 3 cases without a significant change of the diameter of the stenosis myocardial perfusion improved, too, in 2 cases combined with an improvement of the electrocardiogram and of the clinical symptoms. In 2 patients myocardial perfusion was unchanged in spite of successful dilatation.

If angiographically demonstrated dilatation of the stenosis of the vessel is

182

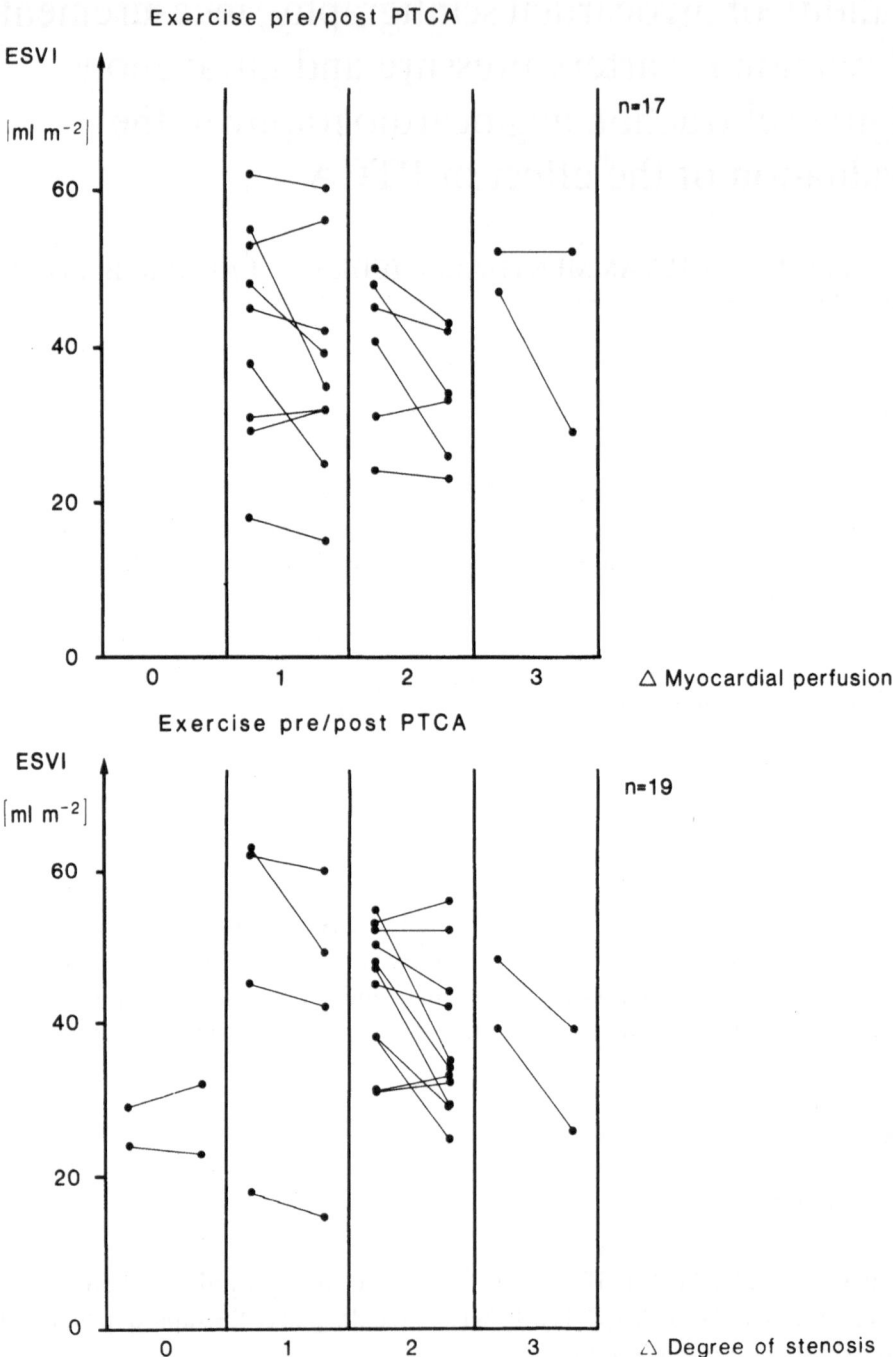

Figure 1a. Endsystolic volume index versus changes of myocardial perfusion/degree of stenosis. Marked improvement or normalization of myocardial perfusion (upper diagram) and of the degree of coronary stenosis (lower diagram), respectively, are frequently combined with a reduction of endsystolic volume index. 0: No change; 1: Slight change; 2: Marked change; 3: Normalization.

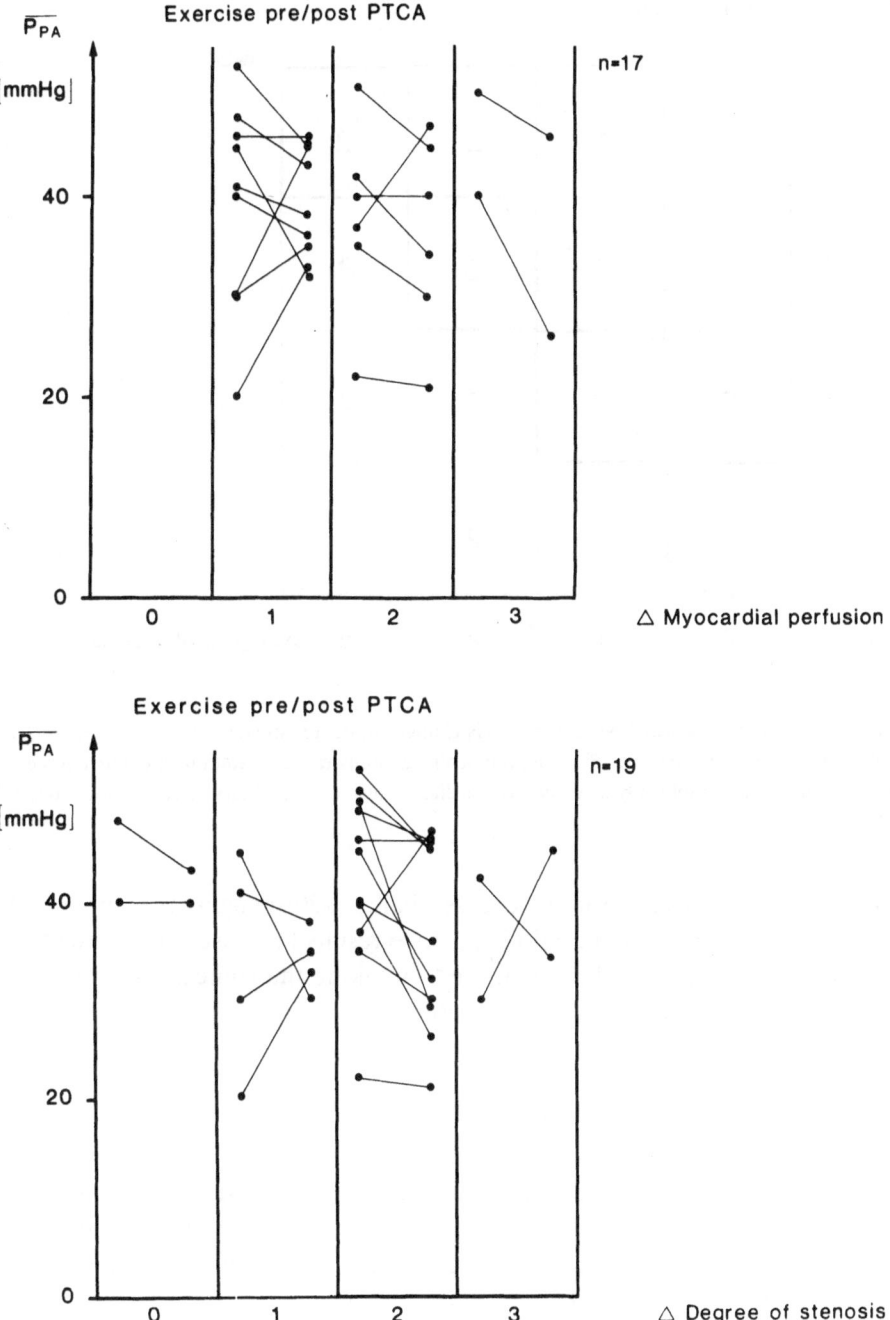

Figure 1b. Pulmonary artery pressure versus changes of myocardial perfusion/degree of stenosis. Marked changes of myocardial perfusion (upper diagram) and of the coronary artery stenosis (lower diagram) are combined with a reduction of pulmonary artery pressure only in few cases. Abbreviations see Figure 1a.

184

△ Myocardial perfusion

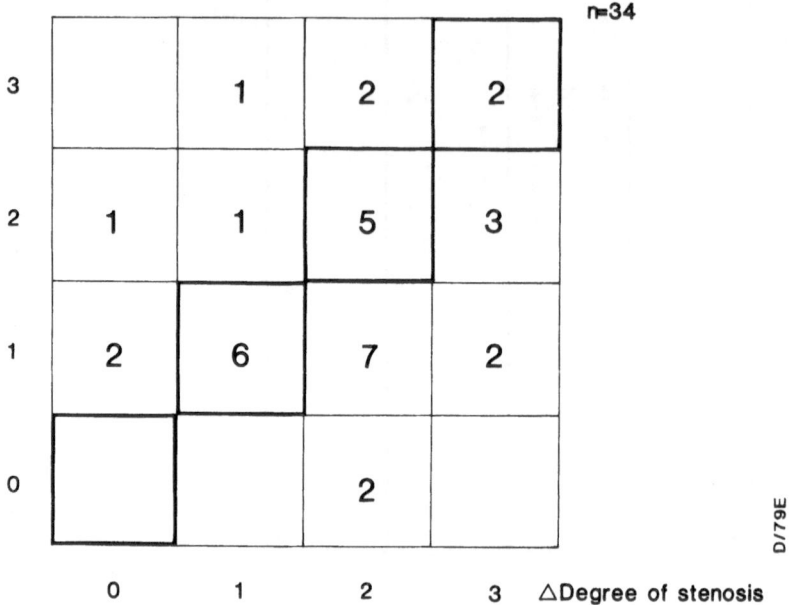

Table 1. Changes of myocardial perfusion versus changes of degree of stenosis. There was no clear correlation between the degree of angiographically demonstrated dilatation and the degree of improvement of scintigraphically assessed myocardial perfusion (probability of error about 60% $\times$ ^{2} McNamara-Test).

regarded as the only criterion of success, thallium-201-imaging presents falsely negative results in 2 cases and falsely positive results in 3 cases. The rate of the falsely positive results can be diminished by taking the clinical symptoms and exercise electrocardiograms into consideration.

Digital subtraction angiocardiography

After successful PTCA left ventricular function (determined from ejection fraction or endsystolic volume index) during exercise improved in 10/17 = 58%. Left ventricular function was unchanged in 2 patients with unsuccessful and in 7/17 (41%) patients with successful dilatation.

Measurement of pulmonary artery pressure

Successful PTCA resulted in a marked reduction of pulmonary artery pressure during exercise only in 41% (10/28).

Despite an improvement of left ventricular function, determined angiocardiographically, pulmonary artery pressure remained pathological in 59% (10/17). After unsuccessful dilatation pulmonary artery pressure was unchanged.

Discussion

The lack of correlation between the angiographic result of PTCA or the change of myocardial perfusion and the improvement of left ventricular function may be explained by the following reasons:
1. Methodological problems: errors of the angiographic and scintigraphic methods
2. Inadequate classification: problems to quantify angiographic or scintigraphic changes
3. Biologic differences: the degree of functional improvement is influenced to a greater extent by factors as: degree of impairment of left ventricular function before PTCA, one- or multi-vessel – disease, myocardial infarction prior to the intervention.

Conclusion

After successful PTCA
1. Thallium-201 – imaging during exercise presented falsely negative results in about 10% and falsely positive results in about 10% of the cases.
2. Despite an improvement of myocardial perfusion in 90%, digital subtraction angiocardiography revealed a distinct improvement of left ventricular function in only about 60%.
3. Measurement of pulmonary artery pressure seems to be only of limited value in evaluating the effect of PTCA.

Monitoring of myocardial ischaemia during PTCA improved sensivity with 12 – Lead ECG

TH. VON ARNIM, B. KEMKES, B. HÖFLING

Introduction

In the treatment of coronary heart disease, percutaneous transluminal angio-plasty (PTCA) is well established as alternative and additive to coronary bypass graft surgery. The indications are rapidly expanding and can include unstable angina, evolving infarction, occluded vessels, stenosed bypass grafts and multi-vessel disease [1–5]. The potential risk of complications increases with complex lesions and critically ill patients.

Improved monitoring during PTCA is mandatory and can also help to avoid acute complications. Moreover, accurate analysis of presseure readings, con-tractility parameters, echo- and electrocardiographic changes and metabolic studies during PTCA can help to understand basic events during acute ischaemia.

In an effort to improve monitoring of electrocardiographic changes we com-pared the recording of two bipolar chest leads with conventional limb leads and common V1–V6 chest leads during dilatations of varying duration.

Methods

In addition to conventional limb leads we recorded two bipolar chest leads (Oxford Medilog system) in 22 consecutive patients as discribed elsewhere [6]. In 12 patients we placed electrodes in the common V1–V6 positions and developed thin wound-wire electrodes in order not to disturb the fluoroscopic view signifi-cantly.

During 42 balloon insufflations we monitored all electrocardiographic readings and noted the onset of chest pain. In addition, the aortic pressure and distal coronary pressure were continuously measured.

Results

Specially designed thin wound-wire electrodes can be placed in common V1–V6 position for continous tracing of the classical chest lead ECG during PTCA without significant disturbance of the fluoroscopic view (Figure 1). Only 10/22

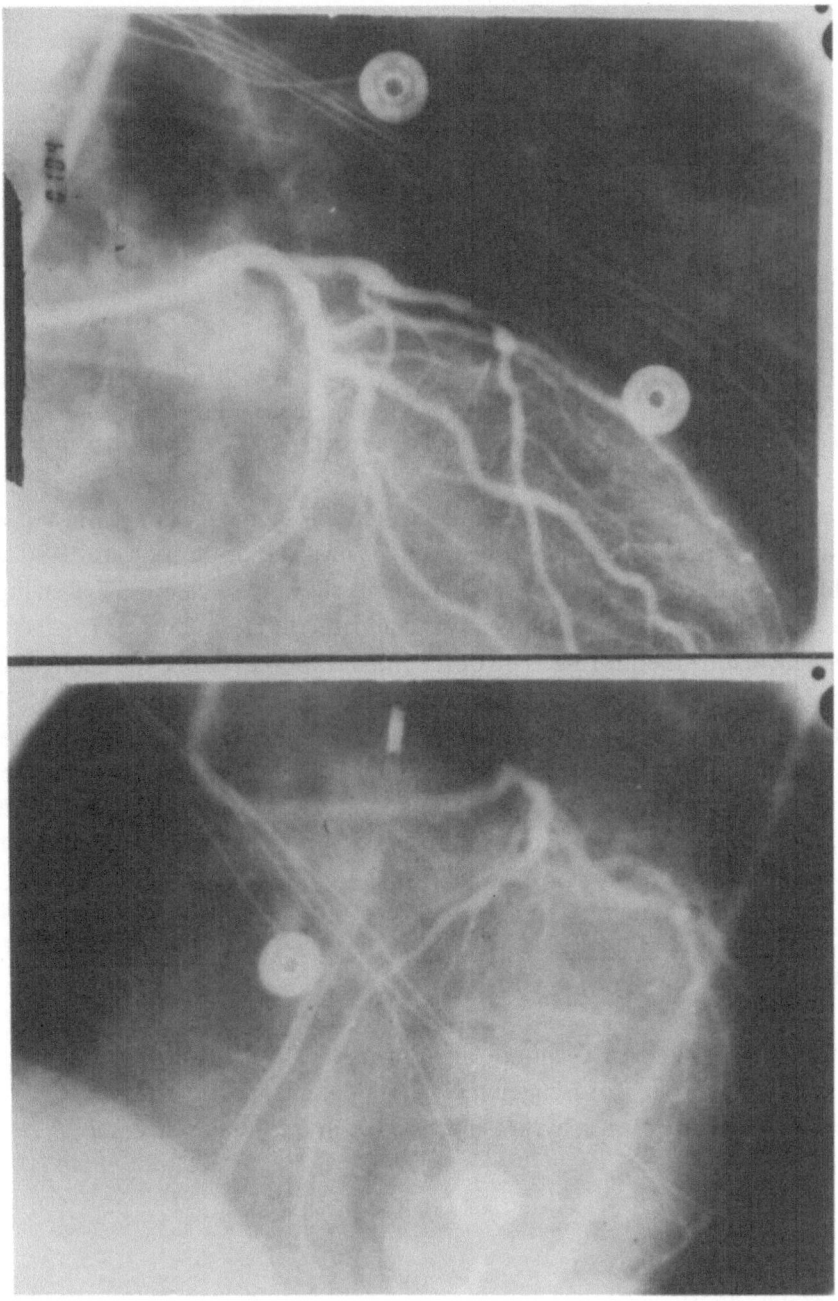

Figure 1. 40° LAD and 15° RAD view of a coronary angiography with a proximal LAD lesion. The small electrodes and thin wires of common chest leads do not disturb the fluoroscopic view significantly.

188

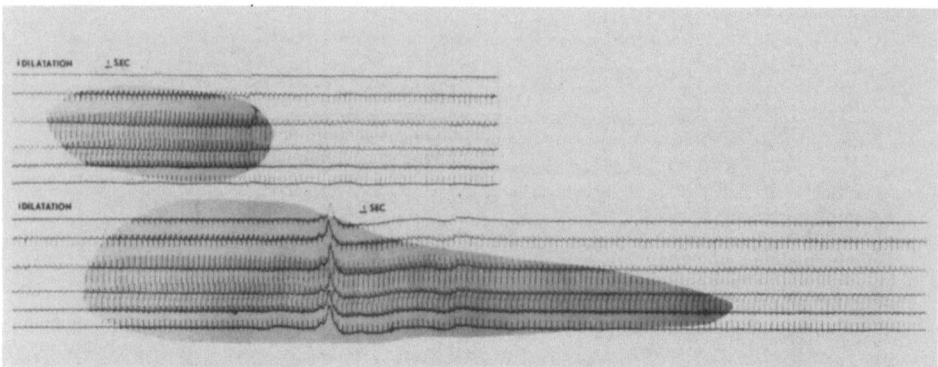

Figure 2. Two examples of different temporal and regional electrocardiographic appearance of ischaemia in leads V1–V6 (shadowed field). Insufflation periods were 22 or 35 sec respectively.

consecutive patients showed ischaemia related ST segment changes in bipolar chest leads or conventional limb leads when the insufflation period was 20–30 sec. By additional use of 12-lead ECG, 12/12 patients showed ischaemie ST-T changes with a mean duration of 53.8 ± 16.9 sec as compared to 17.9 ± 15.4 sec (p<0,0001) for a single lead II monitoring. The onset and duration of ischaemic changes can be considerably different in each chest lead (Figure 2) so that a complete V1–V6 monitoring is more sensitive to PTCA-related ST-segment changes than limb lead and single or bipolar chest lead monitoring. During 42 dilatations with mean duration of 31.6 ± 8 sec signs of ischaemia in precordial chest lead began after 18.3 ± 2.8 sec. ECG changes always preceded chest pain with a medium time intervall of 15 ± 5 sec.

Conclusions

1. Continous 12 – lead ECG monitoring during PTCA is possible.
2. It improves sensivity for ischaemic ST-segment changes considerably.
3. Pain is a late and less sensivitive indicator of myocardial ischaemia.

References

1. Meyer J et al. (1982) Percutaneous transluminal coronary angioplasty immediately after intracoronary streptolysis of transmural infarction. Circulation 5: 905–913
2. Schmutzler H, Rutsch W (1983) Die transluminale Koronar-Dilatation. Internist 24: 402–407
3. Meier B, Grüntzig A (1984) Indikationen der transluminalen Koronardilatation. Dtsch med Wschr 109: 673–677
4. Dorros G et al. (1984) Percutaneous transluminal coronary angioplasty in patients with prior coronary artery bypass grafting. The Journal of Thoracic and Cardiovascular surgery 87: 17–26

5. Jones EL, Murphy DA, Craver JM (1984) Comparison of coronary artery bypass surgery and percutaneous transluminal coronary angioplasty including for failed angioplasty. American Heart Journal 107: 830–835
6. v Arnim Th, Höfling B, Schreiber M, Bolte HD (1983) Beziehungen zwischen ST-Segment-Veränderungen im Langzeit-EKG und Angina pectoris. Verh Dt Ges f Inn Med 89: 477–480

Results of percutaneous transluminal coronary angioplasty assessed by TL-201 perfusion scintigraphy

S. MARRA, V. PAOLILLO, P.F. ANGELINO, T. VARETTO,
G. PICCIOTTO, P.G. DEFILIPPI, B. DORONZO, R. SCHMITT,
M. SABATIER and V. DOR

Introduction

It has been well shown [1, 2] that percutaneous transluminal coronary angioplasty (Ptca) improves the anatomy of the degree of stenoses in most patients (Pts) who undergo this procedure. The subjective symptomatic improvement experienced by Pts after a successful Ptca procedure may well be explained by the improved coronary blood flow to ischemic myocardium even if some placebo effect cannot be ruled out. Considering that 96.3% of our population had 1 vessel disease, the low sensitivy of the bycicle stress test, evaluating the ST segment depression, was anticipated [3]. Our Pts underwent a TL-201 perfusion scintigraphy (TLS-201) before and after the Ptca procedure [4]; Pts with unstable angina, before the Ptca, had a TLS-201 at rest to have a baseline. We compared results of the ST segment response under stress and for the TLS-201 after the procedure with the coronary angiography perfored within six months after the Ptca; a comparison was done between the TLS-201 before and after Ptca as well.

Methods

From March 81 to January 84, 27 Pts underwent a Ptca procedure; they were 25 males and 2 females aging from 31 to 62 (mean: 51.2). 14 Pts were in anginal class IV and 13 in class III or II. 15 Pts over 24 with a successful Ptca procedure had a TLS-201 study before and after Ptca.

Bycicle exercise test

Twelve standard leads were monitored and steps of 30 watts increased every 3 minutes. An exercise was considered positive with the usual criteria [3].

Thallium scintigraphy

It was performed at rest before Ptca in 5 Pts with anginal class IV and after the maximal bycicle exercise in 10 Pts with anginal class III or II. All 15 Pts after Ptca had a TLS-201 under stress [5].

Results

The primary Ptca success was 88% (24 Pts); 3 Pts had elective coronary by pass grafting (Table 1). Within 6 months 19 Pts (79.1%) were still asymptomatic, while 4 Pts had restenosis and 1 was controversial. 15 Pts over the 24 with a primary success underwent a TLS-201 before and after (mean 4.6 months) the Ptca procedure. Before Ptca 10 Pts had an exercise TLS-201 and 5 Pts a TLS-201 at rest because of anginal class IV. All Pts had either during exercise or at rest a TLS-201 perfusion defect, while 3 (over 10) had a negative ST segment response on exercise (Table 2).

After Ptca all 15 Pts had an exercise TLS-201: 1 Pt had a normal ST segment response but a TLS-201 defect; 4 Pts had a diagnostic ST segment depression without a TLS-201 defect; 1 Pt had both and 9 Pts had a normal ST segment response and a negative TLS-201.

All 15 Pts evaluated had a new coronary angiography performed within 6 months from the Ptca procedure. Sensitivity and specificity of the ST segment response was summarized in Table 2.

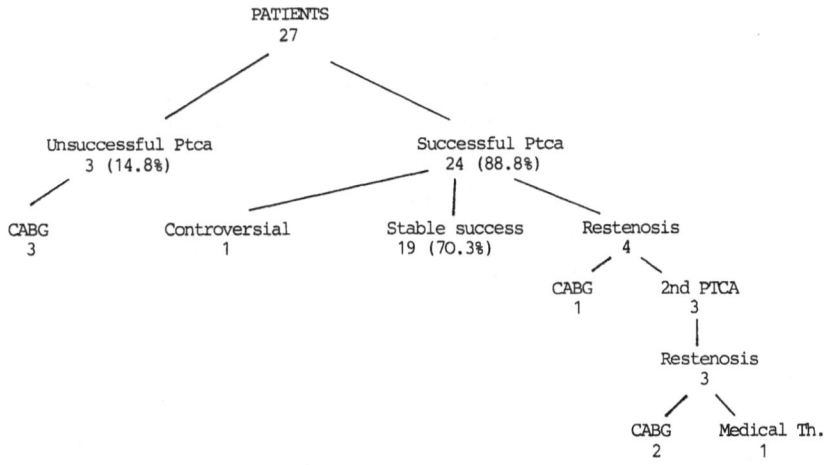

Table N.1

Table 2. Sensitivity and specificity of the ST segment response in comparison to thallium 20: scintigraphy.

Population	TL-201	Before PTCA ST		Sensitivity	Specificity
10 stress	10+	7+	3−	70%	100%
5 rest	5+	/		/	/

− = negative, + = positive.

Population	Angiocontrol	TL-201	After PTCA ST	Sensitivity	Specificity
15 stress	13 <75%	13−	4+		
			9−		
				93%	69%
	2 >75%	2+	1+		
			1−		

− = negative, + = positive.

Discussion

To visualize the primary effect of dilatation and the ongoing changes in the dilated segment of the coronary artery, selective coronary arteriography is the most direct approach but it is invasive and so, it has limited use for serial studies [1, 4]. The findings of this study clearly show that thallium-201 exercise permits documentation of changes in regional myocardial activity after Ptca, documenting either the success or not of the intervention [4, 5].

Considering the very high incidence of Pts with 1 vessel disease in our population, the low sensitivity [3] of the ST segment response and the low specificity of the anginal symptom was clearly stated. Even if we don't have a large group of patients, our results confirm the reliability and the reproducibility of the TLS-201 study [6] following up Pts after a Ptca procedure.

The high sensitivity of the TLS-201 test and its acceptance from Pts suggest to be a reliable technique in the evaluation of the long term Ptca results.

References

1. Gruntzig AR, Semcing A, Siegenthaler E, (1979) nonoperative dilatation of coronary artery stenosis. Percutaneous transluminal coronary angioplasty. N Engl J Med 301: 61–68
2. Meier B, Gruentzig AR, Siegenthaler WE, Schlumpf M (1983) Long term exercise performance

after percutaneous transluminal coronary angioplasty and coronary artery bypass grafting. Circulation 68: 796–802

3. Goldschlager N, Selzer A, Cohn K, San Francisco, California (1976) Treadmill stress tests ad indicators of presence and severity of coronary artery disease. Annals of Internal Medicine 85: 277–286

4. Hirzel HO, Nuesch K, Gruentzig AR, Lurtolf U, (1981) Short- and long-term changes in myocardial perfusion after percutaneous transluminal coronary angioplasty assessed by Thallium-201 Exercise scintigraphy. Circulation 63: 1001–1007

5. Wainwright RJ (1981) Scintigraphic anatomy of coronary artery disease in digital thallium-201 myocardial images. Br Heart J 46: 465–477

6. Rosing DR, van Raden MJ, Mincemoyer RM, Bonow RO, Bourassa MG, David PR, Ewels CJ, Detre KM, Dr Ph, Kent KM, (1984) Exercise, electrocardiographic and functional responses after percutaneous transluminal coronary angioplasty. Am J Cardiol 53: 36C–41C

Automated computer- assisted quantitative assessment of stenosis geometry and hemodynamics pre and post PTCA

H. BAHAWAR, M. GOTTWIK, J. LANG, M. KINDLER, G. STAEMMLER and M. SCHLEPPER

Introduction

Visual interpretation of coronary arteriograms is limited in its prediction of the physiologic importance of a coronary stenosis for several reasons: multiple complex factors relating to stenosis geometry and its projection on an image are important sources of error. In addition substantial inter- and intra observer variation has been described. As a consequence conventional methods of clinical coronary routine angiographic evaluation have to be considered inadequate for determination of changes of coronary stenoses pre and post pharmacological or mechanical interventions [1].

Therefore a computer assisted graphic method has been described in order to quantify coronary lesions in a monoplane or biplane approach [2, 3]. Recently this method was associated with a system for automated border recognition. Accordingly the geometry of coronary arteries on angiograms can be quantified by a reproducible observer independant automated method. This facility was used to evaluate the effect of percutaneous transluminal angioplasty on the angiograms of ten patients.

Methods

The solution to the problem of vascular border recognition is based on infinitesimal calculation specifically on differentiation. This is under the assumption that the difference of two values (i.e. grey levels) of a digital image is highest at a sudden change. The calculations are performed in a karthesian coordinate system by utilisation of a reference line in direction of the third, first, fourth and second quadrants respectively. For determination of significant points differential quotients dgr/ds* and dg/ds are used. Dgr/ds is the absolute differential in relation to the relative differential of two neighbouring points. The resolution of 40 micro meter per pixel allows the assumption $dg/ds = \lim (\text{delta } s \to 0 \text{ delta } g/\text{delta } s)$. The determination of the maximum of both differentials results in a koordinate with the highest difference which represents the border.

The hardware consists of a custom built unit equipped with a PDP 11/23 and a hard disk (30MB) and Ampex magnetic tapes for storage. The image processing unit includes three image stores with a matrix of 512×512 pixels.

As a clinical application of the system ten coronary arteries were digitized pre and post PTCA. Normal diameter proximal and distal of ten stenoses and the minimal diameter were determined in absolute and relative measurements. The pressure drop across the stenoses was estimated on the basis of the geometry of the lesions and a presumed flow of 60 ml/min (Figure 1 and 2).

Results

The diameters of the vessels proximal and distal to the stenoses measured 3.7 ± 0.8 mm and 3.6 ± 1.0 mm respectively. The minimal diameter was 1.1 + 0.5 mm, the stenosis in relative measurements amounted to an area reduction of 81%. After dilatation the stenoses diameter was twice original size with 2.0 + 0.6 mm (p 0.01). The area reduction was calculated and resulted in an average residual stenosis of 56 + 19% (p 0.01). Pressure drop across the stenoses was estimated on the basis of the stenosis geometry at a flow volume of 60 ml/min (2,3): Before dilatation pressure drop across the stenoses was calculated to be 12 + 14 mm/Hg. This pressure difference was reduced to 0.68 + 6 mm/Hg after dilatation (Table 1).

```
COMPUTER ANGIOGRAM ANALYSIS                REPORT DATE: 06-JUL-84
================================

          PROXIMAL  DISTAL   MIN    REDUCTION   AR   11.55  KV   4487.
LAO (CM)   0.219    0.256   0.082    65.3%      L/D  3.34
RAO (CM)   0.245    0.225   0.058    73.7%      AV   0.2296 ALPHA1 13.1
AREA       0.042    0.045   0.004    91.3%      B    0.0078 ALPHA2 15.3

FLOW (ML/MIN)  VISC RES (CRU)  ORIFICE RES (CRU)  PRESSURE DROP (MM HG)
    60.           0.2296          0.4684                 41.9
   120.           0.2296          0.9369                140.0
   180.           0.2296          1.4053                294.3
   240.           0.2296          1.8738                504.8
```

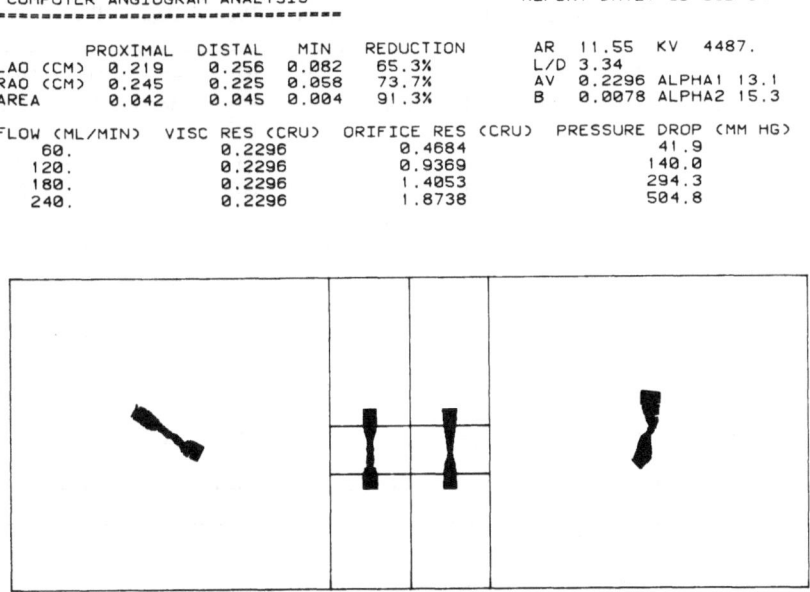

Figure 1. Example of automated border recognation of coronary lesion.

```
COMPUTER ANGIOGRAM ANALYSIS                    REPORT DATE: 05-JUL-84
-------------------------------

          PROXIMAL  DISTAL   MIN   REDUCTION     AR   1.25  KV   170.
LAO (CM)   0.238    0.281   0.228    12.1%       L/D  3.41
RAO (CM)   0.252    0.206   0.207     6.6%       AV   0.0074 ALPHA1 ****
AREA       0.047    0.045   0.037    20.0%       B    0.0000 ALPHA2 ****

FLOW (ML/MIN)  VISC RES (CRU)   ORIFICE RES (CRU)   PRESSURE DROP (MM HG)
     60.          0.0074            0.0002                 0.5
    120.          0.0074            0.0004                 0.9
    180.          0.0074            0.0006                 1.4
    240.          0.0074            0.0008                 2.0
```

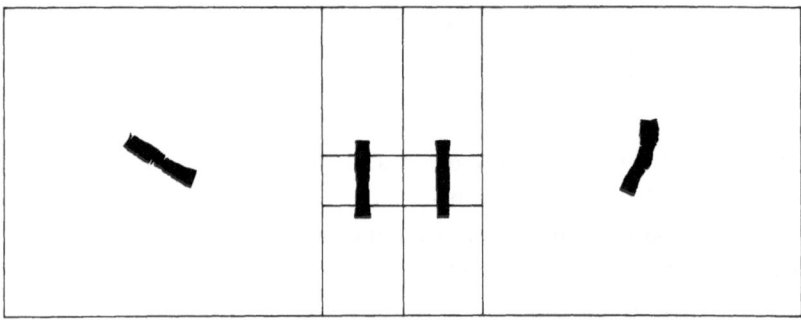

Figure 2. Example of Quantitative evaluation of coronary lesion in two orthogonal planeds pre an post PTCA.

Table 1. Quantitative evaluation of 10 coronary stenoses pre and post PTCA.

Patient	Prox		Dist		Min		% Area		DP	
	Pre	Post	Pre	Post	Pre	Post	Pre	Post	Pre	Post
1	3.3	2.9	3.4	3.1	2.1	2.3	62	45	0.7	0.4
2	2.0	1.9	1.8	2.1	0.4	1.3	95	58	24	2.1
3	3.7	3.8	3.0	2.7	1.3	0.9	85	66	3.1	0.7
4	4.1	4.6	3.3	3.4	1.0	2.1	93	73	9.3	0.5
5	3.8	2.5	3.4	2.1	0.7	1.9	96	28	43	0.5
6	4.6	4.8	3.9	3.5	1.5	2.4	88	67	2.4	0.4
7	3.9	4.2	3.5	2.8	1.1	2.6	91	52	7.1	0.4
8	4.5	4.7	3.2	3.7	0.7	1.6	96	85	33	1.4
9	4.0	3.6	4.4	4.0	0.9	2.4	95	60	16	0.3
10	2.9	2.9	2.3	2.5	1.3	2.4	77	24	3.0	0.1
Mean	3.7	3.6	3.2	3.0	1.1	2.0	81	56	12	.68
SD+/−	0.8	1.0	0.7	0.7	0.5	0.6	27	19	14	0.6
p	(p>0.05)		(p>0.05)		(p<0.01)		(p<0.01)		(p<0.05)	

The data indicate

1. A method was developed capable of processing images of angiographic films and of determining the geometry of vascular stenoses in absolute and relative measurements.

2. Application of the method to a collective of coronary films pre and post PTCA revealed a significant reduction of vascular narrowings by an 62% average increase of the minimal surface area.

References

1. White CW et al. (1984) Does visual interpretation of the coronary arterigram predict the physiologic importance of a coronary stenosis. NEJM 310: 819–24
2. Siebes M et al. (1982) Quantitative Angiography: Experimental studies on the representation of model coronary angiographies in angiographic films. Proc. ISM3 Computer Society Press
3. Kirkeeide RL et al. (1981) Computerassisted evaluation of angiographic findings. In: K. Breddin (ed) Thrombose und Atherogenese. Gerhard Witzstrock Verl. Baden-Baden, Koeln, New York: 414–417

Relationship of the occlusion pressure during PTCA to collaterals

PETER PROBST, WALHEIDE ZANGL and OTMAR PACHINGER

Patients and methods

To investigate the relationship of the gradient of a coronary artery stenosis and the pressure distal to the stenosis after proximal occlusion during PTCA to the amount of angiographically estimated collaterals 63 patients were studied. All patients had single vessel disease (54 LAD, 8 RCA, 1 CX) and there were 55 males and 8 females. All patients had documented ischemia and PTCA was carried out within 4 weeks after the initial angiogram. The patients were divided according to their initial angiogram into 4 groups: O = no collaterals (n = 35), + = just visible collaterals (n = 8), ++ = collaterals without reaching the contralateral vessel (n = 10), +++ = filling of the contralateral vessel (n = 10).

PTCA was carried out by a G 20/30 balloon catheter and only perfect undamped pressure tracings were used. The gradient across the stenosis was defined as systolic pressure measured by the guiding catheter minus the systolic pressure measured by the balloon catheter. The occlusion pressure was defined as the systolic pressure measured by the balloon catheter after reaching a steady state after inflation of the balloon.

Results

There was no difference in age within the 4 groups. There was a significant negative relationship of the gradient versus the amount of collaterals (Figure 1). There was a significant positive relationship of the occlusion pressure (in absolut terms and in per cent of the proximal systolic pressure) versus the amount of collaterals (Figure 2). There was a sharp dividing line of the occlusion pressure between O collaterals and good visible collaterals (++, +++) at 45 mmHg and 45% of the proximal systolic pressure. The occlusion pressure remained constant during one occlusion up to 40 seconds and was reproducible in 3 successive occlusions.

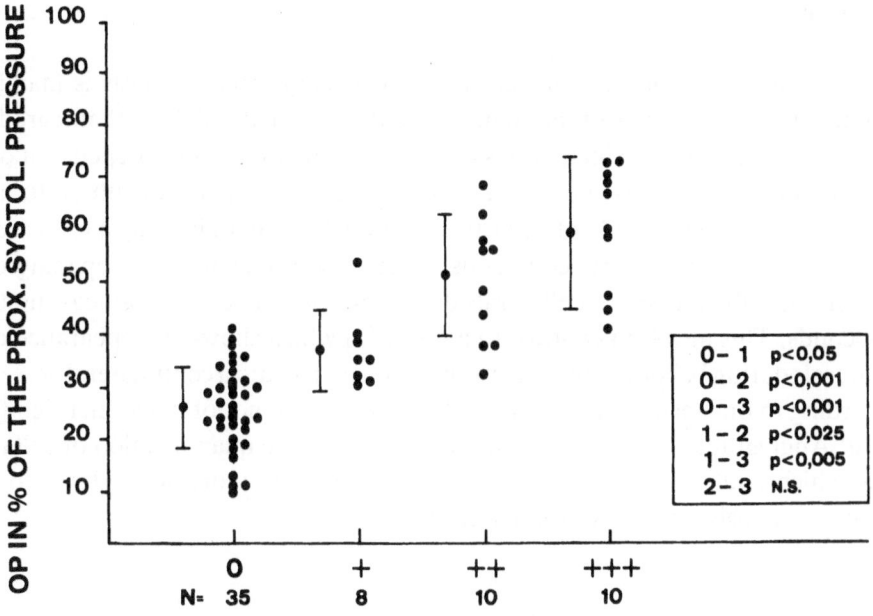

Figure 1. Demonstration of the single values and the respective mean value and the standard diviation of the 4 patient groups without (O) and with collaterals (+, ++, +++). For explanation see text. There is a significant difference of the systolic gradient of patients without collaterals vs patients with collaterals.

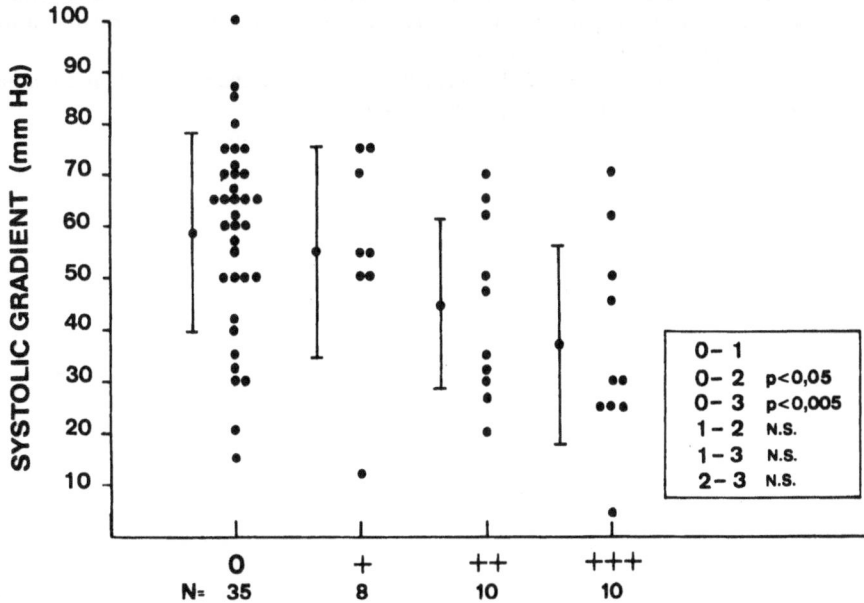

Figure 2. Demonstration of the relationship of the relativ occlusion pressure (occlusion pressure in % of the proximal systolic pressure) vs the amount of collaterals. There is a significant relationship according to the amount of collaterals.

Conclusion

We conclude thath the pressure distal to a coronary artery stenosis is mainly dependent on the severity of the stenosis and on the collateral flow. If antegrade flow is eliminated by proximal occlusion the distal pressure is only dependent on the amount of collaterals showing almost no overlap. This is in contrast to an other study [1] which could not show this relationship, but only using a few cases and no quantification of the collaterals. There also seems to be no opening of angiographically not visible collaterals during prolonged occlusion at least up to 40 seconds. This also is in contrast to a paper [2] which shows an appearance of collaterals during balloon inflation and injection of dye into a contralateral vessel. According to our results these collaterals obviously are not of functional significance. Angiography seems to be a sufficient tool for the quantification of collaterals which could be also shown by intraoperative measurements distal to a coronary stenosis during bypass surgery [3, 4].

References

1. Feldman RL, Pepine CJ (1984) Evaluation of coronary collateral circulation in conscious humans. Am J Cardiol 53: 1233–38
2. Rentrop P, Cohen M, Phillips R, Blanke H (1984) Acute changes in collateral filling during transluminal coronary angioplasty. Eur Heart J 5: Suppl I-464
3. Goldstein RE, Stinson EB, Scherer JL, Seninger RP, Grehl TM, Epstein SE (1974) Intraoperative coronary collateral function in patients with coronary occlusive disease. Nitroglycerin responsiveness and angiographic correlations. Circulation 49: 298–308
4. Parker FB, Neville JF, Hanson EL, Webb WR (1974) Retrograde and antegrade pressures and flows in preinfarction syndrome. Circulation 49, 50: Suppl II: 122–6

Changes in creatine phosphokinase after coronary angioplasty

STÉPHANE BERCLAZ, BERNHARD MEIER, JEAN-CLAUDE BARTHÉLÉMY and WILHELM RUTISHAUSER

Introduction

Several studies have shown that creatine phosphokinase (CPK) levels may be altered by uncomplicated cardiac catheterization [1–6]. Values exceeding the normal limit, however, are rare and commonly associated with special circumstances [4–6]. This study examines CPK changes caused by percutaneous transluminal coronarory angioplasty (PTCA) and the usefulness of routine serial CPK samples in this context.

Methods

The study was planned prospectively on 150 consecutive patients undergoing PTCA at our institution. It entailed CPK samples before PTCA, and about 6 and 20 hours after PTCA. CPK was determined enzymatically. The upper normal limit of the method employed is 250 U/l. If CPK exceeded this limit, CPK-MB fraction was determined enzymatically after immunologic reaction with antigen M. CPK-MB fractions of <10% of total CPK were considered non-significant.

There were 132 males and 18 females patients with a mean age of 54 years (range 23–71 years). Ten patients were excluded because the stenosis could not be reached, four because they had PTCA for ongoing infarction, four because they needed emergency bypass surgery for complications of PTCA, and 20 because CPK sampling was incomplete.

Results

Of the 112 remaining patients all baseline CPK levels were normal. Both postinterventional CPK levels were normal in 104 patients (Group A) and at least one was elevated in 8 patients (Group B). Table 1 depicts the pertinent angiographic and clinical characteristics of both groups. Elevation of CPK-MB, a valid indicator for myocardial necrosis, was only found in patients with angiographically unsuccessful PTCA and with permanent ECG changes. Two of those patients also had chest pain for >1 hour. Table 2 shows the CPK values of group A and B.

Table 1. Outcome of patients without (A) and with (B) CPK elevations.

	A (104)	B (8)	
		CK-MB normal 2	CK-MB elevated 6
PTCA – successful*	95	2	0
– failed*	9	0	6
Chest pain after PTCA	11	0	2
– <1 hour	11		0
– >1 hour	0		2
Permanent ECG changes	0	0	6

*Angiographic assessment. Figures denote number of patients.

Table 2. CPK values of patients without (A) and with (B) CPK elevation.

	A (104)	B (8)
Before PTCA	67 ± 35	84 ± 33
After – 6 hours	88 ± 42*	244 ± 174*
–20 hours	97 ± 59	486 ± 196*

* $p < 0.05$ compared to values before PTCA.
Values are mean ± standard deviation. Figures in parentheses denote number of patients.

Baseline values were similar. Postinterventional values in both groups wei significantly higher than baseline values.

Discussion

A slight rise in CPK levels was found after PTCA. It is similar to that found aftε diagnostic cardiac catheterization and may be multi-factorial e.g. myocardiε reaction to contrast medium or to episodes of ischemia caused by the ballooi trauma to sceletal muscles due to position on hard table. Values exceeding tℏ normal limit, however, were only found in <2% of uneventful procedures an were not accompanied by an elevated CPK-MB fraction. Elevated CPK-M fractions were found exclusively in patients with problems during and after PTC, apparent already angiographically and by clinical and electrocardiographic signs of myocardial infarction. Serial CPK sampling is unnecessary with uneven ful PCTA. Solely obvious problems during or after PCTA are an indication for CPK determinations.

Summary

On the basis of serial samples in 112 patients with coronary angioplasty (PTCA) the changes of creatine phosphokinase (CPK) levels and their usefulness for the management of the patients were examined. Abnormal CPK values were found in less then 2% of uneventful procedures. Abnormal CPK-MB fractions were only found in patients with obvious problems during and after PTCA. CPK samples are only indicated in case of problems with PTCA.

References

1. Edmiston WA, Bornheimer J, Takiff H (1980) Serum enzyme changes after cardiac catheterization and angiographic procedures. Angiology 31: 39–44
2. Rettig G, Keller HE, Schieffer H, Hoffmann W, Bette L (1976) Einfluss von Herzkatheter-Untersuchung und Angiokardiographie auf die Enzymaktivitäten im Serum. Münch Med Wochenschr 118: 997–1000
3. Baltaxe HA, Sos TA, McGrath MB (1976) Effects of the intracoronary and intraventricular injections of commonly available vs. a newly available contrast medium. Invest Radiol 11: 172–181
4. Hori M, Inoue M, Fukui S, Furukawa T, Abe H (1976) Significance of serum enzyme changes after cardiac catheterization and selective coronary arteriography. Br Heart J 38: 97–103
5. Lucena GE, Scheftel M, Azar M, Adicoff A, Gobel FL (1974) Serum enzyme activity following cardiac catheterization and endomyocardial biopsy. Lab Clin Med 84: 6–19
6. Chahine RA, Eber LM, Kattus AA (1974) Interpretation of the serum enzyme changes following cardiac catheterization and coronary angiography. Am Heart J 87: 170–174

Antiischemic properties of intracoronary Diltiazem

P. SCHANZENBÄCHER, H. KAHLES, G. LIEBAU and K. KOCHSIEK

Introduction

The intracoronary administration of calcium channel blocking agents may potentially be useful during interventional procedures. During reperfusion of acute myocardial infarction it may allow to rule out coronary arterial spasm as the major cause of myocardial ischemia. During PTCA it may facilitate easier passage of the ballon catheter through a tight stenosis and may additionally exert regional cardioplegia with increased tolerance to myocardial ischemia. Consequently, the coronary hemodynamic and metabolic effects of Diltiazem (2 mg intracoronarily) were evaluated in 13 patients with angina pectoris.

Methods

The study was performed on 13 patients (11 male, 2 female) during routine cardiac catheterization. Coronary angiography was performed by the Judkins technique using Iopamidol (Solutrast 370, Byk Gulden Company) as contrast material. Coronary sinus blood flow was measured by the constant infusion thermodilution technique [1]. Arterial and coronary venous blood samples were simultanously drawn for determination of oxygen content (LexO$_2$-Con-K). Myocardial oxygen consumption was calculated from the product of the arterio-venous oxygen content difference and coronary sinus blood flow [1]. Before the intracoronary bolus injection of 2 mg Diltiazem (Gödecke AG) two baseline coronary arteriograms and coronary sinus blood flow measurements were obtained. Coronary blood flow was determined 2 and 5 minutes after the bolus injection. Coronary arteriography in multiple projections was performed, when coronary blood flow had returned to preinjection values. Two non-obstructed coronary arterial segments were selected for quantitative evaluation [2].

Results

The results are summarized in Table 1. The intracoronary injection of Diltiazem led to a transient decrease in mean aortic pressure and a decrease in heart rate.

Table 1. HR = heart rate, P_{Ao} = mean aortic pressure, CSBF = coronary sinus blood flow, MVO_2 = myocardial oxygen consumption, CVR = coronary vascular resistance, CA-D = diameter of epicardial conductance vessels, Co = control, D2, D5 = 2 and 5 minutes after the intracoronary injection of Diltiazem, * * = $p<0.01$; * = $p<0.05$.

	Co	D2	D5
HR (min^{-1})	74 ± 10	68 ± 11* *	71 ± 11*
P_{Ao} (mmHg)	109 ± 10	102 ± 13* *	106 ± 11
CSBF (ml/min)	98 ± 24	191 ± 59* *	116 ± 36
MVO_2 (mlO$_2$/min)	13.2 ± 3.6	10.9 ± 3.2* *	12.2 ± 2.7
CVR (mmHg/ml/min)	1.08 ± 0.26	0.56 ± 0.10* *	0.96 ± 0.18
CA-D (mm)	2.03 ± 0.45		2.40 ± 0.44* *

Coronary blood flow increased due to a considerable reduction in coronary vascular resistance. Myocardial oxygen consumption was significantly reduced by Diltiazem. Relaxation of epicardial conductance vessels persisted, when coronary flow had returned to basal levels.

Discussion

The decrease in heart rate and mean aortic pressure are probably related to a negative chronotropic and negative inotropic action of Diltiazem, which are unmasked by indirect peripheral effects [3, 4]. As a consequence of both effects, myocardial oxygen consumption decreased significantly. The increase in coronary blood flow is primarily related to a relaxation of small intramural resistance vessels. The transient increase in coronary flow is followed by a persistent dilation of the epicardial conductance in the presence of maintained autoregulation. The intracoronary application of Diltiazem is therefore potentially useful during interventional procedures, by increasing the tolerance of the myocardium to ischemia and probably preventing a reflex increase in vascular tone of epicardial conductance vessels due to mechanical manipulation.

References

1. Schanzenbächer P, Liebau G, Deeg P, Kochsiek K (1982) Effect of intracoronary nifedipine on coronary sinus blood flow and myocardial oxygen consumption in patients with coronary artery disease Z Kardiol 71: 393–397
2. Schanzenbächer P, Göttfert G, Kahles H, Liebau G, Maisch B, Riegger G, Kochsiek K (1984) Effect of nifedipine and nitroglycerin on epicardial coronary arteries in coronary heart disease. Dtsch Med Wschr 109: 656–660
3. Schanzenbächer P, Liebau G, Deeg P, Kochsiek K (1983) Effect of intravenous and intracoronary nifedipine on coronary blood flow and myocardial oxygen consumption. Am J Cardiol 51: 712–717

4. Schanzenbächer P, Göttfert G, Liebau G, Kochsiek K. Coronary hemodynamic and metaboli effects of nifedipine in betablocked patients with coronary artery disease. Am J Cardiol (in pres January 1985)

Cardio-computertomography for assessing regional myocardial perfusion abnormalities in coronary heart disease

K.-H. SANDRING, V. GLIECH, W. DÄNSCHEL, CHRISTINE MÜLLER and K.H. GÜNTHER

Myocardial perfusion may be an important determinant as well as from the diagnostic and therapeutic point of view, especially in coronary heart disease. At present, there are existing several methods being usable noninvasively or invasively for assessing myocardial perfusion. Most widely used in the general cardiological practice is the Thallium-201-scintigraphy [1, 2]. There are limitations however concerning quantitative evaluation [3]. Recently also computertomography (CT) became available for determination of perfusion abnormalities [4, 5]. An interesting modification seemed us to be cardio-CT in combination with intracoronary injections of contrast medium [6].

Aim of this study is therefore testing this method in patients with ischemic heart disease.

Patients and methods: As pilot study we have been investigated 10 males with coronary heart desease determined angiographically. CT investigations were carried out with a whole body scanner Somatom SF, Siemens, Scanning time is 5 seconds, slice thickness 8 mm and distance between two consecutive slices likewise 8 mm. The investigation is performed in supine position after maximum inspiration. Selective injection of contrast medium into the left and right coronary artery is done manually.

Results: In normal subjects (coronary artery disease excluded) regional myocardial attenuation shows typical distributions after intracoronary injections of contrast medium, which are however clearly differing in the different planes from apex to basis. Separate analysis of the attenuation values of the subendocardial or subepicardial layers normally show the same regional distribution. In cases of coronary artery stenosis on the other hand typical abnormalities in the regional distribution of myocardial attenuation could be found (see Figure 1 and 2). In the investigated patients without coronary heart disease none has perfusion abnormalities. On the other hand patients with significant coronary artery stenosis a reduced attenuation in the poststenotic areas is found (see Table 1). Conclusion: Assessment of regional myocardial perfusion has been considered to be partially an unsolved problem. Computertomography has become increasingly interesting when equipments became available providing short scan time. Our preliminary results show, that cardio-CT can be used for evaluating perfusion abnormalities

208

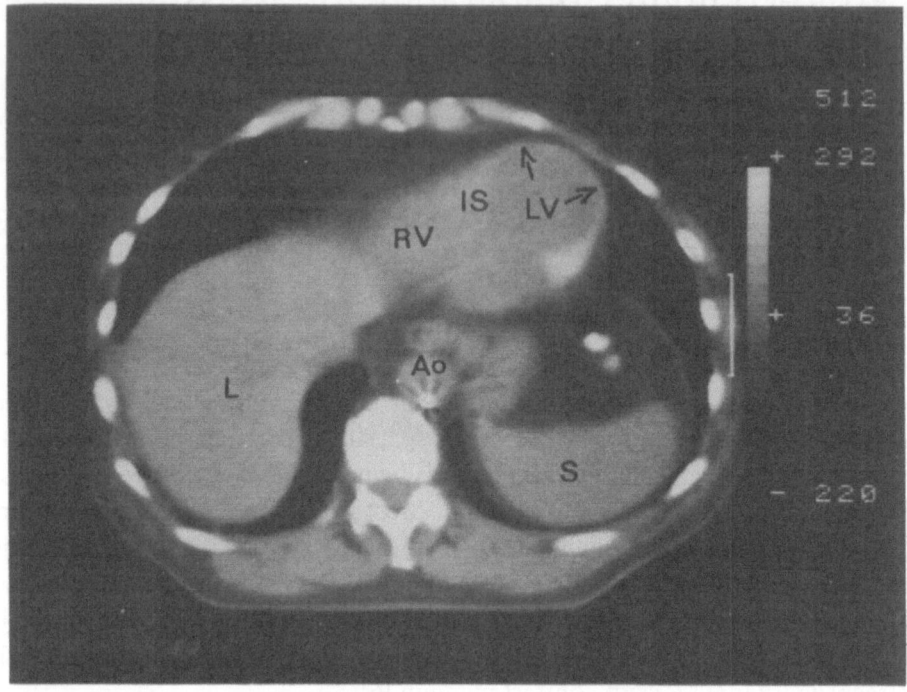

Figure 1. Significant LAD stenosis. Unchanged perfusion lateral, significant underperfusion anterior and septal (↑). RV = right ventricle, LV = left ventricle, IS = interventricular septum, Ao = descending aorta, Vc = vena cava inferior, L = liver, S = spleen.

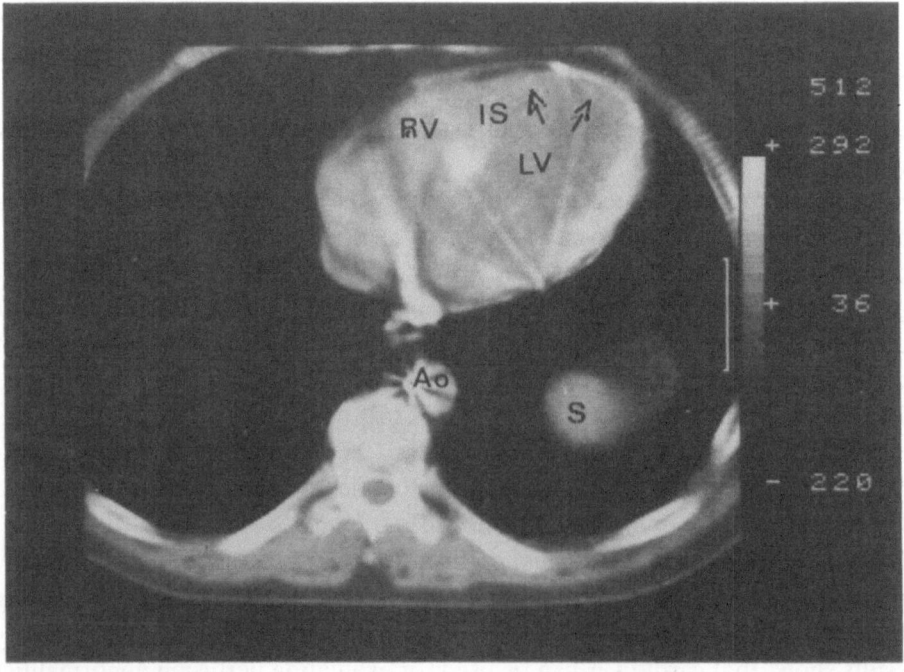

Table 1. Cases report.

Pat. no.	Coronary angio abnormalities	Selective cardio-CT perfusion reduced
1	None	None
2	(LAD), (LCX)	ant., (sept.) (Fig. 2)
3	None	None
4[T.A]	LAD, (RCA)	ant., sept.
5	None	None
6[A]	LAD	ant., sept.
7[A]	LAD	ant., sept., lat.
8	LAD, LCX, RCA	ant., sept.
9	LAD	ant., sept. (Fig. 1)
10	None	None

LAD, LCX, RCA = significant stenosis, None = nothing or plaques only, (...) = insignificant stenosis, T = Thrombus, A = Aneurysma of left ventricle.

in cases of coronary heart disease, even at rest. The method also makes visible the subendocardial and subepicardial layers which may be of special interest in some instances. Disadvantage of the intracoronary injection of contrast medium may be its invasive character. Advantages of this method are however considered its higher sensitivity by using very small amounts of contrast medium.

References

1. Botvinick EH, Dunn RF, Hattner RS, Massie BM (1980) A consideration of factors affecting the diagnostic accuracy of thallium-201 myocardial perfusion scintigrams in detecting coronary artery disease. Semin Nucl Med 10: 157
2. Hamilton GW (1979) Myocardial imaging with thallium-201: the controversy over its clinical usefulness in ischemic heart disease. J Nucl Med 20: 1201
3. Ritchie JL, Zaret BL, Strauss HW, Pitt B, Berman DS, Schelbert HR, Ashburn WL, Berger HJ, Hamilton GW (1978) Myocardial imaging with thallium-201: A multicenter study in patients with angina pectoris or acute myocardial infarction. Amer J Cardiol 42: 345
4. Carlsson E, Lipton MJ, Berninger WH, Doherty P, Redington RW (1977) Selective left coronary myocardiography by computed tomography in living dogs. Invest Radiol 12: 559
5. Sandring K.-H, Gliech V, Dänschel W, Müller C, Günther KH (1983) Beurteilung der regionalen Myokardperfusion mittels Computertomographie, Dt Gesundh-Wesen 38: 2017

←

Figure 2. LAD (+ LCX) plaques only, no stenosis, rarefication of branches Prominently amplified LAD (artifact), unchanged perfusion lateral, underperfusion anterior and septal (↑). RV = right ventricle, LV = left ventricle, IS = interventricular septum, Ao = descending aorta, Vc = Vena cava inferior, L = liver, S = spleen.

Clinical significance of microsphere myocardial scintigraphy in coronary artery disease

PAOLO MARZULLO, OBERDAN PARODI, CLARA CARPEGGIANI,
DANILO NEGLIA, CLAUDIO MARCASSA, CALOGERO BELLINA,
NICOLA MAZZUCA and ANTONIO L'ABBATE

Introduction

The application of ECG-gated reconstruction to myocardial images obtained by the use of intraventricular injected 99m-Tc labeled human albumin microspheres (G-HAM) ensures the simultaneous assessment of myocardial perfusion and contractility in man [1–2].

In contrast to ungated images, such as those obtained with Thallium-201, G-HAM allow a distribution strictly proportional to regional blood flow, not affected by metabolic interference and tracer redistribution. The technique provides high quality end-diastolic and end-systolic perfusion images allowing long-term monitoring of left ventricular function in different clinical conditions [3].

Methods

Four millions of HAM (TCK5s by CIS) averaging 15 microns in diameter, labeled with 25 mCi of 99m-Tc are injected via a pig-tail catheter into the LV during routine cardiac catheterization. LV hemodynamics and ECG are monitored throughout the study. Gated acquisition is performed in multiple views with a large field Anger camera equipped with a dedicated nuclear medicine computer (Medusa 12b, Sepa, Italy). Gated acquisition is used to improve the detection of small and/or localized perfusion defects which could be masked from cardiac motion and wall systolic thickening.

Study population

In the past eight years we applied G-HAM to a large group of patients with various degrees of coronary artery disease.

Fifteen additional patients who underwent coronary angiography and ventriculography for atypical chest pain provided control population both for regional myocardial perfusion and wall motion.

In transmural myocardial infarction G-HAM provided the true anatomical location of necrosis and the functional evaluation of poorly perfused sectors to be medically or surgically treated (Figure 1).

In myocardial infarction without QRS changes (so called subendocardial infarction) G-HAM were able to identify large nontransmural and/or transmural perfusion defects; neither coronary anatomy nor impairment of LV function were able to identify this subset of patients [4].

Furthermore in acute myocardial infarction (transmural and nontransmural) G-HAM provided information on the reperfusion and function of acutely ischemic segments following intracoronary thrombolysis (Figure 2).

In transient ischemia, at rest or following exercise, G-HAM allowed the study of very short lasting ischemic episodes freezing myocardial blood flow distribution at the moment of the injection (short lasting ischemic episodes represent a severe challenge for conventional radioisotopic techniques).

In combination with coronary angiography, G-HAM allowed a better evaluation of the efficacy of coronary collateral circulation.

Recently, HAM were complemented by single photon emission computed tomography; the technique provides a better spatial definition hardly appreciable using planar and even gated imaging.

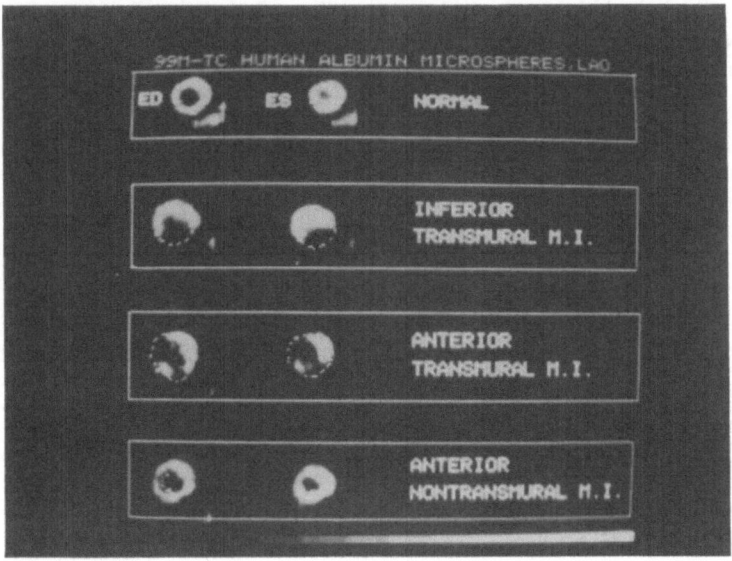

Figure 1. Myocardial end-diastolic (ED) and end-systolic (ES) ECG-gated scintigraphy obtained in left anterior oblique projection (LAO) following intraventricular injection of labeled albumin microspheres in normal subject and in different types of myocardial infarctions. Dotted lines outline the contour of the heart in correspondence of the perfusion defect. Micosphere scintigraphy, reflecting a distribution strictly proportional to coronary blood flow, allows the functional evaluation of poorly perfused sectors to be medically or surgically treated.

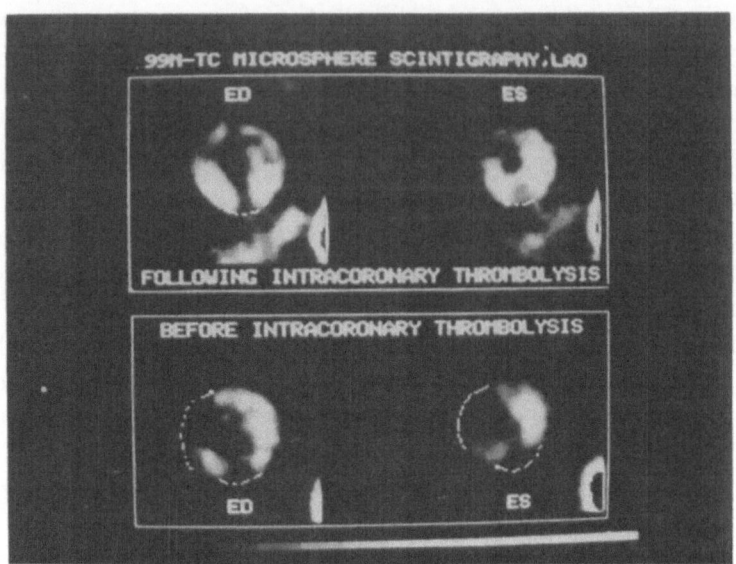

Figure 2. Myocardial scintigraphy obtained in left anterior oblique projection (LAO) following intraventricular injection of labeled microspheres. Before intracoronary thrombolysis (lower panel), both end-diastolic (ED) and end-systolic (ES) frames show evident transmural septal and inferoapical perfusion defects. Following intracoronary thrombolysis (upper panel), significant reperfusion of the septal wall and systolic thickening are evident. In intracoronary thrombolysis, microsphere scintigraphy provides direct anatomical information on regional blood flow and function recovery beyond the information on vessel anatomy provided by coronary angiography.

Conclusions

The clinical applicability of G-HAM in the study of coronary heart disease is widely exploitable. On this basis we feel that the systematic application of G-HAM and/or single photon emission computed tomography in patients with infarction and ischemia who undergo routine angiographic evaluation may provide useful additional parameters for short and long term correlation with cardiac events [5].

References

1. Ashburn W, Braunwald E, Simon A, Peterson K, Gavet J (1971) Myocardial perfusion imaging with radioactive-labeled particles injected directly into the coronary circulation of patients with coronary artery disease. Circulation 44: 851–865
2. Bencivelli W, Parodi O, Marzullo P, Camici P, Davies G, Pisani P, Riva A, L'Abbate A, Maseri A (1981) A new technique for gated reconstruction applied to microsphere myocardial imaging. Computers in Cardiology, IEEE Computers Society, Long Beach, California, pp 95–100
3. Parodi O, Bencivelli W, Marzullo P, Galli M, Neglia D, L'Abbate A (1983) Gated myocardial

imaging with 99m-tc albumin microspheres. In: Salvatore M and Porta E (eds) Radioisotopes in cardiology, Plenum Publishing Corporation, New York, p 163–169

4. Marzullo P, Carpeggiani C, Parodi O, Neglia D, L'Abbate A (1984) Scintigraphic assessment of myocardial infarction in absence of ECG Q waves. Proceedings of the 7th European Congress of Nuclear Medicine, Helsinki 1983. Schattauer Verlag Edt, Stuttgart (in press)

5. Krone R, Friedman E, Thanavaro S, Miller P, Kleiger R, Oliver C (1983) Long term prognosis after first Q-wave (transmural) and non-Q-wave (nontransmural) myocardial infarction: analysis of 593 patients. Am J Cardiol 52: 223–239

Current aspects of transluminal coronary angioplasty

PIERRE P. LEIMGRUBER and ANDREAS R. GRUENTZIG

Introduction

In the United States, atherosclerotic coronary vascular disease remains the most common cause of death. Despite tremendous emphasis on diagnosis and disease prevention, most advances have come in the form of palliative therapy of overt disease.

The medical treatment of coronary artery disease has seen many advances with the introduction of beta blockers and calcium blockers. In addition, bypass graft surgery has undergone numerous refinements since Favaloro first described coronary saphenous vein graft in 1967 [1]. Bypass graft surgery has been effective in symptomatic relief of patients with obstructive coronary disease.

The origin of percutaneous transluminal angioplasty can be traced back to the work of Dotter and Judkins, in 1964, who introduced a catheter technique for therapeutic intervention in peripheral vascular disease [2], which was subsequently modified to a distensible (balloon) tip in 1974. Further changes led to its experimental use in the coronary circulation in 1976 [3]. Finally, on September 16, 1977 in Zurich, Switzerland, the procedure was first performed on a patient with obstructive coronary artery disease [4]. PTCA has undergone many changes and improvements in material and technique. Today it is considered the therapy of choice in selected patients with coronary artery disease and as a distinct alternative in patients who would require bypass graft surgery.

Indications

Single vessel disease: well-defined, hemodynamically significant single vessel disease remains the classic indication for PTCA. Patients in this group would otherwise require bypass graft surgery because of the severity of symptoms which are refractory to medical treatment. Also, the anatomy should be favorable for dilatation and the length of the stenosis should not exceed 15–20 mm. We do exclude patients with left main stenosis due to the potential hazard of life-threatening dissection of this vital vessel and unfavorable long term results. Patients who have had prior bypass graft surgery are also candidates for PTCA. However, this group of patients is at higher morbidity and mortality if emergency bypass surgery is required [5]. Angioplasty has been performed successfully on saphenous vein grafts. Even though initial success is comparable to single vessel angioplasty, the recurrence rate of dilated vein grafts is higher than what we see after angioplasty of native coronary arteries. One exception to this rule is stenosis of vein grafts involving the distal anastomosis site, which has an excellent long-term prognosis.

Multi-vessel disease: High success rates and low complication rates have led to the inclusion of patients with double or triple vessel disease such as discrete stenosis in two or more major arteries. Criteria for selection of patients in this group should be stricter than those outlined for single vessel disease since there is increased potential for having complications. Further work needs to be done regarding the timing and strategy of dilatation in patients with multivessel diseases.

Other indications: Percutaneous angioplasty seems to be effective in combination with streptokinase in patients with acute infarction. In addition, intraoperative angioplasty has been used to dilate small vessels otherwise not amenable to bypass grafting.

Procedure

PTCA demands more concise angiographic information than that afforded by many laboratories. High resolution and rapid visualization of multiple projections is required for catheter manipulation. The radiological capabilities considered optimal for performing PTCA include 1) an X-ray tube image intensifier capable of multiangular projections, including cranial and caudal angulation, easy to position and preferably biplanal; 2) a high resolution image intensifier and monitor chain providing definition of the steerable 0.4 mm diameter guidewire; 3) multimode image intensification including 10–13, 15–18, 30–23 cm field sizes; 4) capacity for increasing dose rates that allow for brief periods of increased penetration and definition; 5) high resolution freeze frame video recorder of this so that at least 2 guide projections can be displayed constantly for comparison with real-time images. Four TV monitors are thus necessary.

The equipment to perform PTCA essentially consists of two catheters. The larger, guiding catheter is available in modified Judkins, Amplatz and Brachial size #8 and #9 French. The tip of these catheters is not tapered for allowing the passage of the balloon catheter. The dilatation catheter has two lumen. The central lumen allows contrast injections, pressure measurements and passage of a small 0.4 mm steerable guidewire over which the balloon dilatation catheter can be advanced once the guidewire is placed in the appropriate coronary artery. The second lumen is used to inflate the balloon. This is done using a mixture of dilated contrast material in a 50/50 ratio with sterile, normal saline. This allows for visualization of the balloon and also prevents air embolism in event of balloon rupture. The outer diameter of the balloon is predetermined and almost constant over a wide range of inflation pressures (5–10 atmospheres). At present, balloons with inflated sizes are available from 2–4.2 mm in outer diameter.

The dilatation catheter is inserted into the guiding catheter through a Y-connector. This makes it possible to continuously monitor relative pressure at the tip of the guiding catheter and to inject contrast material into the coronary ostium for visualization of the corresponding coronary arteries.

After functional capacity is defined with exercise testing and surgical backup arranged, informed consent is obtained. The patient is taken to the catheterization laboratory. Tranquilizers are used for pre-medication. Local anesthesia is accomplished with 2% Lidocaine. The femoral vein is cannulated and a pacing catheter is advanced into the right ventricular apex. This is used to control bradyarrhythmias and to serve as a spatial marker between contrast injections. The femoral artery is then punctured and a sheath is inserted. Using a 1.6 mm diameter guidewire, the selected guiding catheter is advanced retrogradely into the ascending aorta. Several medications are administered at this point to prevent thrombosis (10,000 units Heparin intravenously) and to minimize spasm (nitrates and calcium blockers). Angiograms of the vessel are obtained to define 1) anatomy and to assess the stable seating of the guiding catheter in the coronary ostium, without wedging and its hemodynamic consequences; 2) the lesion's geometry, including its eccentricity; 3) vascular path to the stenosis so that the origins of side branches are displayed; 4) identification of compromised branches at risk of closure at the time of balloon inflation; and 5) the distal vessel and its ramifications.

Subsequently, the dilatation catheter is advanced in the guiding catheter with the movable, steerable J guidewire extending from the catheter tip about 10–15 cm. Since the guidewire can be rotated 360°, it is possible to selectively advance the wire and subsequently maneuver the balloon catheter into the appropriate coronary artery. Aortic pressure and the pressure at the distal tip of the balloon catheter are continuously and simultaneously recorded. A sharp drop in the distal pressure can be noticed when the lesion has been crossed with the balloon catheter. At this point, the balloon is inflated for 20–30 seconds. Often several inflations are necessary to obtain satisfactory angiographic enlargement of the stenosis. Whenever possible the pressure gradient across the stenosis is reduced to below 15–20 mmHg for a satisfactory dilatation. Once an adequate result has been obtained with several inflations, the procedure is terminated and the pullback pressures are recorded. A post-interventional angiogram is then performed in 3 different views. Residual percent diameter stenosis is measured using a digital electronic caliper system from the mean value of the 3 projections. Approximately 3 hours after the procedure the femoral sheaths are removed after the patient returns to his room and appropriate local hemostasis applied. Patients are routinely monitored with telemetry and CPK after the procedure. Medications after the procedure include nitrates, calcium blockers, and acetylsalicylic acid.

Results

The success rates have risen and frequency of complications has lessened as experience with angioplasty increases (Table 1).

Between 1980 and July 1984, 3383 patients have undergone balloon dilatation at Emory University Hospital. Since several patients had dilatations in more than 1 artery, a total of 3774 lesions were attempted. The primary success rate overall on those lesions was 90%. Emergency coronary bypass surgery was necessary in 2.8% of the patients. MI defined by Q-waves or significant R loss was present in 2% of the patients. Mortality was 0.2%.

The primary success rate increased steadily over the years and showed a significant increase with the advent of the steerable balloon catheter in 1982.

Recently, the National Heart, Lung and Blood Institute PTCA Registry reported the results of 3079 patients. The reported primary success rate was 67%. Emergency coronary artery bypass graft surgery was neccessary in 6.6%, MI occurred in 5.3%, deaths related to PTCA occured in 0.9%. In the same report, PTCA involvement was associated with a significantly lower success rate, higher complication rate, mortality rate in women than in men. The sex difference was attributed to the high age of woman and more severe symptomatic status [6].

The long-term efficacy of PTCA is also very encouraging. After one year, 78% of patients remained improved [7]. According to the data from the National Heart, Lung and Blood Institute PTCA Registry, successful PTCA alone results in sustained improvement in 84% of patients. The angiographic recurrence rate in our institute is currently 32%. However, many patients who are asymptomatic do not undergo repeat angiogram because of their clinical well-being. Recurrence happens most commonly within the first 6 months after PTCA. A second PTCA carries a smaller complication rate and better primary success rate. Recurrence after the second dilatation is similar to the first procedure.

It is estimated that approximately 15–20% of patients requiring revascularization can be treated with PTCA. When carefully chosen, this therapeutic alternative not only has many benefits comparable with those of surgery but has additional advantages as well. This includes functional outcome, reduction in

Table 1. Emory university experience.

	Patients N	Lesions N	Primary success	Patient (%)		
				CABG	MI	Death
1980–81	518	540	82%	5.6	3.7	0
1982	813	896	91%	2.8	1.7	.1
1983	1260	1424	91%	2.1	2.0	.2
1984 (July)	792	914	92%	2.1	1.1	.4
Total	3383	3774	90%	2.8	2.0	.2

physical and emotional suffering, substantial economic savings, and reduced time lost from work.

In conclusion, the role of PTCA in the management of coronary artery disease has evolved over the past six years as experience has grown and technical advances have been made. As has been clearly demonstrated in its relatively short history, it offers an effective means of immediate palliation in symptomatic coronary artery disease. The natural history of coronary artery disease is one of progression and therapy should be of a type that can be used on a repeated basis through the years. Technical advances in our diagnostic skills hopefully will enable physicians to intervene earlier in the course of the disease prior to the compromise of ventricular function which often accompanies triple vessel disease. The main question, however, is still unanswered and that is whether PTCA is an alternative approach to coronary artery bypass graft surgery in patients with multivessel disease. Preliminary reports indicate the safety and good results of PTCA performed in multivessel coronary artery disease but the true usefulness and exact role needs to be carefully determined in a randomized study comparing coronary artery bypass surgery and PTCA. Hopefully in the future, patients with coronary artery disease can be diagnosed early before their disease progresses to severe triple vessel disease, when it may be too late for PTCA.

References

1. Favaloro RG (1968) Saphenous vein autograft replacement of severe segmental coronary occlusion: Operative technique. Am Thorac Surg 5: 334–339
2. Dotter CT, Judkins MP (1964) Transluminal treatment of atherosclerotic obstruction: Description of a new technique and a preliminary report of its application. Circulation 30: 654–670
3. Gruentzig AR, Turina MI, Schneider JA (1976) Experimental percutaneous dilatation of coronary artery stenosis (abstr). Circulation (Suppl II): 81
4. Gruentzig AR, Senning A, Siegenthaler WE (1979) Non-operative dilatation of coronary artery stenosis. NEJM 301: 61–68
5. Dorros G, Cowley MJ, Simpson J, Bentivoglio LG, Block PC, Bourassa M, Detre K, Gosselin AJ, Gruentzig AR, Kelsey SF, Kent KM, Mock MB, Mullin SM, Myler RK, Passamani ER, Stertzer SH, Williams DO (1983) Percutaneous transluminal coronary angioplasty: Report of complications from the National Heart, Lung, and Blood Institute PTCA Registry. Circulation 67: 730
6. Cowley MJ, Mullin SM, Bentivoglio LG, Block PC, Bourassa M, Detre K, Dorros G, Gosselin A, Gruentzig A, Kelsey S, Kent KM, Myler RK, Passamani ER, Simpson J, Stertzer SH, Williams DO (1983) Sex differences in results with coronary angioplasty: NHLBI PTCA Registry experience. (abstr) Circ 68 (Suppl III): 97
7. Kent KM, Bentivoglio LG, Block PC, Bourassa MG, Cowley M, Dorros G, Detre K, Gosselin AJ, Gruentzig A, Kelsley SF, Mock M, Mullin S, Passamani E, Myler RK, Simpson J, Stertzer SH, Williams DO (1983) Long-term efficacy of percutaneous transluminal coronary angioplasty (PTCA): Report from NHLBI-PTCA Registry. (abstr) Circ 68 (Suppl III): 6

Treatment of unstable angina by transluminal coronary angioplasty PTCA

J. MEYER, R. ERBEL, H.J. SCHMITZ, T. POP, K. v. OLSHAUSEN,
B. HENKEL, H.J. RUPPRECHT, H. KOPP and S. EFFERT

Abstract

The transluminal coronary angioplasty is successfully used in stable and unstable angina. If possible the first angiography and PTCA are performed within the same cath-lab procedure. By this the patient does not need to be exposed to the cath-lab situation twice. Moreover the cost for personnel and material is reduced. Out of 142 patients admitted because of unstable angina 29% were treated medically, 27% operatively, and 51% by angioplasty. In a total of 127 patients treated in Aachen and Mainz the stenosis diameter was improved from $75.9 \pm 11.7\%$ obstruction to $23.3 \pm 17.1\%$ (improvement $52.6 \pm 17.9\%$) without significant differences between concentric and eccentric or right and left coronary artery stenoses. The absolute diameter of the stenoses was improved from 0.69 ± 0.29 mm to 2.07 ± 0.48 mm (improvement 1.4 ± 0.55 mm). The primary successrate did not differ between unstable and stable angina (87% vs. 86%).

In 75 successfully treated patients a control angiography has already been performed after six months. The recurrance rate was significantly higher than in stable angina (43.9% vs. 28%). The vessel stenosis had deteriorated from $24.8 \pm 15.1\%$ immediately after the dilatation to $43.9 \pm 29.7\%$ at the six months control study. There were no significant differences between the group with lasting success and that with a restenosis with respect to the degree of the initial stenosis and the immediate result after dilatation.

The number of pathologically contracting segments was diminished from 5.1 ± 4.8 to 2.5 ± 4.1 segments in the group with good results and from 7.0 ± 5.6 to 7.0 ± 4.6 segments in patients with restenosis.

Angioplasty can be used with good results and a low complication rate in unstable as well as in stable angina. Since the trauma for the patient and the costs for personnel and material are much lower than in bypass surgery it is an alternative to it in quite a remarkable percentage of patients.

Percutaneous transluminal coronary angioplasty (PTCA) was initially used in patients with stable angina pectoris, in whom isolated stenoses of the major coronary arteries has been demonstrated [1]. It has been shown that PTCA can successfully apply both to patients with stable and with unstable angina [2–8]. The balloon technique can also be used after successful thrombolytic therapy in patients with acute myocardial infarction in order to remove the underlying

220

coronary artery stenosis [9, 10]. The aim of this study is to demonstrate the early and the late results of PTCA in patients with unstable angina.

Methods

Patients

One hundred and twenty-seven patients with the clinical picture of unstable angina were selected for PTCA. Most of them were transferred from other institutions. Eighty-three patients were treated in the years 1978–1982 in Aachen, while 44 were treated between January 1983 and July 1984 in Mainz.

Since we are a large referal center for patients with unstable angina between 1983 and 7/1984 a total of 142 patients with this syndrom were admitted to our hospital (Table 1). According to the clinical picture and the angiographical findings 31 patients (pts) (22%) were treated medically, 39 pts (27%) with bypass surgery and 72 pts (51%) by PTCA.

All patients with unstable angina had had attacks of increasingly frequent or severe pain either of recent onset or superimposed on previous by milder angina within the last three months. All patients had experienced anginal attacks at rest or during the night. The ECG's which were recorded in at least one instance from each patient in the unstable phase showed reversible ST-segment elevations or depressions and/or negative T-waves without development of new Q-waves. These patients did not show enzymatic changes. In all patients the clinical symptoms could not be sufficiently stabilizied by medical treatment consisting of nefidipine, isosorbiddinitrat, betablockers, and some times nitroglycerin-infusions.

Before the PTCA operation the principal investigator explained the protocol, the possible advantages and the risks of the method. All patients received a detailed written information form, which had been approved by the university's legal advisers. Written consent was obtained not only for PTCA but also for an immediate bypass operation, should this be necessary. All operations were scheduled at a time, when the surgical team was available for a possible emergency bypass operation.

Table 1. Patients with unstable angina admitted to the Medical University Clinic Mainz 1983 – 7/1984. Treatment according to the clinical picture and the angiographical findings.

Unstable angina 1983–7/1984
n = 142

Conservative therapy	n = 31 (22%)
Operative therapy	n = 39 (27%)
Dilatation	n = 72 (51%)

Technique of PTCA

The patient population consisted of those in whom the initial coronary angiography was performed in another hospital and who were referred to our institution for PTCA. These patients received 1,5 g of acethylsalicylic acid and 3 × 10 mg of nifedipine the day before and 500 mg acethylsalicylic acid as well as 20 mg of nifedipine the morning before PTCA. Those patients who were directly admitted to our hospital were prepared by the application of 500 mg acethylsalicylic acid and 20 mg nifedipine before the coronary angiography. If during this angiography a highgrade stenosis suitable for PTCA was found, this treatment was immediately performed within the same cath-lab session. The initial coronary angiography for these patients was always scheduled at noon-time, in order to have a surgical team in stand-by position.

Since these 127 patients were treated between October 1978 and July 1984 the PTCA technique as well as the material of the guiding catheters and the balloons was different according to the development stage. The size of the dilatation balloon was always chosen according to the diameter of the prestenotic part of the diseased coronary artery.

After PTCA all patients were monitored for 24 h in the coronary care unit, where ECG's and blood samples for enzyme levels were taken every six hours. The introducing sheeth was left in place for 24–36 h for quick access in case of late complications. Heparin was administered for 24 h after the operation at a rate of 800–1200 IU/h. The patients were usually discharged three days after the operation when after withdrawel of the sheeth the puncture side had been observed for 48 h and the control bicycle ergometry has been performed. Until 1981 the patients were put on oral coumadine-treatment, after that date on 500 mg acethylsalicylic acid until the routine repeat coronary angiography six months later the patients additionally received 3 × 10 mg of nifedipine daily.

Seventy-five of the successfully treated patients had a repeat arteriographic study. They received 1 × 10 mg of nifedipine the day before and 20 mg of nifedipine plus 1.6 mg of nitroglycerin sublingually 30 min before the control procedure. This control arteriography was performed with the whole cath-lab prepaired for an eventual repeat PTCA within the same session.

Calculation of stenosis

The degree of the stenosis was measured from a twentyfold magnified projection of the cine film. The vessel contours were outlined by hand with an ultrasonic pen and analyzed by the computer system. The degree of obstruction was calculated as the mean of the narrowest segments of all projections, in which the stenosis was clearly seen. Results were given in terms of percent stenosis of the luminal diameter. In the follow-up studies the same radiographic projections were used.

Statistics

Statistical analysis was performed using student's T-test for unpaired samples. A p value <0.05 was considered significant. All numbers given represent mean values ± standard deviation.

Results

Out of the whole group of 127 patients PTCA was successful in 99 patients (success rate 77,9%). Until early 1983 the successrate was lower. Since low-profile balloon catheters with stearable guides were available, the successrate in 1983 and 1984 has risen to 82%.

The stenosis diameter in unsuccessfully treated patients was significantly higher (p<0,02) than in those with successful treatment (82.3 ± 11.6 vs. 75.9 ± 11.7%; Figure 1). After successful treatment the luminal diameter was reduced to 23.3 ± 17.1%, the improvement being 52.6 ± 17.9%.

In 64 out of the 127 pts the obstruction was also calculated in absolute numbers (Figure 2). The stenosis diameter in unsuccessfully treated patients (0.48 ± 0.23 mm) was significantly smaller than in those with successful treatment (0.69 ± 0.29 mm, p<0.02). After successful PTCA the vessel was enlarged to 2.07 ± 0.48 mm. With the dilatation the narrowed segment was enlarged by 1.4 ± 0.55 mm.

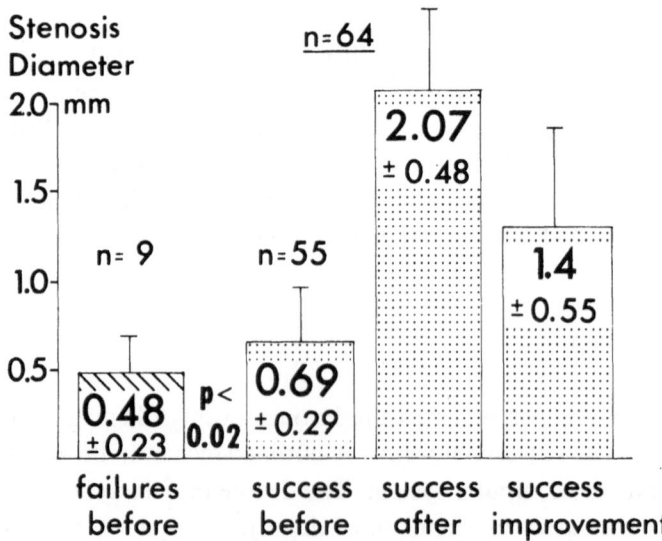

Figure 1. Improvement of coronary stenoses (percent of luminal diameter) by PTCA.

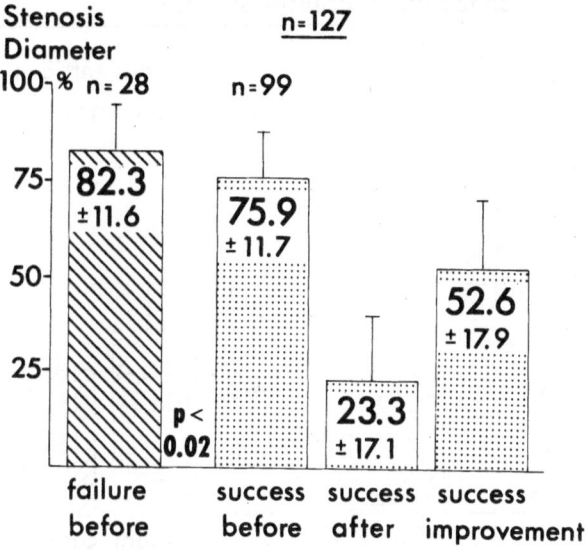

Figure 2. Improvement of coronary stenoses (absolute values, mm) by PTCA.

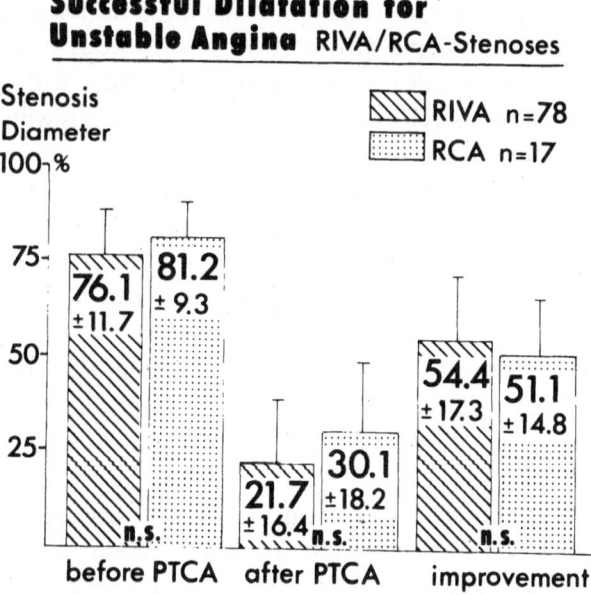

Figure 3. Improvement of vessel stenosis (percent luminal diameter). Comparison between left anterior descending artery (RIVA) and right coronary artery (RCA).

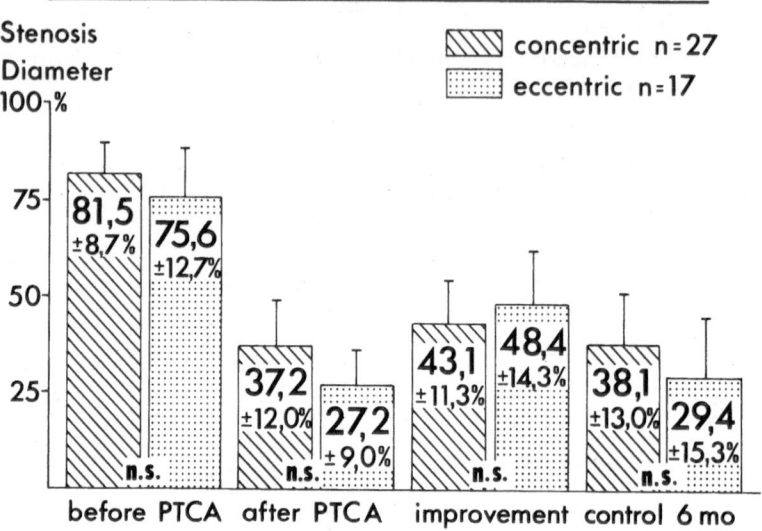

Figure 4. Comparison between concentric and excentric coronary artery stenosis (percentage of luminal diameter). Before PTCA, after PTCA, improvement and control after six months.

In order to compare the successrate in different segments of the coronary artery tree the results in 78 pts with obstructions of the left anterior descending artery (RIVA) was compared to 17 pts with obstructions of the right coronary artery (RCA) (Figure 3). There were no significant differences with respect to the degree of diameter stenosis before and after PTCA as well as with respect to the degree of improvement of the stenosis.

In a small subgroup of 44 pts with successful dilatation the behaviour of concentric stenoses was compared to eccentric stenoses. The differences of the vessel obstruction before and after PTCA were not different. Neither the immediate improvement nor the degree of obstuction at the control study six months later showed significant differences (Figure 4).

Seventy-five out of the 99 pts with successful PTCA-procedure returned for a control coronary arteriography (Figure 5). The diameter stenosis before PTCA in this subgroup was not significantly different from a total group (75.0 ± 12.4% vs. 75.9 ± 11.7%).

After PTCA the resting stenosis was calculated by 24.8 ± 15.1% (degree of the whole group 23.3 ± 17.1%). The degree of improvement was at least 20% of luminal diameter. In some cases nearly no residual stenosis was found. At the six months control study a wide scatter of measurements was found with an average diameter obstruction of 43.9 ± 29.7%. While in some patients the luminal diameter had slightly enlarged spontaneously a reobstruction occurred in others.

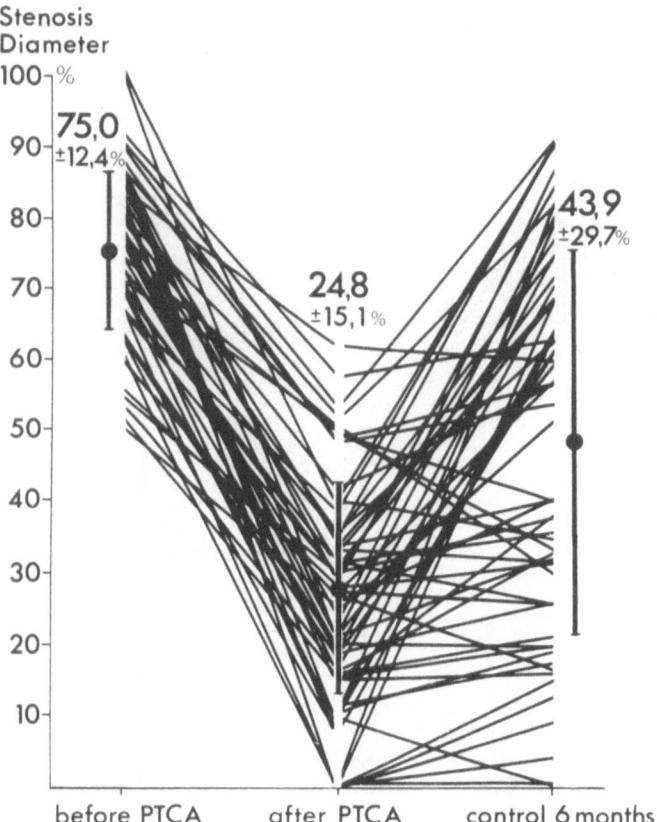

Dilatation for Unstable Angina n=75

Stenosis Diameter

Figure 5. Development of coronary stenosis in 75 patients (percentage of luminal diameter), before and after PTCA and at the control study (six months).

In 29 patients (39%) a relapse was found (73.5 ± 12.3%). In 46 pts the dilatation success was permanent (24.4 ± 18.3%). If more than 50% of the initially reached improvement had disappeared at the control study the case was regarded to be a relapse.

If the stenosis diameters of the patients with permanent success and those with a relapse were compared (Figure 6) there was no significant difference in the angiographic situation before PTCA (76.9 ± 10.9% vs. 71.9 ± 13.1%). Immediately after PTCA both groups did also not differ significantly (26.1 ± 15.7% vs. 23.0 ± 16.1%).

In 34 out of 75 pts we were able to compare left ventricular angiograms before PTCA to those at the six months control study (Figure 7). In this group the heart

Dilatation Unstable Angina n=75

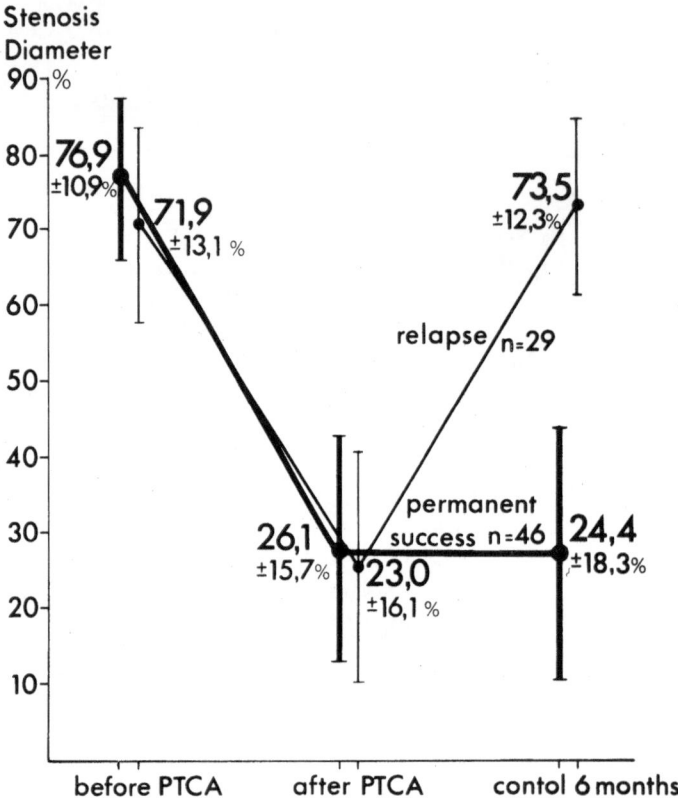

Figure 6. Comparison between patients with permanently patent vessels and those with relapse of coronary stenosis.

rate between both studies was comparable (frequency difference ± 5 beats/min). There were also no extrasystoles or tachyarrhythmic episodes during the angiography. In 20 pts with good angiographical late results 5.1 ± 4.8 wall segments showed a pathological contraction pattern in the acute phase. At the control study only 2.5 ± 4.1 segments were abnormal. Despite a good coronary angiographic result two pts at the control study showed al larger hypokinesia than in the acute phase. In the group with angiographically proven restenosies there were no significant differences between the acute phase and the control study.

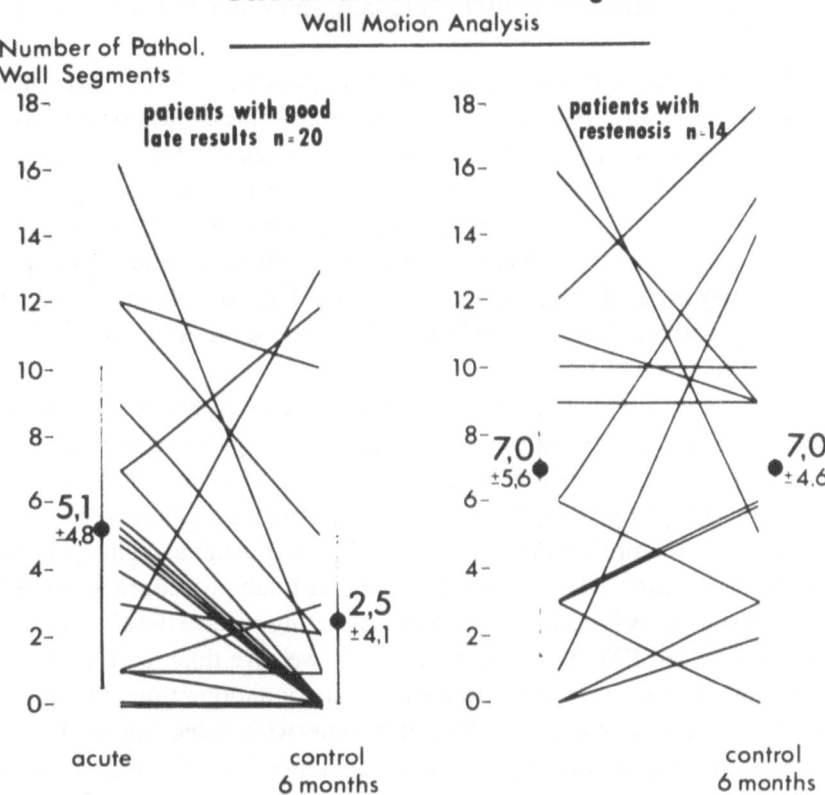

Dilatation for Unstable Angina
Wall Motion Analysis

Number of Pathol.
Wall Segments

patients with good late results n = 20

patients with restenosis n - 14

Figure 7. Analysis of number of pathological wall segments before PTCA and at the control study after six months. Improvement in patients with good late results. Non significant variations in patients with restenosis.

Discussion

The clinical syndrom of unstable angina has attracted great interest over the last 10 years with respect to diagnosis, follow-up, and medical as well as surgical treatment [2–6, 11]. The rate of total vessel obstruction within the first six months after diagnosis is quite remarkable [11]. Despite an initial stabilisation of symptoms the mortality rate during the first year after the first unstable phase is high. At least 30% of patients with unstable angina show a single vessel disease, approximately an other 30% a double vessel disease with mostly isolated, proximal subtotal stenoses of a major coronary artery. Such patients often between 30 and 40 years of age are potential candidates for PTCA. The stenoses are more often located in the LAD than in the RCA. As we have shown, however, they can be treated equally good [3, 4]. There were no significant differences with respect to the degree of stenosis before and after treatment. Patients with isolated stenoses of the left circumflex artery seldomly show symptoms requiring angiography.

To exclude coronary spasms we pretreated the patients with nitroglycerin and nifedipine. From reasons that are not fully understood, the clinical symptoms and apparently also the degree of arterial obstruction often change very rapidly in patients with unstable angina. This may be the reason why despite the full clinical picture of unstable angina during angiography in some patients the degree of vessel obstruction is only between 50 and 70%. Probably additional spastic components may occur during the anginal phases [12]. Possibly the patho-physiologic process and the kind of organic material of the stenosic area are different from that in the chronic stable form [13].

Since 1978 we have extended the indication for PTCA also to patients with unstable angina. During the following years coronary angioplasty has become an established treatment for this threatening form of the coronary artery disease. It has been shown [2–4], that PTCA can be performed with equally good results and with the same low complication rate as in patients with stable angina pectoris.

We prefer to perform PTCA within the same cath-lab procedure in which the coronary arteriography is done. The patients therefore receive the same pretreatment as in scheduled PTCA procedures. By this we save time, cost, and equipment. The patient has not to return to the cath-lab for another time. In our hands the complication rate was similar to that of patients with stable angina [4]. In the whole series, despite all our early results beginning from the year 1978 were included, the rate of infarction plus vessel obstruction was only 2,1%. The mortality rate was 0.8%. These numbers are quite comparable to those in good series of bypass surgery in unstable angina.

Up to now there is no good explanation why in some patients despite an initially good angiographical result the coronary vessels show a restenosis after six months, while in others the permanent success can be noted [14–21]. From this series we do not have the impression that the degree of the initial stenosis plays a role. There is also no difference in the percentage of vessel obstruction immediately after dilatation nor in the amount of improvement [21]. These differences are also not explained by the pre-, intra-operative or post-operative treatment [22]. The follow-up treatment during the six months interval until the control study was also comparable. It consisted of nifedipine and acetylsalicylic acid, until 1980 also in coumadine.

While the initial PTCA results were quite satisfying and the rate of complication was low, the restenosis rate is too high. Despite a redilatation during the control angiography does not pose too much molestation to the patient, the high restenosis rate is disappointing [23]. Up to now there is no satisfactory explanation for this. Probably the coronary artery disease in these patients is in another phase of its development. Further studies have to show why the disease changes from the stable to the unstable phase and why the rapid development occurs.

The study has shown that PTCA can effectively and economically [24, 25] dilate highly stenotic coronary vessels and improve coronary perfusion in unstable angina. In double and triple vessel diseases the dilatation should be performed first in the vessel with the highest obstruction [26, 27]. According to the clinical picture further stenoses in separate vessels may be dilated within the same cath-lab procedure or after watching the patient carefully for 24 h on the next day.

With the newly available improved catheter material the success rate at the moment exceeds 90%. In case of recurrent stenosis PTCA can easily be repeated. It can postpone the time of bypass graft surgery in a number of cases. It will at least gain time in critical clinical situations, until bypass surgery is available. The trauma for the patient is much less than with bypass surgery. The costs for equipment, material, and personnel staff is about 20% of that for bypass surgery [24, 25]. After a total hospital stay of five days the patient can return to work one week later.

It is to be expected, that the indications and possibilities of angioplasty will be influenced by further technical developments of the catheter material [5, 16, 23, 26, 27]. The method is still in a developmental phase. Its possibilities and limitations therefore must be thought over and defined critically within the future.

References

1. Grüntzig AR, Senning A, Siegenthaler WE (1979) Nonoperative dilatation of coronary artery stenosis: Percutaneous transluminal coronary angioplasty. N Engl J Med 301: 61–68
2. Meyer J, Böcker B, Erbel R, Bardos P, Messmer BJ, Effert S (1980) Treatment of unstable angina with transluminal coronary angioplasty (PTCA). Circulation 62/III: 160
3. Meyer J, Schmitz H, Erbel R, Kiesslich T, Böcker-Josephs B, Krebs W, Braun PC, Bardos P, Minale C, Messmer BJ, Effert S (1981) Treatment of unstable angina pectoris with percutaneous transluminal coronary angioplasty. Cath Cardiov Diagnosis 7: 361–371
4. Meyer J, Schmitz HJ, Kiesslich T, Erbel R, Krebs W, Schulz W, Bardos P, Minale C, Messmer BJ, Effert S (1983) Percutaneous transluminal coronary angioplasty in patients with stable and unstable angina pectoris: Analysis of early and late results. Am Heart J 106: 973–980
5. Meyer J, Erbel R, Schmitz HJ, Pop T, Meinertz T, Schreiner G, Henkel B, Henrichs HJ, Rupprecht HJ, Effert S (1984) Transluminale Angioplastik – Unstabile Angina, frischer Infarkt. 50 Jahrestg Dtsch Ges Herz-und Kreislaufforschg, Mannheim, 1984. Z Kardiol 73/II: 167–176
6. Williams DO, Riley RS, Singh AK, Gewirtz H, Most RS (1981) Evaluation of the role of coronary angioplasty in patients with unstable angina pectoris. Am Heart J 102: 1–9
7. David PR, Waters DD, Scholl JM, Crepeau J, Szlachcic J, Lespérance J, Hudon G, Bourassa M (1982) Percutaneous transluminal coronary angioplasty in patients with variant angina. Circulation 66: 695–702
8. Faxon DP, Detre KM, McCabe CH, Fisher L, Holmes DR, Cowley MJ, Bourassa MG, van Raden M, Ryan TJ (1984) Role of percutaneous transluminal coronary angioplasty in the treatment of unstable angina: Report from the National Heart, Lung, and Blood Institute percutaneous transluminal coronary angioplasty and coronary artery surgery study registries. Am J Cardiol 53: 131–135
9. Meyer J, Merx W, Schmitz H, Erbel R, Kiesslich T, Dörr R, Lambert H, Bethge C, Krebs W,

Bardos P, Minale C, Messmer BJ, Effert S (1982) Percutaneous transluminal coronary angioplasty immediately after intracoronary streptolysis of transmural myocardial infarction. Circulation 66: 905–913

10. Serruys PW, Wijns W, Van den Brand M (1983) Is transluminal coronary angioplasty mandatory after successful thrombolysis? Quantitative coronary angiographic study. Br Heart J 50: 257–265

11. Moise A, Thereoux P, Taeymans Y, Descoings B, Lespérance J, Waters DD, Pelletier GB, Bourassa MG (1983) Unstable angina and progression of coronary atherosclerosis. New Engl J Med 309: 685

12. Grüntzig AR Douglas Jr JS, King III SB (1983) Coronary artery spasm at the site of angioplasty in the first 2 months after successful percutaneous transluminal coronary angioplasty. J. Amer Coll Cardiol 2: 1039

13. Kramer JR, Matsuda I, Mulligan JC, Aranow M, Proudfit WL (1981) Progression of coronary atherosclerosis. Circulation 63: 519–526

14. Meier B, Grüntzig AR, Siegenthaler WE, Schlumpf M (1983) Long-term performance after percutaneous transluminal coronary angioplasty and coronary artery bypass grafting. Circulation 68: 796–802

15. Kaltenbach M, Kober G, Schmidt-Moritz A, Scherer D (1983) Rezidivhäufigkeit nach erfolgreicher transluminaler Koronarangioplastik. Dtsch med Wschr 108: 1387–1390

16. Grüntzig AR (1984) Percutaneous transluminal coronary angioplasty: 6 years experience. Am Heart J 107: 818

17. Holmes DR Jr, Vlietstra RE, Smith HC, Vetrovec GW, Kent KM, Cowley MJ, Faxon DP, Grüntzig AR, Kelsey SF, Detre KM, van Raden MJ, Mock MB (1984) Restenosis after percutaneous transluminal coronary angioplasty (PTCA): A report from the PTCA registry of the National Heart, Lung, and Blood Institute. Am J Cardiol 53: 77–81

18. Kent KM, Bentivoglio LG, Block PC (1984) Long-term efficacy of percutaneous transluminal coronary angioplasty (PTCA): Report from the National Heart, Lung, and Blood Institute PTCA registry. Am J Cardiol 53: 27–31

19. Swan MJC (1982) Thrombolysis in acute myocardial infarction: Treatment of the underlying coronary artery disease. Circulation 66: 914–915

20. Faxon DP, Kelsey SF, Ryan TJ, McCabe CH, Detre K (1984) Determinants of successful percutaneous transluminal coronary angioplasty: Report from the National Heart, Lung, and Blood Institute Registry. Am Heart J 108: 1019

21. Schmitz HJ, Meyer J, Kiesslich T, Effert S (1982) Greater initial dilatation gives better late angiographic results in percutaneous coronary angioplasty (PTCA). Circulation 66/II: 123

22. Thornton MA, Grüntzig AR, Hollman J, King SB, Douglas JS (1984) Coumadin and aspirin in prevention of recurrence after transluminal coronary angioplasty: a randomized study. Circulation 69: 721–727

23. Meier B, King III SB, Grüntzig AR, Douglas JS, Hollman J, Ischinger T, Galan K, Tankersley R (1984) Repeat Coronary Angioplasty. J Am Coll Cardiol 4: 463

24. Jang GC, Block PC, Cowley MJ, Grüntzig AR, Dorros G, Holmes Jr DR Kent KM, Leatherman LL, Myler RK, Sjolander SME, Stertzer SH, Vetrovec GW, Willis Jr WH, Williams DO (1984) Relative cost of coronary angioplasty and bypass surgery in a one-vessel disease model. Am J Cardiol 53: 52–55

25. Holmes DR, van Raden MJ, Reeder GS, Vlietstra RE, Jang GC, Kent KM, Vetrovec GW, Cowley MJ, Dorros G, Kelsey SF, Detre KM, Mock MB (1984) Return to work after coronary angioplasty: A report from the National Heart, Lung, and Blood Institute percutaneous transluminal coronary angioplasty registry. Am J Cardiol 53 (1984): 48–51

26. Hartzler GO (1983) Percutaneous transluminal coronary angioplasty in multivessel disease. Cath Cardiov Diagn 9: 537

27. Dorros G, Stertzer SH, Cowley MJ, Myler RK (1984) Complex coronary angioplasty: Multiple coronary dilatations. Am J Cardiol 53: 126–130

Coronary angioplasty in multivessel disease

GEOFFREY O. HARTZLER, BARRY D. RUTHERFORD, DAVID R. McCONAHAY and WARREN L. JOHNSON, JR.

Introduction

During the past five years, the indications for coronary angioplasty have changed dramatically. In many centers, the procedure is no longer restricted to patients with single coronary stenoses but is being applied more aggressively by experienced and skilled interventional Cardiologists to patients with multiple vessel disease requiring multiple lesion PTCA [1–2]. With modification, Dr. Gruentzig's initial therapeutic procedure has been refined and applied successfully to patients with multiple vessel disease, left main coronary stenoses, previous bypass surgery, poor left ventricular function, acute myocardial infarction and other clinical circumstances previously felt to contraindicate the procedure [1–6].

With increased experience and improved catheter technologies, it was inevitable that PTCA would come to play a more important role in the mangements of patients with coronary artery disease than the predicted 5% of patients undergoing coronary angiography. In our own experience, approximately 50% of patients who would have otherwise been considered candidates for coronary bypass surgery are alternatively treated with coronary angioplasty. In fact, previous contraindications for PTCA (e.g. acute infarction, poor left ventricular function) now serve as indications for the procedure.

Results

Total experience

Between July of 1980 and July of 1984, a group of four Cardiologists at the Mid-America Heart Institute of St. Luke's Hospital in Kanses City, Missouri, performed 2500 consecutive PTCA procedures, attempting to dilate 4453 coronary stenoses. There were 1972 males and 528 females with age range 22–84 years, mean age 59 years. Utilizing the original NHLBI criteria, 91% over of all stenoses attempted were successfully dilated.

The total experience is one of marked evolution. Initially, we utilized standard 'fixed wire' angioplasty catheters for the first approximate 800 patients followed by a transition to movable wire systems and ultimately directionally changeable catheters. In the past two years, we have utilized a wide variety of guiding catheters, balloon catheters and guide catheters representing products of the two major manufacturers of angioplasty products within the United States. Based on this experience and at the time of this writing, the authors acknowledge that successful complex and multiple vessel angioplasty requires the availability and use of multiple guiding catheters having differing configurations and physical properties, multiple balloon catheters of differing deflated and inflated dimension, and guide wires with varying properties of torque control and flexibility. In the authors' opinion, the most important technical innovation facilitating the performance of multiple vessel angioplasty was the creation of a freely moving, directionally changeable yet extremely flexible guide wire – polyethylene balloon catheter system (Advanced Cardiovascular Systems, Inc., Mountain View, California).

Within the total experience, the left anterior descending coronary artery and its branches comprised 41% of lesions attempted with a 91% primary success rate. The right coronary artery and its branches comprised 30% of this series with a 90% primary success rate. The circumflex artery and its branches comprised 25% of this series with a 92% primary success rate. In addition, 171 vein graft dilatations were attempted with a 91% success rate and 32 left main coronary artery dilatations were attempted with a 78% success rate. Virtually all segments of the coronary circulation have been dilated including right and left internal mammary artery bypass grafts, native coronary vessels through internal mammary bypass grafts and through previously placed saphenous vein grafts, anomalous circumflex arteries arising from the right coronary artery, anomalous right coronary arteries, septal perforators, conus and acute marginal branches. Recently, a small balloon catheter was passed through a collateral communication from the left AV groove branch of the circumflex artery into the posterolateral branch of the right coronary artery to dilate a stenosis in this otherwise inaccessible branch because of a proximal right coronary occlusion.

We have performed angioplasty in patients with chronic renal failure on dialysis, 'inoperable' patients with malignancy and other severe systemic illnesses, patients with unstable neurologic syndromes resulting from severe cerebrovascular disease, and patients with active systemic infections with unstable angina.

Multiple lesion PTCA experience (Table 1)

One thousand-one hundred-eleven (44%) of the first 2500 PTCA procedures included dilatation of 2 or more stenoses. There were 889 males and 222 females with an age range of 22–84 years, mean age of 58 years. Two lesions were attempted in 614 procedures, 3 lesions were attempted in 296 procedures, 4 lesions were attempted in 108 procedures and from 5–10 lesions were attempted in

Table 1. Multiple lesion PTCA Mid America Heart Institute* St. Luke's Hospital Kansas City, Missouri U.S.A.

Population	
Males	889 (80%)
Females	222 (20%)
Age – 22–84 yrs (m = 58 yrs)	
	1111 (44%)
Lesions Attempted	
Two	614 (25%)
Three	296 (12%)
Four	108 (4%)
Five-Ten	93 (3.7%)
Success	
2873/3064 (94%) lesions attempted	
Complete revascularization	953 (86%)
Partial revascularization	155 (14%)
Complications	
Urgent surgery	17 (1.5%)
Transmural infarction	15 (1.4%)
Death	9 (0.8%)

*Cardiovascular Consultants, Inc.

93 procedures. Of 3064 stenoses attempted during multiple lesion PTCA, 2873 or 94% were successfully dilated. However, only 953 patients (86%) had 'complete' revascularization defined as successful dilatation of all lesions attempted. One hundred-fifty-five or 14% of patients had partial revascularization. Still, approximately 90% of those patients having partial revascularization were rendered asymptomatic or improved by the procedure. In part, this reflects our general policy of commencing the multiple lesion PTCA procedure by attempting to dilate the clinically most significant stenosis first. Of course, many exceptions exist to this general directive, particularly in the setting of prior occlusion of one or more coronary arteries with collateral circulation present. In those circumstances we generally first attempt to recanalize the totally obstructed artery and create a situation where collateral flow may reverse from the previously obstructed artery to the narrowed yet patent vessel undergoing primary dilatation.

Discussion

This brief communication summarizes the results of a large and continuing experience with multiple lesion and multiple vessel coronary angioplasty. It clearly establishes that multiple lesion PTCA can be accomplished with relatively low risk and a high degree of technical success. Further, 'palliative' multiple lesion PTCA without complete revascularization may benefit a majority of patients, at least for the short term.

Vital long-term follow-up data is incomplete at the present time. Consequently, multiple lesion and multiple vessel PTCA has not yet been fully characterized and its application cannot yet be recommended on a widespread basis.

The incidence of restenosis in patients with predominantly single vessel disease undergoing single lesion dilatation has been described by numerous authors in multiple reports including one from the NHLBI registry [1]. However, this data cannot be extrapolated to patients undergoing multiple lesion dilatation. Although one might conclude that if two or three lesions are dilated, the patient should experience a two to threefold increase in the incidence of restenosis, this pattern has not been observed in our clinical practice. Patterns of restenosis in multiple vessel PTCA patients have been unpredictable. When symptoms recur following multiple vessel PTCA, we have frequently observed the recurrence of a single stenosis only, or the presence of a new lesion in a coronary segment previously not dilated. Obviously, much clinical investigation will be required to fully characterize and define the long-term results of multivessel PTCA.

Clinical follow-up data is being obtained on the 1111 patients described in this report but at the present time is incomplete and not supported by a high level of late, routine follow-up angiography. In our institution, several trials are underway with the multiple vessel population of patients including a randomized quantitative angiographic study assessing the true incidence of late restenosis and the potential benefit of certain medications.

Ultimately, a randomized trial comparing multiple vessel PTCA with multiple vessel bypass surgery may be appropriate. However, at the present time, the widespread lack of experience and technical skills allowing the rigorous performance of multiple vessel PTCA do not exist. Such a comparison may be further skewed by failure to compare procedural costs, procedure related morbid events other than myocardial infarction and death, length of hospital stay, procedure-related psychological trauma and the ability to resume productive work following PTCA or coronary bypass surgery.

The future of coronary angioplasty resides within our ability to safely and effectively apply this technique to patients with multiple vessel disease, and to establish or create a satisfactory long-term result.

References

1. Dorros G, Stertzer SH, Cowley M, Kent K, Williams D (1982) Complex transluminal coronary angioplasty: Multivessel disease and multiple dilatations. Circulation (suppl 11): 2–329, (abstr)
2. Hartzler GO, Rutherford BD, McConahay DR, McCallister SH (1982) Simultaneous multiple lesion coronary angioplasty. A preferred therapy for patients with multiple vessel disease. Circulation 66 (suppl 11): 11–5 (abstr)

3. Douglas JS, Gruentzig AR, King SB, Holman J, Ischinger T, Meier B, Craver JM, Jones EL, Waller JL, Bone DK, Guyton R (1983) Percutaneous transluminal coronary angioplasty in patients with prior coronary bypass surgery. JACC 2: 745–54

4. Meyer J, Merx W, Doerr R, Lambertz H, Bethge C, Effert S (1982) Successful treatment of acute myocardial infarction shock by combined percutaneous transluminal coronary revascularization (PTCR) and percutaneous transluminal coronary angioplasty (PTCA). Am Heart J 103: 132–137

5. Hartzler GO, Rutherford BD, McConahay DR, Johnson WL, McCallister BD, Gura GM, Conn RD, Crockett JE (1983) Percutaneous transluminal coronary angioplasty with and without thrombolytic therapy for treatment of acute myocardial infarction. Am Heart J 106: 965–973

6. Hartzler GO, Rutherford BD, McConahay DR (1984) Percutaneous transluminal coronary angioplasty: Application for acute myocardial infarction. Am J Cardiol 53: 177C–121C

7. Holmes DR, Vlietstra RE, Smith HC, Vetrovec GW, Cowley MG, Kent KM, Detre KM, Myler R (1982) Restenosis following percutaneous transluminal coronary angioplasty (PTCA): A report from the NHLBI PTCA registry. Am J Cardiol 49: 905 (abstr)

Effect of coronary occlusion during percutaneous transluminal angioplasty on systolic and diastolic left ventricular function

PATRICK W. SERRUYS, WILLIAM WIJNS, MARCEL VAN DEN
BRAND, CORNELIS SLAGER, JOERG GRIMM, BRIAN E. JASKI,
RONALD W. BROWER, OTTO M HESS and PAUL G. HUGENHOLTZ

Abstract

The response of left ventricular function, was studied in a series of patients undergoing percutaneous transluminal coronary angioplasty (PTCA). From 4 to 6 balloon inflations procedures per patient were performed with an average duration per occlusion of 51 ± 12 sec (mean $\pm$ sd) with a total occlusion time of 252 ± 140 sec. Analysis of LV hemodynamics showed that the relaxation parameters peak negative rate of change of pressure and the early time constant of relaxation responded earliest to acute coronary occlusion while other parameters such as peak P, LV end-diastolic pressure, and peak positive rate of change of pressure responded more gradually and suggested a progressive depression in myocardial mechanics during the entire procedure. LV angiograms available in 14 patients indicated an early onset of asynchronous relaxation concurrent with the early response in peak $-dP/dt$ and the time constant of early relaxation.

Similarly, ischemia induced by complete occlusion of the left anterior descending artery in as little as 20 seconds increased the chamber stiffness of the anterior wall which resulted in an alteration of the global diastolic properties of the left ventricle. Fifteen minutes after the end of the procedure, the constant of global chamber stiffness had returned to control values despite a persisting increase in regional stiffness in the core of the ischemic zone. The latter finding contrasts with the perfect reversibility of the abnormalities in global and regional systolic function, as shown from the indices of isovolumic contraction and relaxation and segmental wall motion. This may suggest that complete recovery of a normal diastolic regional function after repeated ischemic injuries is delayed after restoration of a normal systolic function.

Introduction

Until recently, the measurement in man of left ventricular geometry and hemodynamics early after an abrupt occlusion of a major coronary artery had not been feasible. Percutaneous transluminal coronary angioplasty (PTCA) however, now provides a unique opportunity to study the time course of these variables during the transient interruption of coronary flow in the balloon occlusion sequence in patients with single vessel disease and without angiographically demonstrable collateral circulation [1, 2]. We report here the dynamic changes in left ventricular hemodynamics and the concurrent left ventricular geometry changes assessed by angiography in 14 patients during PTCA. This study was undertaken in order to investigate the sequence of events during transient ischemia induced by trans-luminal angioplasty and to determine whether the effects of ischemia after repeated occlusions were reversible or not.

Study population and protocol

Fourteen patients were selected from 356 consecutive attempted angioplasty procedures. These patients met the criteria of an isolated obstructive lesion of one coronary vessel (left anterior descending artery in ten patients, right coronary in four, left circumflex in one) having a normal resting left ventricular function and wall motion. Four patients had mild essential hypertension and elevated left ventricular filling pressures (EDP >25 mmHg). During the PTCA procedure the number of transluminal occlusions performed per patient was 4.9 ± 2.2 (mean $\pm$ SD).

The average duration of each occlusion was 51 ± 12 sec (mean $\pm$ SD) and the total occlusion time during the whole procedure was 252 ± 140 sec (mean $\pm$ SD). With a tipmanometer 8F pigtail catheter, pressures were recorded and derived variables were calculated off-line by a computer system [3, 4].

Three to four ventriculograms (30 degrees RAO at 50 frames/sec) were obtained by injection of 0.75 ml/kg of a non ionic contrast medium (metrizamide, Amipaque [R]). The hemodynamic and angiographic investigations were performed before the PTCA procedure was begun, after 20 sec of occlusion during the second dilatation, after 50 sec of occlusion during the fourth dilatation, and again 5 minutes after completion of the PTCA procedure. These sequential LV angiograms were made only after the values for left ventricular end-diastolic pressure and the various isovolumic parameters had returned to those recorded before the initial angiogram. In all cases, the interval between any two angiograms was at least 10 minutes. Care was taken to maintain the patient's position unchanged in relation to the X-ray equipment during the consecutive angiograms. Diaphragm movement was reduced to a minimum by instructing the patient to take a shallow inspiration with care to prevent the Valsalva manoeuvre.

Methods

A. Analysis of pressure derived indices during systole and diastole

Left ventricular pressure was measured with a Millar micromanometer catheter and digitized at 250 samples/sec. Combined analog and digital filtering resulted in an effective time constant of less than 10 msec. This employed an updated version of the beat-to-beat program described previously [3, 4].

Peak LV pressure, LV end-diastolic pressure, peak negative dP/dt, peak positive dP/dt and the relation between dP/dt/P and P linearly extrapolated to P = 0 (V_{max}) were computed on line after a data acquisition of 20 seconds.

Determination of relaxation parameters
A new technique has been implemented for the off-line beat-to-beat calculation of the relaxation parameters [5, 6, 7], using a semilogarithmic model:
$P(t) = P_oe^{-t/T}$ The Po and T parameters are estimated from a linear least squares fit of $LnP = -t/T + LnP_o$, starting from the time of peak $-dP/dt$.
a) fit of first 40 msec   (n >8), T_1, bi-exponential [7]
b) fit after the first 40 msec   (n >8), T_2, bi-exponential [7]
c) fit of all points   (n >8), T, mono-exponential

B. Analysis of global and regional left ventricular function, during systole and diastole

A complete cardiac cycle was analyzed frame by frame from all cineangiograms. The ventricular contour was detected automatically [8]. For each analyzed cineframe left ventricular volume was computed according to Simpson's rule. After the end-diastolic and end-systolic frames were determined, stroke volume, global ejection fraction and total cardiac index were computed. End-diastolic (ED) pressure was defined at that point on the pressure trace at which the derivative of the pressure first exceeded 200 mmHg/sec [3] and in all cases coincided with the maximal measured LV volume.

End-systole (ES) was defined, with reference to the pressure tracing, at the occurrence of the dicrotic notch of the central aortic pressure. To analyze the regional left ventricular function, the computer generated a system of coordinates along which the left ventricular wall displacement is determined frame by frame in 20 segments (Figure 1). The definition of the 20 segmental coordinates was derived from the mean trajectories of endocardial sites in 23 normal individuals [9] and generalized as a mathematical expression amenable to automatic data processing [10, 11].

Segmental wall velocity was computed as the first derivative of the instantaneous displacement function. Mean ejection phase wall velocity (V) for each

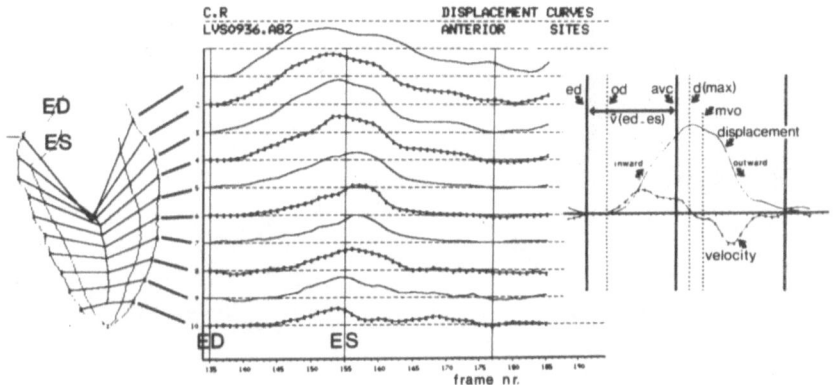

Figure 1. End-diastolic and end-systolic left ventricular contours, as detected by the automated analysis system. On these silhouettes is superimposed a system of coordinates along which segmental left ventricular wall displacement is detected. Left ventricular wall velocity – first derivative of wall displacement – is derived from these data. Abbreviations: ed: end-diastole; es: end-systole; od: onset of displacement; v(ed-es): mean ejection phase wall velocity; d(max): maximal inward wall displacement; mvo: mitral valve opening.

segment was calculated from end-diastole to end-systole (V_{ed-es}), (Figure 1). Segmental volume was computed from the local radius (R) and the height of each segment (1/10 of left ventricular long axis length L) according the formula:

$\frac{1}{20} \Pi R^2 L$, when normalized for end-diastolic volume, the systolic segmental volume change can be considered as a parameter of regional pump function (Figure 2). During systole this parameter expresses quantitatively the contribution of a particular segment to global ejection fraction, termed regional contribution to global ejection fraction or CREF [10]. The sum of the values for all 20 segments equals the global ejection fraction.

For the evaluation of the global chamber stiffness, the left ventricular pressure (P) and volume (V) data obtained every 20 msec starting at the lowest diastolic pressure and ending at the end-diastolic pressure were fitted by a simple elastic model: $P = ae^{bv} + c$, where a = intercept (mmHg), b = constant of elastic chamber stiffness and c = baseline pressure (mmHg). The three constants of this equation (a, b, c) were determined using an iteration procedure until the best non-linear curve fit was obtained [12].

As mentioned above, left ventricular wall displacement was determined along a system a 20 coordinates derived from the previously described 'endocardial land marker model' [9, 10]. The length of these 20 segmental coordinates was measured frame by frame and among them, we selected 3 pairs of segments located in the core of the ischemic zone (anterolateral and apical segments), in the non-ischemic zone (anterobasal and posterobasal segments) and immediately adjacent to the ischemic zone (inferior and anterior segments), as shown in Figure 3.

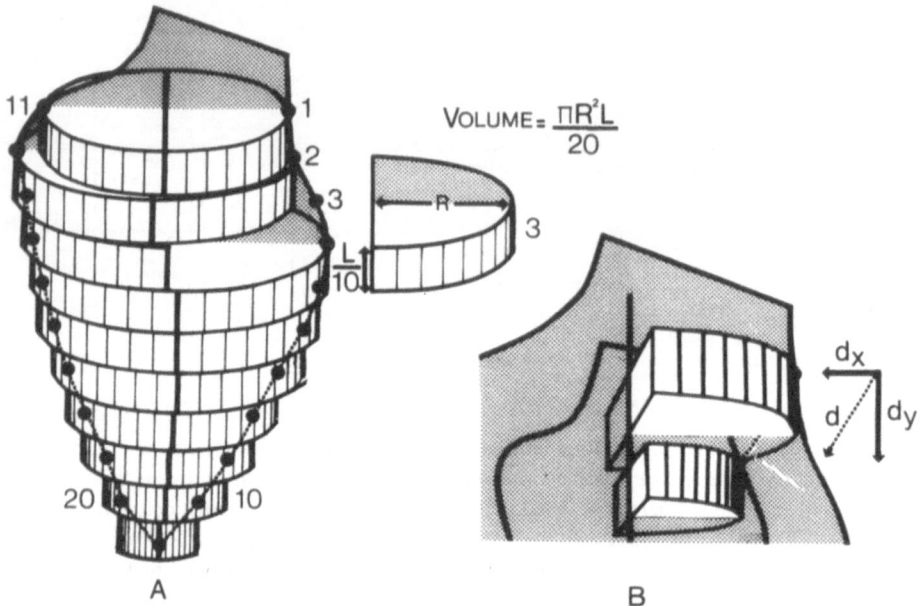

Figure 2. Method for computing regional contibution to ejection fraction (CREF): volume of each segment (slice volume) is computed according to the formula shown in the figure. The systolic volume change is derived from the regional displacement and is mainly a consequence of the decrease of radius (R) of a half slice, which is expressed by the x-component (dx) of the displacement vector (d). L: left ventricular long axis length extending from base to apex.

For the evaluation of the regional chamber stiffness the left ventricular pressure and the segment length (L) data were fitted in a similar way for each of the six analyzed segmental coordinates: $P = ae^{bl} + c$, where b represents the regional elastic stiffness for a given segment. The latter approach was applied previously by others to pressure-length [13] and pressure-circumference [14] relations.

Statistical analysis
Results are given either as mean ± standard deviation or as median values. Comparisons between pre-PTCA, post-PTCA, 20 sec, and 50 sec occlusion conditions were performed using two way analysis of variance with orthogonal contrast.

Results

A. Global left ventricular function during systole and diastole

The left ventricular pressures and volumes measured before, during, and after angioplasty are shown in Table 1. There was no important change in heart rate

REGIONAL CHAMBER STIFFNESS

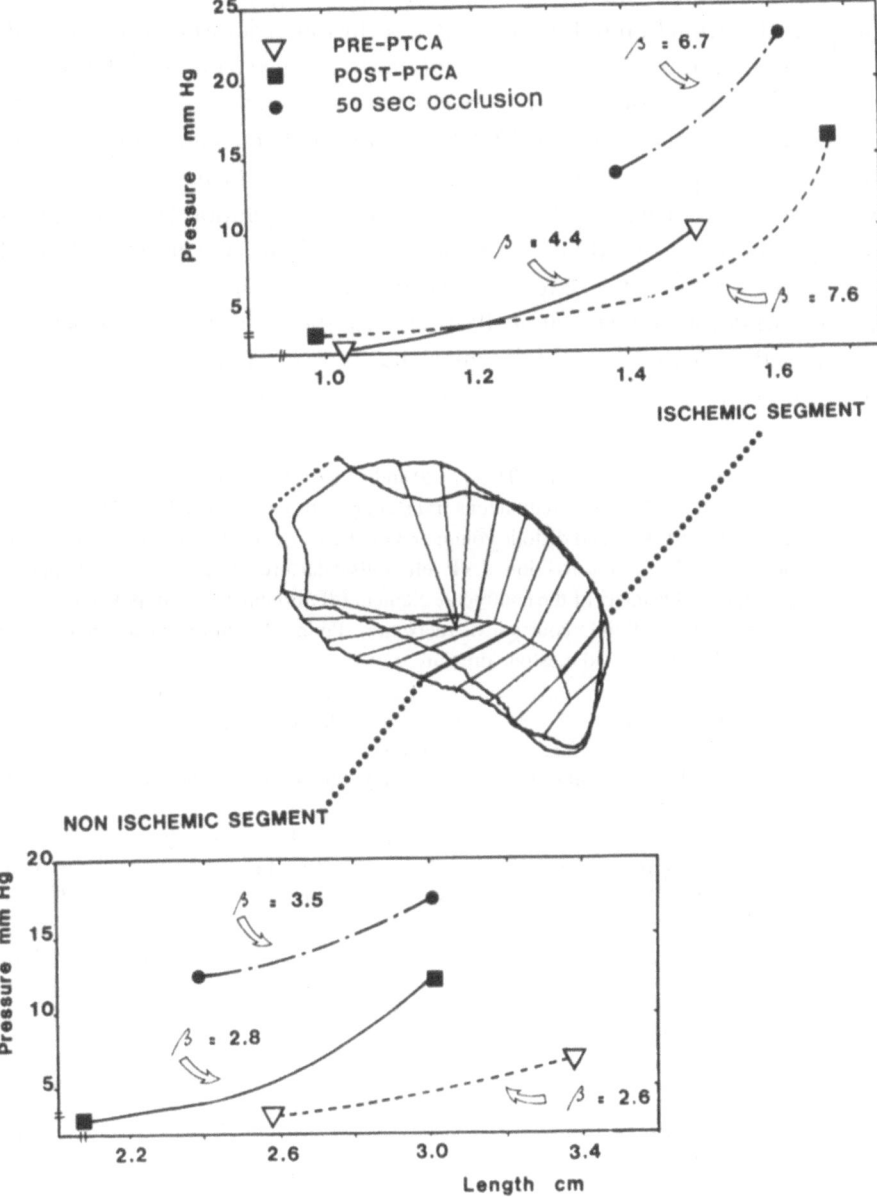

Figure 3. For the evaluation of the regional chamber stiffness pairs of segments located in the core of the ischemic (anterolateral and apical segments) or in the non-ischemic zone (anterobasal and posterobasal segments) were selected. For each of the analyzed segmental coordinates the left ventricular pressure (P) and the segment length (L) data were fitted according to the following formula: $P = ae^{bl} + c$, where b represents the regional elastic stiffness constant for a given segment.

during the PTCA procedure. The pattern of change in peak LVP, LVEDP, peak
+ dP/dt, and V_{max}, however, suggests a progressive depression in myocardial
mechanics without any indication of an early peak (Figure 4).

In contrast, within four of five beats after occlusion, a deformation appeared in
the ascending limb of the negative dP/dt curve (Figure 5) and in the next ten
seconds this deformation in the negative dP/dt curve gradually increased so that
the irregularity in the negative dP/dt curve reached the same height as peak
−dP/dt which has progressively decreased to its nadir. In the next 20–50 sec, peak
−dP/dt began to return towards control levels with a resolution of the irregularity
in the ascending limb of −dP/dt. At 50 sec, peak −dP/dt recovered to 77% of the
preocclusion value and the deformity was no longer present.

This deformation of the negative dP/dt signal at the early phase of the occlusion
means that the time course of left ventricular pressure decay deviates substantially from the mono-exponential model usually proposed and it means also that

Table 1. Hemodynamic variables before PTCA, at 20 and 50 sec after occlusion, and after the PTCA
procedure. Abbreviations: PTCA Percutaneous transluminal coronary angioplasty, HR heart rate,
bpm beats per minute, EDV = end distolic volume index, ESV = end systolic volume index, SV =
stroke volume index, EF ejection fraction, LVP left ventricular pressure, dP/dt rate of change of
pressure, Vmax maximal velocity of the contractile element (dP/dt/P linearly extrapolated to P = 0),
ESP end systolic pressure, T time constant of relaxation, Pmin left ventricular minimal diastolic
pressure, EDP left ventricular end diastolic pressure.

	Pre PTCA		20 sec occlusion	50 sec occlusion	Post PTCA	
	Total group	Subgroup	total group	subgroup	subgroup	total group
	n = 14	n = 9	n = 14	n = 9	n = 9	n = 14
HR, bpm	62 ± 16	59 ± 18	61 ± 13	62 ± 14	63 ± 11	64 ± 11
EDV, ml/m²	81 ± 15	79 ± 14	81 ± 15	81 ± 16	78 ± 11	77 ± 11
ESV, ml/m²	31 ± 9	29 ± 7	$37 \pm 9°$	$41 \pm 9°$	26 ± 15	$27 \pm 7*$
SV, ml/m²	50 ± 11	49 ± 11	$44 \pm 12*$	$39 \pm 14*$	52 ± 10	50 ± 9
EF, %	61 ± 8	62 ± 6	$54 \pm 8°$	$48 \pm 12°$	66 ± 6	64 ± 7
peak LVP, mmHg	154 ± 30	151 ± 35	142 ± 29	145 ± 37	148 ± 25	147 ± 21
peak +dP/dt, mmHg.s⁻¹	1403 ± 304	1356 ± 257	1312 ± 320	1278 ± 317	1442 ± 384	1412 ± 333
Vmax, s⁻¹	39 ± 9	40 ± 8	39 ± 9	$34 \pm 10*$	43 ± 12	42 ± 11
ESP, mmHg	95 ± 18	92 ± 22	90 ± 19	98 ± 24	91 ± 15	90 ± 14
peak −dP/dt, mmHg.s⁻¹	1727 ± 322	1614 ± 267	$1268 \pm 355°$	$1404 \pm 370*$	1665 ± 296	1664 ± 243
T_1, msec	55 ± 8	55 ± 6	$79 \pm 17°$	$68 \pm 16°$	56 ± 7.5	54 ± 7
T_2, msec	44 ± 7	43 ± 7	$51 \pm 8*$	$59 \pm 8°$	45 ± 8	45 ± 9
Pmin, mmHg	10 ± 5	8 ± 3	11 ± 4	$16 \pm 6°$	8 ± 5	8 ± 4
EDP, mmHg	22 ± 8	18 ± 6	22 ± 7	$29 \pm 5°$	21 ± 5	20 ± 6

* .05 with respect to preop PTCA, paired T-test of Student.
° .005 with respect to preop PTCA, paired T-test of student.

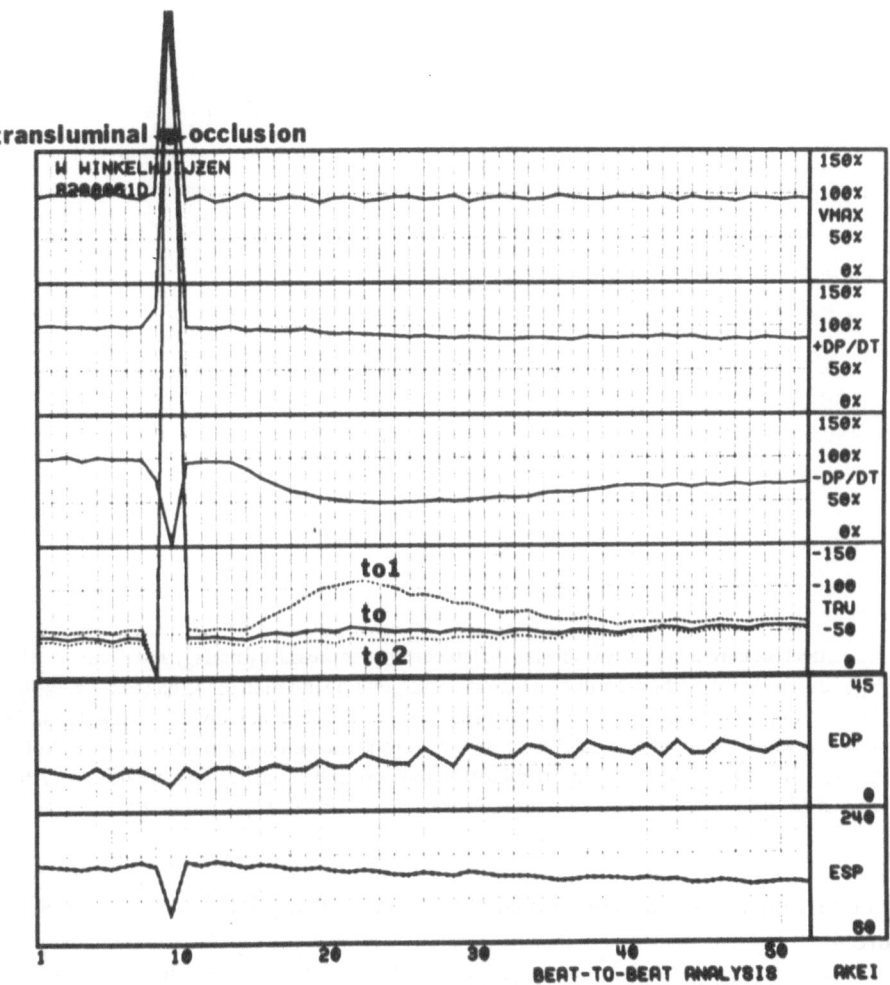

Figure 4. Hemodynamic measurements in a patient during percutaneous transluminal coronary angioplasty. From top to bottom, maximal velocity of the contractile elements (Vmax), peak − and + dP/dt expressed as a percentage of control values, the time constants of relaxation To$_1$ dashed line, To solid line, TO$_2$ dotted line (scale 50 msec), end-diastolic pressure (EDP, scale 15 mmHg), peak systolic pressure (ESP, scale 60 mmHg, with 60 mmHg offset). The break in the data at beat 10 corresponds in inflation of the PTCA balloon.

asynchronous contraction or relaxation may be involved at the very beginning of the transluminal occlusion. Therefore bi-exponential fitting of the pressure curve was computed during the isovolumic relaxation, primarily on the basis that the pressure curve when plotted on semilogarithmic paper was noted to follow two straight lines rather than the one predicted by the mono-exponential mode.

The second half of Table 1 summarizes the results of the relaxation parameters.

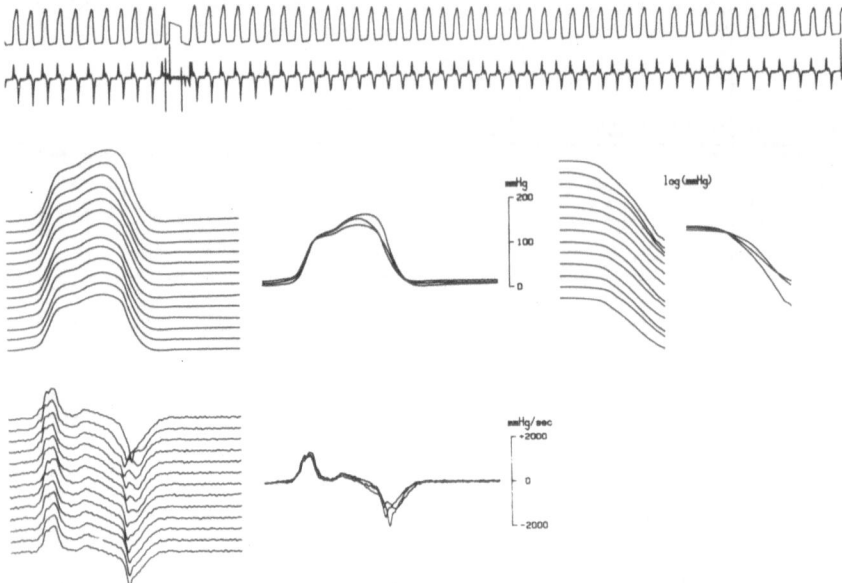

Figure 5. Effects of coronary artery occlusion on left ventricular pressure (mmHg) and + and − dP/dt (mmHg/sec). The break in the recording at beat 15 corresponds in inflation of the balloon. On the left hand side are displayed the left ventricular pressure and + and − dP/dt of individual beats (15, 18, 21, and so forth) while the natural logarithm of the pressure is shown on the right hand side. Notice decrease in − dP/dt associated with an irregularity in the upstroke of the negative dP/dt curve. After 30 sec (beat 42) peak − dP/dt starts to return toward a more normal shape of the signal.

The behaviour of the two time constants (T_1, T_2) during PTCA is illustrated in Figure 4.

An occlusion of a major coronary artery during 20 sec already resulted in a significant ($p < 0.005$) increase in end-systolic volume (from 31 ± 9 to 38 ± 9 ml/m^2) while the end-diastolic volume remained unchanged after 20 sec and even after 50 sec of transluminal occlusion.

At 50 sec, the ejection fraction decreased from 62% to 48% ($p < 0.005$) and this decrease was essentially due to an increase in end-systolic volume from 29 ± 7 to 41 ± 9 ml/m^2 ($p < 0.005$).

The relationship between left ventricular diastolic pressure and volume during transluminal occlusion is illustrated by one example (Figure 6). It is evident that the entire diastolic pressure-volume relationship during transluminal occlusion is gradually shifted upward and to the right so that at any given volume, diastolic pressure was higher. This effect was consistently observed after 50 sec of occlusion.

In the subgroup of patients studied after 20 as well as after 50 sec of LAD occlusion the calculated parameters of global chamber stiffness showed a increased constant of eleastic stiffness (b) (Figure 6). The baseline pressure in-

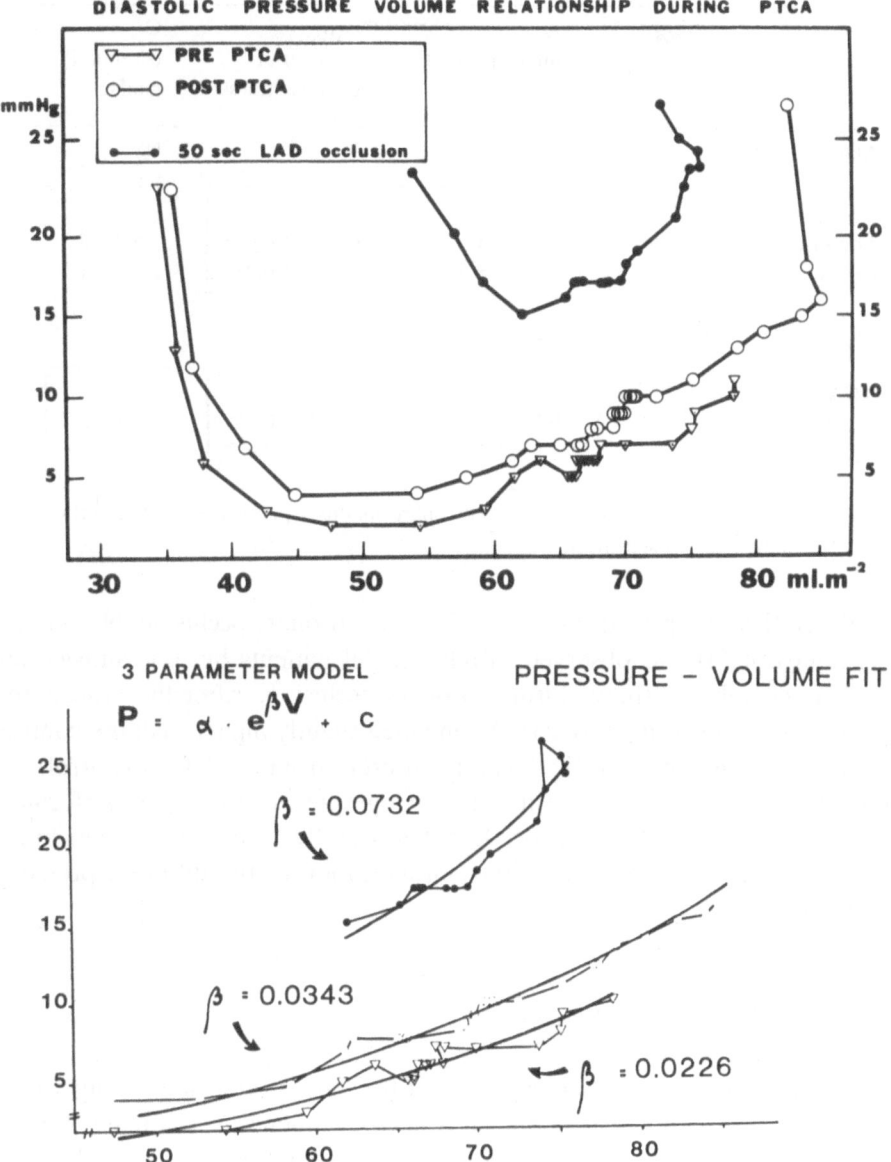

Figure 6. Diastolic pressure volume relationships during percutaneous transluminal angiloplasty (PTCA). During occlusion, there is a shift upward and to the right of the diastolic pressure volume relationship. Abbreviations: LAD: left anterior descending artery.

Table 2. Global left ventricular chamber stiffness.

	A intercept mmHg	B constant of elastic stiffness	C baseline P mmHg
all patients (n = 9)	NS	*	NS
pre PTCA	4.6 ± 4.9	0.0273 ± 0.017 ⎤	−1.4 ± 9.5
20 sec occlusion	1.2 ± 3.3	0.0621 ± 0.026* ⎟	5.2 ± 8.3
post PTCA	1.2 ± 1.5	0.0529 ± 0.037 ⎦	2.8 ± 4.7
subgroup (n = 5)	NS	°	°
pre PTCA	5.3 ± 5.9	0.0214 ± 0.007 ⎤	−5.8 ± 7.4 ⎤
50 sec occlusion	0.2 ± 0.3	0.0605 ± 0.015* ⎟	9.4 ± 2.7° ⎟
post PTCA	1.9 ± 1.8	0.0396 ± 0.027 ⎦	0.8 ± 5.6 ⎦

Values are mean $\pm$ 1 s.d.; * = p <0.05; ° = p <0.01; abbreviations as previously; defined vertical bars refer to orthogonal contrast statistics).

creased significantly (p <.01) only after 50 sec of coronary occlusion. No change in the intercept (a) was observed (Table 2). All patients but one showed an increase in chamber stiffness during coronary occlusion. After the procedure, although in 6 patients the post-PTCA remained slightly higher than the control value, mean values were not significantly different from pre-PTCA control.

In addition, the hemodynamic and cineangiographic investigations performed after completion of the PTCA procedure demonstrated the perfect reversibility of the systolic function as well as the normalization of the different pressure derived indices.

B. Regional left ventricular function

The profound effect of a 20 sec occlusion of the left anterior descending artery (LAD) on left ventricular wall motion and its time sequence is shown in Figure 7. The delay in onset of displacement with respect to end-diastole as well as the timing relationship between the aortic valve closure and the occurrence of the maximal wall displacement is illustrated in Figure 8. The onset of displacement of the anterior and inferior wall was not significantly affected after 20 sec of LAD occlusion. On the contrary, the moment of maximal wall displacement for the anterior wall shifted from end-systole to early diastole. The anterolateral segment (no 6 and 7) and the apical segment (no 9 and 10) of the anterior wall, as well as the apical segment (no 20 and 19) of the inferior wall appeared to be most affected.

The measurement of mean ejection phase velocity, after 20 and 50 sec of LAD occlusion, showed a decrease which was again more pronounced in the anterior

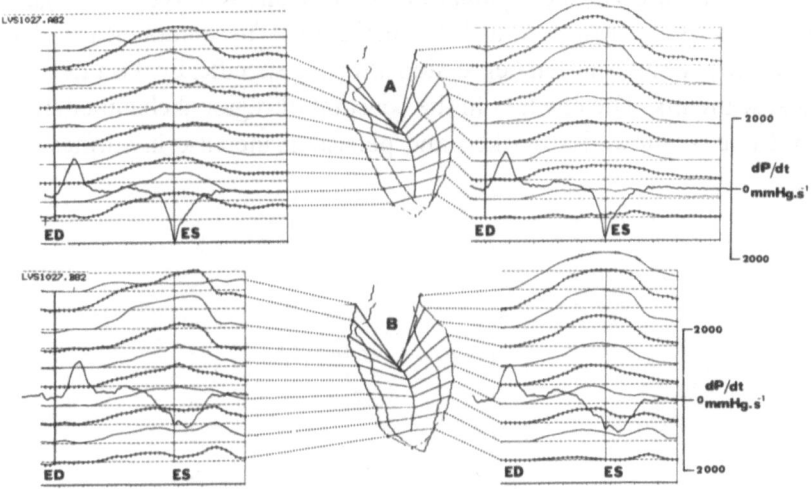

Figure 7. Left ventricular wall displacement studied in twenty separate segments, ten in the anterior (right) and ten in the infero posterior wall (left). A typical example of the relation between segmental wall displacement and dP/dt curve is observed before PTCA (A) and after 20 sec (B) of left anterior descending artery occlusion: after 20 sec of occlusion, the notch in the dP/dt curve corresponds to a second wave of inward wall displacement in the antero- and infero-apical segments.

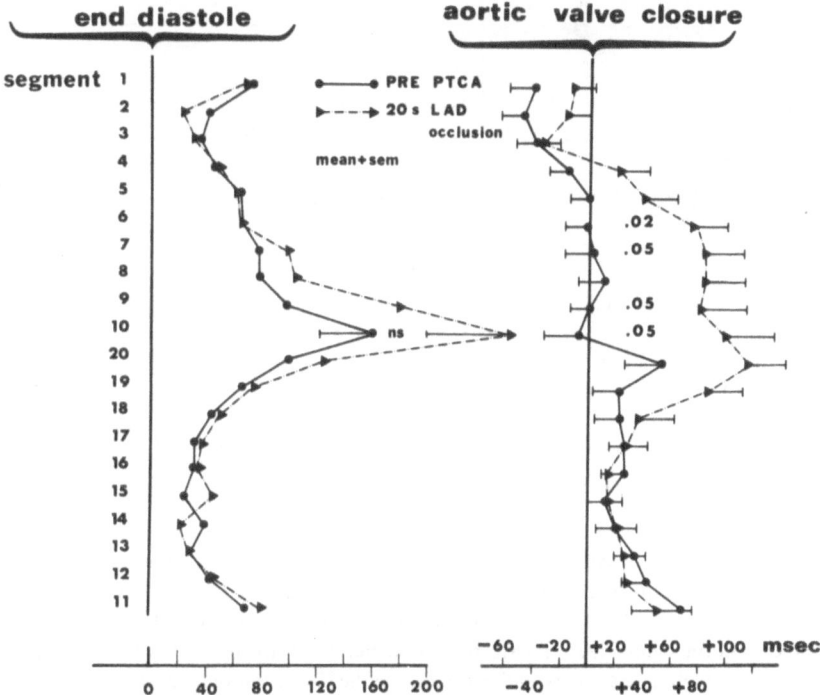

Figure 8. Delay (msec) in onset of displacement for the 20 individual wall segments with respect to end-diastole (time zero) before and after 20 sec of LAD occlusion. Time relationship between aortic valve closure (time zero) and the occurrence of maximal wall displacement before and after 20 sec of LAD occlusion.

wall segments (Figure 9). The regional wall motion and wall velocity (Figure 9A and B) show a similar response to LAD occlusion. These data clearly demonstrate a progressive myocardial depression affecting specifically the anterolateral and apical segments. The changes in the constant of regional chamber stiffness, given in Table 3, showed a marked and persistent increase in stiffness in the

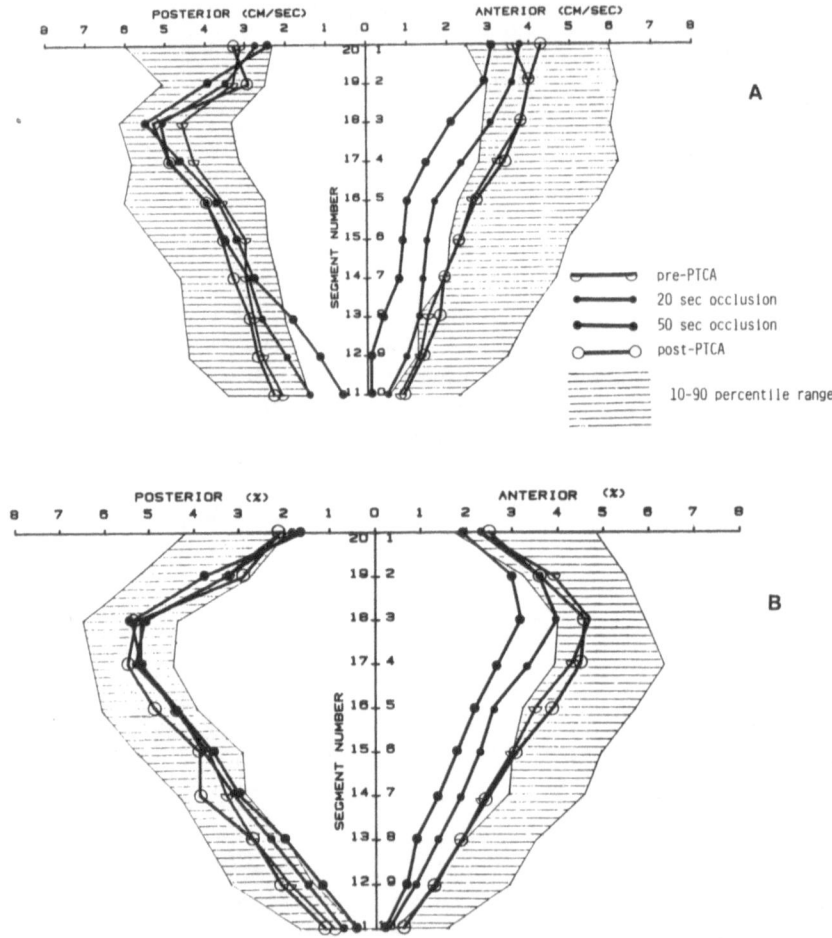

Figure 9. A) Display of the computed CREF values after a 20 or 50 sec occlusion of the left anterior descending artery. On the X-axis the CREF values of the anterior and infero-posterior wall areas are displayed (%), while on the Y-axis the segment numbers of the anterior wall (1–10) and of the infero posterior wall (11–20) are depicted. The shaded zones represent the 10th–90th percentile area of CREF values in normal individuals. B) Mean ejection phase velocity: pre PTCA versus 20 sec and 50 sec occlusion of the left anterior descending artery. On the X-axis the velocity values of the anterior and infero-posterior wall areas are displayed (cm/sec) while on the Y-axis the segment numbers of the anterior wall (1–10) and of the infero-posterior wall (11–20) are depicted. The shaded zones represent the 10th–90th percentile area in normal individuals.

Table 3. Regional left ventricular chamber stiffness (B') = constant of regional elastic stiffness).

Zone	non-ischemic	adjacent	ischemic		adjacent	non-ischemic
Segment	antero-basal	anterior	antero-lateral	apical	inferior	postero-basal
all patients (n = 9)	NS	NS	*	NS	NS	NS
pre-PTCA	1.59	3.92	3.11 ⎤	2.93	2.76	4.03
20 sec. occl.	3.03	4.03	5.63 ⎢	4.97	6.59	5.01
post-PTCA	2.73	2.59	6.45* ⎦	7.16	5.98	3.64
subgroup (n = 5)	NS	NS	>0.05[1]	>0.05[1]	°	NS
pre-PTCA	1.59	3.45	2.81	1.09	1.52 ⎤	2.59
50 sec. occl.	4.13	4.81	5.39	6.16	7.56* ⎢	5.54
post-PTCA	1.98	3.71	5.59	7.16	6.93 ⎦	4.35

Given are medican values; [1] the statistical significance was borderline at the 0.05 level; * = $p < 0.05$; ° = $p < 0.01$; vertical bars refer to orthogonal contrast; abbreviations as previously.

ischemic zone as well as in the adjacent inferior segment (Figure 3).

The regional stiffness in the non-ischemic zone and in the adjacent anterior segment was not affected by the coronary occlusions (Figure 3). No significant changes in the non-linear elastic constant (a) were observed for the regional pressure-length relations. Similar shifts in the baseline pressure as for the global diastolic function were measured since the left ventricular pressure data were used for both calculation of global and regional stiffness.

The latter findings contrast with the perfect reversibility of the abnormalities in global and regional systolic function, as shown from the indices of isovolumic contraction, relaxation and segmental motion. This may suggest that complete recovery of a normal diastolic regional function after repeated ischemic injuries is delayed after restoration of a normal systolic function. Global and regional left ventricular chamber stiffness was studied only in the 10 patients who underwent an angioplasty of the left anterior descending coronary artery stenosis. One of these was excluded because of a small number of available data points due to a high heart rate precluded reliable analysis of the diastolic function.

Discussion

Global and regional left ventricular performance

The earliest (1 to 15 sec after occlusion) and most sensitive hemodynamic indicator of regional perfusion deficit proved to be an impairment in early relaxation, with extreme prolongation of T_1, the time constant of the early relaxation phase. If the premise of the two time constant models previously described [7], is correct, then the early change in T_1 with constant T_2 represent an exacerbation in the asynchrony of relaxation.

This is illustrated by the change in negative dP/dt and wall displacement induced by a 20 sec coronary occlusion (Figure 7). Within four or five beats after occlusion, a distinct deformation appears in the ascending limb of the negative dP/dt curve and in the next ten seconds this deformation reaches the same height as peak $-$dP/dt which in the meantime has progressively decreased to its nadir. Accompanying this change in negative dP/dt, the ischemic segments exhibit a biphasic inward-outward wall displacement that occurs after valve closure and peak negative dP/dt. During the remainder of relaxation and rapid filling the ischemic segments display a second wave of inward wall displacement. The beginning of this second wave of inward wall displacement in early diastole corresponds closely in time to the irregularity in dP/dt. In the same way, the peak inward displacement of the control segment is consistently observed near the notching in the dP/dt. Shortly after this point, the pressure ceases to have a relaxation time constant T_1 and abruptly switches to T_2. On the other hand, after 50 sec of occlusion the majority of the ischemic segments were akinetic exhibiting an increased regional stiffness, whereas T_1, the time constant of the early relaxation phase tended to return toward less abnormal values. At 50 sec, the deformity in $-$dP/dt was no longer present.

The connection between transient asynergy, myocardial ischemia and alteration in the time course of relaxation was pointed out as early as 1969 by Tyberg et al. [16] who designed an experimental model consisting of two papillary muscles in series; they demonstrated that when one muscle of the pair was hypoxic, but still contracting, it was disturbing the time course of the total tension fall generated by the two muscles, much more than when one of the muscles in series was not contracting at all and infinitely stiff [16]. More recent studies in conscious animals after experimental coronary occlusion have indicated that ventricular dyssynchrony due to late systolic contraction and relaxation in different regions can produce marked effects on the linearity and maximal rate of pressure fall in the left ventricle [14, 15, 16].

The present study suggests that a similar phenomenon may occur in the intact human heart during acute ischemia. At 20 sec, the late systolic outward displacement of the ischemic segment is probably passive and due to a simultaneously increased and active inward displacement of the non-ischemic segments. Conversely the early diastolic inward displacement of the ischemic segments must correspond to an accelerated outward displacement of the normal segment. Ultimately the ischemic zone after 20 sec of ischemia appears to act as an additional elastic element, in series with the actively contracting and relaxing non-ischemic segment. This mechanism is consistent with the model of LV pressure relaxation recently proposed by our group [7] which assumes that the observed time constant T_1 results from the combined action of that fraction of the myocardium in the process of relaxing and the remainder yet to initiate relaxation.

Another finding of the present study was that ischemia induced by complete occlusion of the LAD as short as 20 seconds increased the chamber stiffness of the anterior wall, which resulted in an alteration in the global diastolic properties of the left ventricle.

Fifteen minutes after the end of the procedure including repeated (4 to 6) and brief (20 to 60 sec) occlusions, the constant of global chamber stiffness had returned toward control values despite a persisting increase in regional stiffness in the core of the ischemic zone. The latter finding contrasts with the perfect reversibility of the abnormalities in global and regional function, as shown from the indices of isovolumic contraction and relaxation and segmental wall motion. This may suggest that completerecovery of a normal diastolic regional function after repeated ischemic injuries is delayed after restoration of a normal systolic function. It is also shown that the shift in the diastolic pressure-volume curve of the left ventricle occurring during coronary occlusion is dependent on the duration of regional myocardial ischemia. It cannot be inferred from our data that the intrinsic diastolic properties of the myocardium are affected since analysis of wall stress and strain is required to assess myocardial properties as distinct from ventricular chamber properties. Forthis, regional wall thickness measurements are needed which cannot be obtained accurately at 20 msec intervals from the angiographic technique. Also, at least for interpatient comparison, stress-strain data should be normalized for a reference unloaded muscle length, i.e. at a transmural pressure of 0 mmHg, and this data cannot be obtained easily during cardiac catheterization in man. Thus, extrinsic factors such as the right ventricular loading conditions [20, 21] and pericardial constriction [20, 15] may have contributed to the apparent increase in chamber stiffness. The socalled 'erectile effect' [20] is not likely to account for the increased stiffness; during coronary occlusion, inflation of the dilatation balloon results on average in a 44% decrease in regional blood flow [2, 22], thereby reducing the myocardial blood volume.

Likewise, the post-PTCA measurements were obtained 10–15 minutes after completion of the procedure, at which time an increased myocardial turgor due to reactive hyperhemia is no longer expected. It should be emphasized that our findings do not apply to high demand, high flow situations such as pacing-or exercise-induced ischemia, but rather mimic the experimental coronary occlusion in the animal laboratory. Such studies by Hess et al. [14, 23] showed similar abnormalities of the left ventricular pressure volume curve, at least during a complete coronary occlusion. By means of ultrasonic crystals, measurements of wall thickness and short and long axes of the left ventricle were obtained in conscious chronically instrumented dogs [23]. It was concluded that 'myocardial wall stiffness is icreased during complete coronary occlusion when there is systolic thinning of the ischemic wall'. The upward shift of the diastolic pressure volume curve expected from this alteration in the intrinsic diastolic properties of the muscle could be prevented by inferior vena cava obstruction, emphazising the modulation role of the right ventricular loading conditions and the ventricular interaction. In the same study [23], data obtained 10 minutes after a single 1 minute complete coronary occlusion showed a flattened pressure-volume curve, shifted to the left, with a reduced diastolic volume at 0 pressure.

In the present study, recovery of a normal regional diastolic function is not yet observed after 10–15 minutes, despite normalisation of the relaxation parameters, presumably due to the longer period of ischemia since the total occlusion time ranged from 110 sec to 390 sec. A limitation of the present study is that a simple elastic model was used instead of a video-elastic model, which was shown to better characterize the diastolic properties of the left ventricle in dogs [24]. As a consequence, the calculated simple elastic stiffness constant include both elastic and viscous forces.

Experimental data in dogs [25] as well as studies in patients [26] suggest however that viscous forces are negligible at low filling velocity and in the absence of hypertrophy. During coronary occlusion, an increase in viscous resistance during early diastolic filling related to incomplete and prolonged relaxation was observed in dogs [23] and may have contributed to the apparent increase in stiffness in the present study.

Clinical implications

Experimental data on atherosclerotic vessel segments have shown that volume reduction of atherosclerotic tissue is related to the duration of pressure application. These findings have led many clinicians to use longer inflation durations (30–60 sec) during PTCA [27, 28]. On the other hand, Braunwald and Kloner [29] have recently addressed the question whether the myocardium can become chronically, even permanently 'stunned' as a consequence of repetitive episodes of myocardinal ischemia. Although most episodes of transient ischemia occurring in our patients during transluminal angioplasty are not as severe as those of the animal studies [17, 18, 30], the total duration of occlusive episodes during PTCA has increased considerably since our initial experience: the median is now four minutes and a few cases exceed ten minutes in our laboratory [2]. This total occlusion time of four minutes might be excessive since it has been demonstrated in conscious dogs that the return of myocardial function is delayed after periods of coronary occlusion as brief as 100 seconds. Here the reactive hyperemia which occurs normally during reperfusion is prevented by a residual subtotal occlusion [31] a situation which does not apply after successful PTCA. In this respect, the results of the present study seem to be reassuring since there is no evidence of global or regional myocardial dysfunction, even after 4 to 6 coronary occlusions, each of them lasting for 40 to 60 seconds.

References

1. Das SK, Serruys PW, Brand vd M, Domenicuccu S, Vletter WB, Roelandt J (1983) Acute echocardiographic changes during percutaneous coronary angioplasty and their relationship to coronary blood flow. J Cardiovasc Ultrasonography 2: 269–71
2. Serruys PW, Brand vd M, Brower RW, Hugenholtz PG (1983) Regional cardioplegia and cardioprotection during transluminal angioplasty, which role for nifedipine? European Heart Journal 4: 115–21
3. Meester GT, Bernard N, Zeelenberg C, Brower RW, Hugenholtz PG (1975) A computer system for real time analysis of cardiac catheterization data. Catheterization and Cardiovascular Diagnosis 1: 112–23
4. Meester GT, Zeelenberg C, Bernard N, Gorter S (1974) Beat to beat analysis of cardiac catheterization data. In: Computers in Cardiology. Los Angeles IEEE Computer society: 63–65
5. Rousseau M, Veriter C, Detry JMR, Brassuer L, Pouleur H (1980) Impaired early left ventricular relaxation in coronary artery disease. Circulation 62: 764–72
6. Thompson DS, Waldron CB, Juul SM, Naqvi N, Swanton RH, Coltart DJ, Jenkins BS, Webb-Peploe MM (1982) Analysis of left ventricular pressure during isovolumic relaxation in coronary artery disease. Circulation 65: 690–97
7. Brower RW, Meij S, Serruys PW (1983) A model of asynchronous left ventricular relaxation predicting the bi-exponential pressure decay. Cardiovasc Res 17: 482–88
8. Slager CJ, Reiber JHC, Schuurbiers JCH, Meester GT (1978) Contouromat – a hardwired left ventricular angio processing system. Design and application. Comp Biomed Res 11: 491–502
9. Slager CJ, Hooghoudt TEH, Reiber JCH, Booman F, Meester GT (1980) Left ventricular contour segmentation from anatomical landmark trajectories and its application to wall motion analysis. Computers in cardiology. Los Angeles: IEEE Computer society. 347–350
10. Hooghoudt TEH, Slager CJ, Reiber JHC, Serruys PW, Schuurbiers JCH, Meester GT, Hugenholtz PG (1980) 'Regional contribution to global ejection fraction' used to assess the applicability of a new wall motion model to the detection of regional wall motion in patients with asynergy. In: Computers in cardiology; Los Angeles: IEEE Computer society: 253–56
11. Slager CJ, Hooghoudt TEH, Serruys PW, Reiber JHC, Schuurbiers JCH (1982) Automated quantification of left ventricular angiograms. In: Short MD et al. (eds) Physical techniques in Cardiological imaging. Bristol: Hilger A Ltd: 163–72
12. Hess OM, Grimm J, Krayenbruehl HP (1979) Diastolic simple elastic and visco elastic properties of the left ventricle in man. Circulation 59: 1178–87
13. Theroux P, Franklin D, Ross J Jr, Kemper WS (1974) Regional myocardial function during acute coronary artery occlusion and its modification by pharmacologic agents in the dog. Circulation Res 35: 896–908
14. Hess OM, Koch R, Bamert C, Krayenbruehl HP (1980) Regional wall stiffness during acute myocardial ischemia in the canine left ventricle. Eur Heart J 1: 435–43
15. Shirato K, Shabetai R, Bhargava V, Franklin D, Ross J Jr (1978) Alteration of the left ventricular diastolic pressure segment length relation produced by the pericardium: effects of cardiac distension and after load reduction in conscious dogs. Circulation 57: 1191–98
16. Tyberg JV, Parmley WW, Sonnenblick EH (1969) In vitro studies of myocardial asynchrony and regional hypoxia. Circ Res 25: 569–79
17. Theroux P, Ross J Jr, Franklin D, Covell JW, Bloor CM, Sasayama S (1977) Regional Myocardial infarction in the unanesthetized dog. Circ Res 40: 158–65
18. Theroux P, Ross J Jr, Franklin D, Kemper WS, Sasayama S (1976) Regional myocardial function in the conscious dog during acute coronary occlusion and responses to morphine, propranolol, nitroglycerine and lidocaine. Circulation 53: 302–14
19. Kumada T, Karliner JS, Pouleur H, Gallagher KP, Shirato K, Ross J Jr (1979) Effects of coronary occlusion on early ventricular diastolic events in conscious dogs. Am J Physiol 237: H542–H549

20. Glantz SA, Parmley WW (1978) Factors which effect the diastolic pressure-volume curve. Circulation Res 42: 171–80

21. Grossman W, Serisawa T, Carabello BA (1980) Studies on the mechanism of altered left ventricular diastolic pressure-volume relations during ischemia. Eur Heart J 1 (suppl A): 141–7

22. Serruys PW, Wijns W, Brand vd M, Meij S, Slager CJ, Schuurbiers JCH, Hugenholtz PG, Brower RW (1984) Left ventricular performance, regional blood flow, wall motion and lactate metabolism during transluminal angioplasty. Circulation 70: 25–36

23. Hess OM, Osakada G, Lavelle JF, Gallagher KP, Kemper WS, Ross J Jr (1983) Diastolic myocardial wall stiffness and ventricular relaxation during partial and complete coronary occlusion in the conscious dog. Circulation Res 52: 387–400

24. Rankin JS, Arentzen CE, Mc Hale PA, Ling D, Anderson RW (1977) Visco-elastic properties of the diastolic left ventricle in the conscious dog. Circulation Res 41: 37–45

25. Pouleur H, Karliner JS, de Winter MM, Covell JW (1979) Diastolic viscous properties of the intact canine left ventricle. Circulation Res 45: 410–419

26. Hess OM, Grimm J, Krayenbruehl HP (1979) Diastolic simple elastic and visco-elastic properties of the left ventricle in man. Circulation 59: 1178–87

27. Schmitz HJ, Meyer J, Kiesslich T, Effert S (1982) Greater initial dilatation gives better late angiographic results in percutaneous coronary angioplasty (PTCA). Circulation 66 (suppl II): 62

28. Kaltenbach M, Kober G (1982) Can prolonged application of pressure improve the results of coronary angioplasty (PTCA). Circulation 66 (suppl II): 123

29. Braunwald E, Kloner RA (1983) The stunned myocardium: prolonged post-ischemic, ventricular dysfunction. Circulation 66: 1146–49

30. Heijndrickx GR, Millard RW, Mc Ritchie RJ, Maroko PR, Vatner SF (1975) Regional myocardial function and electrophysiological alterations after brief coronary artery occlusion in conscious dogs. J Clin Invest 56: 978–85

31. Pagani M, Vatner SF, Baig H, Braunwald E (1978) Initial myocardial adjustment to brief periods of ischemia and reperfusion in the conscious dog. Circ Res 43 (1): 83–92

Restenosis following successful coronary angioplasty (PTCA): The result of inadequate dilatation? Relation between primary success and late results

HERMANN J. SCHMITZ, JÜRGEN MEYER, RAINER van ESSEN and SVEN EFFERT

Introduction

In a previous study we found indications, that the extent of initial dilatation influences the late outcome of PTCA. For this reason the effect of the primary dilatation was analysed based on a consecutive series of 154 successful angioplasties (stenosis reduction $\geq 20\%$-diameter) for proximal coronary stenoses.

In 81 pts. with concentric short lesions the PTCA procedure was comparable regarding balloon pressure (5,5–6,5 bar), number of inflation (3–5) and inflation time (15–25 seconds). In 41 cases the balloon caliber used was 3,0 mm and in 40 cases 3,7 mm. Control angiograms were performed $5,6 \pm 1,6$ months after angioplasty.

A computer program was employed to determine the prestenotic vessel lumen, stenosis lumen, mean balloon size in the vessel and balloon expansion at the point of maximum narrowing. The rate of restenosis (remaining stenosis reduction $<20\%$ at control) was 26%. In the recurrence group (R, n = 21) the stenosis lumen had decreased from $2,2 \pm 0,3$ mm after PTCA again to $1,1 \pm 0,4$ mm at 6 months control. In the group with continued success (S, n = 60) the average gain in lumen diameter remained unchanged ($2,3 \pm 0,4$ mm).

With similar stenoses before the PTCA was performed ($1,1 \pm 0,5$ mm (R) vs. $1,0 \pm 0,3$ mm (S) n.s.) there were two main differences between the groups: the vessels in which restenosis occurred (Group R) had a larger prestenotic lumen ($3,8 \pm 0,5$ mm vs. $3,4 \pm 0,4$ mm, $p < 0.001$) and the balloon expansion in the stenosis was smaller ($2,3 \pm 0,4$ mm vs. $2,7 \pm 0,5$ mm, $p < 0.005$). In Group R the balloon expansion in the stenosis reached $60 \pm 11\%$ of the normal vessel lumen vs. $81 \pm 15\%$ in Group S ($p < 0.001$).

In conclusion the long-term success of PTCA is mainly determined by the primary dilatation. Apparently the actual balloon expansion in the stenosis in relation to the vessel diameter and stenosis lumen is of decisive importance for the late outcome.

According to concurrent reports from various groups, the rate of recurrent stenosis following successful percutaneous transluminal coronary angioplasty

(PTCA) is approximately 30% [2, 6, 8]. Determinants and predictive criteria for a restenosis appear thus far to elude definition. Investigations currently underway deal specifically with the influence of medicative aftertreatment [3, 5].

In a previous study we found indications that the extent of the initial dilatation is a contributory factor for the long-term results of PTCA [10]. For this reason, the effect of the primary dilatation was analysed based on angiographic investigations taking into consideration the dimensions of the vessels, stenoses, and balloons.

Methods

From a consecutive series of 209 coronary angioplasties performed between October 1979 and October 1982 in 207 patients with high-grade stenoses located in the proximal section of left anterior descending (LAD) or right coronary artery (RCA), those patients who fulfilled the following criteria were included in the further investigation:
1) Concentric stenosis, lesion length <10 mm.
   A stenosis was defined as not being concentric (= eccentric) if the lumen of the stenosis located within only onehalf of the normally assumed vessel lumen in at least one projection. Eccentric lesions, that means stenoses with a normal wall segment were excluded, because here a different mechanism of dilatation might be effective.
2) Successful dilatations, i.e. stenosis reduction ≥20% in diameter.
3) Comparable dilatation procedure regarding:
   a) number of balloon inflations in the stenosis: 3–5
   b) inflation pressure: 5.5–6.5 bar
   c) seperate inflation period: 15–25 seconds
4) Performance of PTCA with a balloon of one size only, either 3.0 or 3.7 mm thickness
5) Angiographic visualization in identical projections before, immediately after, and normally scheduled 6 months after PTCA.

The PTCA was typically performed according to the technique of Grüntzig [4] using a Schneider-Grüntzig-Dilaca[R] balloon catheter. The 9-F guiding catheter was positioned in the coronary ostium via a special insertion dilator according to the method of Judkins. A pacing catheter with a lumen was placed as an orientation marker (intersection with the coronary artery) in the pulmonary artery. It was also used to infuse 100 ml/h of dextran 40%. All patients received 500 mg acetylsalicylic acid and 20 mg nifedipine orally 2 h before the PTCA: during the PTCA, they were given 2 × 5000 IU intravenous heparin and in most cases 0.1–0.2 mg intracoronary nitroglycerin. The balloon catheter was advanced into the stenosis under fluoroscopic control and pressure monitoring and then inflated several times via a pressure pump. The result of dilatation was then evaluated by angiography.

After successful PTCA, the patients received 3×10 mg nifedipine and 500 mg acetylsalicylic acid per day until angiographic follow-up 6 months later.

A 35-mm film, 50 pictures/s, was used for the angiographic documentation. The LAO view, 60 and RAO view, 30 were chosen as the projections for the RCA and the RAO view, 30, LAO view, 60 as well as RAO view 30/30 craniocaudally and LAO view, 60/40 caudocranially for the LAD.

The inflated balloon filled with contrast media was filmed each time during the second half of the inflation period; that projection was chosen in which the pacing catheter crossed the vessel near the stenotic area.

The films were evaluated by two independent investigators. The contoures of the vessel and balloon were traced by hand with a special pencil from a film projection magnified 20-fold and then fed into a computersystem with an x-y coordinate reader. In each case, the contour line was defined as the zone with identical shade of grey. All drawings were from the end-diastolic phase. For the representation of the balloon, only the situation during the last inflation was taken into consideration.

Measurement Data

A computer program was used to measure (Figure 1):
1) The vessel lumen directly before the beginning of the stenosis = 'vessel lumen'

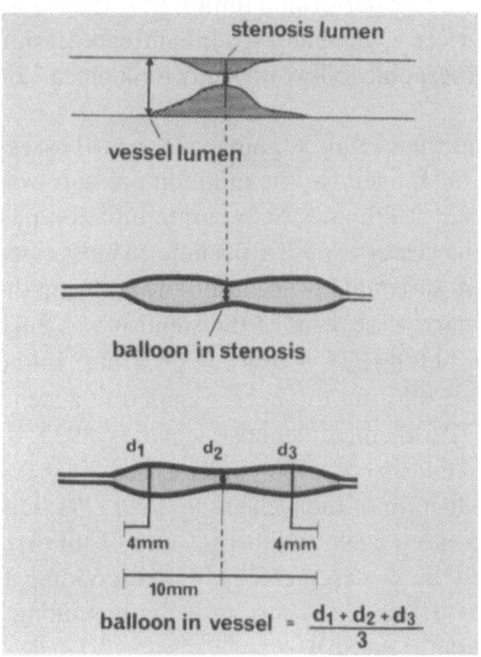

Figure 1.

2) The narrowest site of the vessel lumen in the stenosis = 'stenosis lumen'. (The mean value was determined from the various projections; the percentage degree of stenosis was calculated from points 1 and 2).

3) The 20 mm long balloon both 4 mm before the end and in the geometric center (these 3 data were used to determine the mean balloon size = 'balloon in vessel')

4) The balloon expansion at the narrowest place in the stenosis = 'balloon in stenosis'. (This was determined by its vertex if a clear impression of the balloon by the stenosis could be visualized otherwise it was calculated by geometric relations (distance from the pacing and guiding catheter)).

Calibration was achieved via the shaft of the angiographic or guiding catheter, 7F = 2.2 mm and 9F = 2.9 mm.

Statistical analysis was performed with the t-test for paired and unpaired random samples and with the chi-square test. All numbers given represent mean value and standard deviation.

Results

The above mentioned criteria were fulfilled in 81 cases of coronary angioplasty. Reasons for exclusion from the investigation were: unsuccessful PTCA, n = 55; successful PTCA but stenosis length – 10 mm, n = 7; eccentric stenosis, n = 41; no follow-up examination, n = 5; different PTCA procedure, n = 20.

In 63 cases, dilatation was performed for a LAD stenosis and in 18 cases for a RCA stenosis. There were 77 men and 4 women treated, with an average age of 48 ± 9 years. The angiographic follow-up study took place 5.6 ± 1.6 months after the PTCA.

The PTCA was performed with a 3.0-mm balloon in 41 cases and with a 3.7-mm balloon in 40 cases. On an average, the inflation pressure was 6.1 ± 0.4 bar, the number of inflations 3.8 ± 0.6, and the separate inflation periods 19 ± 3 s. The mean balloon size in the vessel was 3.0 ± 0.4 mm. In most cases, an impression of the balloon by the stenosis could be visualized, whereby on the whole expansion of the balloon at the narrowest point of the stenosis was 2.6 ± 0.5 mm.

The stenosis lumen before PTCA was 1.0 ± 0.4 mm. Based on a prestenotic vessel diameter of 3.5 ± 0.5 mm, this corresponded to a stenosis of $71 \pm 10\%$ in terms of diameter (a 71%-diameter stenosis signifies a 92% area reduction).

The lumen of the stenosis could be expanded to 2.4 ± 0.3 mm with PTCA, corresponding to a reduction of the stenosis by $37 \pm 12\%$. During the follow-up period the lumen decreased again to 2.0 ± 0.7 mm (Table 1).

Restenosis occurred in 21 cases (26%). Corresponding to the criteria for success, a stenosis was defined as recurrent if the remaining stenosis reduction was <20% at the 6 months control.

In the relapse group, after initial reduction to $42 \pm 9\%$ or expansion to

Table 1.

| | Entire group, n = 81 | | |
	Before PTCA	After PTCA	6 months after PTCA
Vessel lumen (mm)	3.5 ± 0.5	3.6 ± 0.4	3.3 ± 0.4
Stenosis lumen (mm)	1.0 ± 0.4	2.4 ± 0.3	2.0 ± 0.7
Stenosis %	71 ± 10	34 ± 10	40 ± 20
Balloon (mm) in vessel	3.0 ± 0.4		
Balloon (mm) in stenosis	2.6 ± 0.5		

2.2 ± 0.3 mm, the stenosis returned to its original level of 69 ± 10% or 1.1 ± 0.4 mm. In the group with long-term success (n = 60), the dilatation achieved remained unchanged: residual stenosis and lumen were 31 ± 8% or 2.4 ± 0.3 mm after PTCA and 29 ± 9% or 2.3 ± 0.4 mm at the follow-up.

The prestenotic vessel diameter was larger during the PTCA (before and immediately afterward) than at the follow-up examination (3.5 ± 0.5 or 3.6 ± 0.4 vs. 3.3 ± 0.4 mm, p<0.001). This difference has to be attributed to the effect of the vasodilative medication; it could be ascertained to the same extent in all subgroups (3.0- vs. 3.7-mm balloon; success vs. recurrence).

Balloon calibers: 3.0 mm–3.7 mm

The mean balloon size in the vessel remained below the levels listed by the manufacturer for both calibers: for the 3.0-mm balloon at 2.8 ± 0.3 mm by 7% and for the 3.7-mm balloon at 3.2 ± 0.5 mm by 14% (Table 2).

With the lumens of the vessels and the stenoses comparable, the 3.7-mm

Table 2.

| 3.0-mm balloon, n = 41; 3.7-mm balloon, n = 40. | | | | |
		Before PTCA	After PTCA	6 months after PTCA
Vessel lumen	3.0	3.5 ± 0.6	3.5 ± 0.3	3.3 ± 0.4
(mm)	3.7	3.5 ± 0.4	3.7 ± 0.4	3.4 ± 0.4
Stenosis lumen	3.0	1.0 ± 0.4	2.3 ± 0.3	1.8 ± 0.7
(mm)	3.7	1.1 ± 0.3	2.4 ± 0.4	2.1 ± 0.7
Balloon in vessel	3.0	2.8 ± 0.3		
(mm)	3.7	3.2 ± 0.5		
Balloon in	3.0	2.4 ± 0.4		
stenosis (mm)	3.7	2.8 ± 0.5		

balloon achieved a larger expansion both in the vessel (p<0.001) as well as in the vertex of the stenosis (2.8 ± 0.5 vs. 2.4 ± 0.4 mm, p<0.001) as could be expected.

In 19 cases, the mean balloon size (3.6 ± 0.4 mm) exceeded the vessel lumen, the diameter of the balloon being larger by maximally 0.8 mm, on the average 0.3 ± 0.2 mm. This was the case 15 times when the 3.7-mm balloon was used and 4 times when the 3.0-mm balloon was used. In none of these cases did a recurrence appear; in one case (5%) a dissection occurred.

The 21 restenosis were to be found in the remaining group (n = 62) in which the size of the balloon did not exceed the vessel dimensions. A dissection occurred in two cases (3%), but did not lead to a recurrence of stenosis.

The lumens of the vessels and the stenoses were not different between the two balloon calibers used, but the rate of recurrence for those dilated with the smaller 3.0-mm balloon was almost twice as high at 34% vs. 18% for the 3.7-mm balloon, (p = 0.08, ns.).

Long-term success rate – recurrence of stenosis

There were some statistically significant differences between the group with long-term improvement (n = 60) and the group with restenosis (n = 21) (Table 3).

Table 3. Long-term improvement (I), n = 60; Restenosis (R), n = 21.

		Before PTCA	After PTCA	6 months after PTCA
Vessel lumen	I	3.4 ± 0.4	3.5 ± 0.3	3.3 ± 0.3
(mm)	R	3.8 ± 0.5	3.9 ± 0.4	3.6 ± 0.4
Stenosis lumen	I	1.0 ± 0.3	2.4 ± 0.3	2.3 ± 0.4
(mm)	R	1.1 ± 0.5	2.2 ± 0.3	1.1 ± 0.4
Stenosis %	I	71 ± 10	31 ± 8	29 ± 9
	R	72 ± 11	42 ± 9	69 ± 10
Balloon in vessel	I	3.1 ± 0.4		
(mm)	R	2.8 ± 0.3		
Balloon in stenosis	I	2.7 ± 0.5		
(mm)	R	2.3 ± 0.4		

There were no differences between the groups in terms of absolute size and percentage stenosis before dilatation, which was 1.0 ± 0.3 mm or $71 \pm 10\%$ in the group without recurrence and 1.1 ± 0.5 mm or $72 \pm 11\%$ in the group with relapse.

		Success	Recurrence	p<
I.	Vessel lumen (mm)			
	a) during PTCA	3.4 ± 0.4	3.8 ± 0.5	0.001
	b) at follow-up	3.3 ± 0.3	3.6 ± 0.4	0.005
II.	Expansion of stenosis (mm)	1.4 ± 0.4	1.1 ± 0.5	0.01
III.	Stenosis after PTCA (mm)	2.4 ± 0.3	2.2 ± 0.3	0.05
IV.	Balloon in stenosis (mm)	2.7 ± 0.5	2.3 ± 0.4	0.005

As can be seen from the above list, those vessels in which stenosis recurred had a larger prestenotic lumen, both the balloon expansion in the narrowest part of the stenosis as well as the dilatation achieved was smaller and the residual stenosis after PTCA was more extensive.

Discussion

The mechanism by which transluminal angioplasty led to enlargement of the lumen of stenosed arteries remained unclear for a long time. The initial assumption that the dilating effect was due to compression of the stenosing atheroma [7] can no longer be supported in the light of more recent findings.

Both Castaneda-Zuniga [1] and Sanborn [9] were able to show in animal experiments that the decisive mechanism consisted of dilation of the entire vessel wall to form an aneurysm. The atheroma, which remains unchanged as to its layer thickness, is displaced outward. This inevitably leads to a rupture of the intima, and the media and adventitia are stretched. If the expansion of the media goes beyond its limit of elasticity, the result is an irreversible, permanent dilatation of the lumen. Thus, restenosis appears to be the consequence of inadequate, reversible expansion of the vessel wall.

Our clinical angiographic findings point in the same direction. On the one hand, dilatation with the larger sized balloon resulted in a higher long-term success rate; on the other hand the results show that when the dilatation of the stenosis was long-lasting a larger widening of the vessel had been achieved. The actual expansion of the balloon in those stenoses with similar lumen size was smaller in the group with restenosis, but the normal vessel lumen was larger. Both these differences were highly significant. Under the justifiable assumption (see above) that the dilatation does not cause compression of the atheroma, the vessel diameter was expanded during balloon inflation by 1.2 ± 0.4 mm in the group with restenosis and by 1.7 ± 0.4 mm in the group with long-term improvement ($p < 0.001$). The diameter increase achieved equals the balloon expansion minus the stenosis lumen (Figure 2). This corresponds to a percentage increase in size

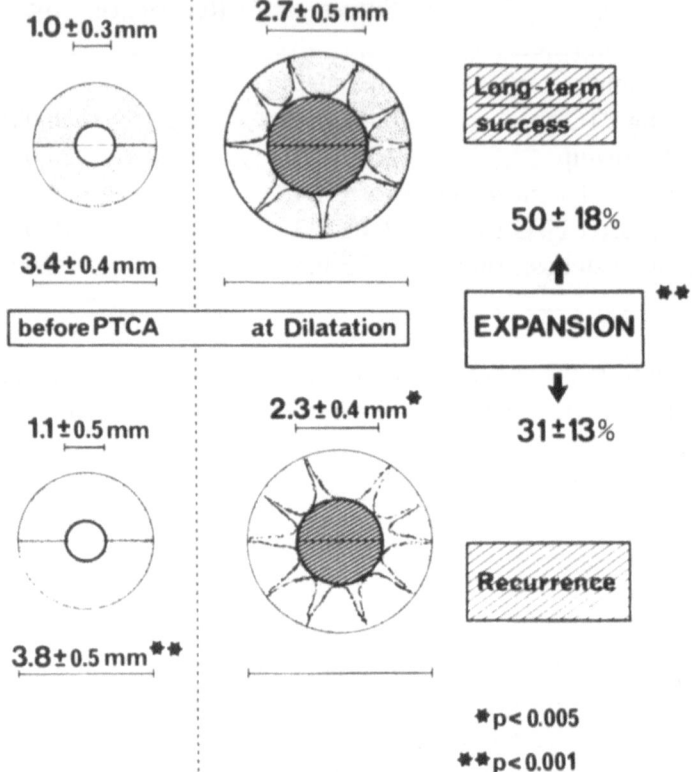

Figure 2.

(increase of vessel diameter × 100%/vessel lumen) and thus an expansion of the wall layer bordering on the lumen of $50 \pm 18\%$ in the group with continued success in comparison to $31 \pm 13\%$ in the relapse group ($p<0.001$). This difference is reflected in the same way by the actual angiographic data: in the recurrence group the balloon expansion in the stenosis reached $60 \pm 11\%$ of the

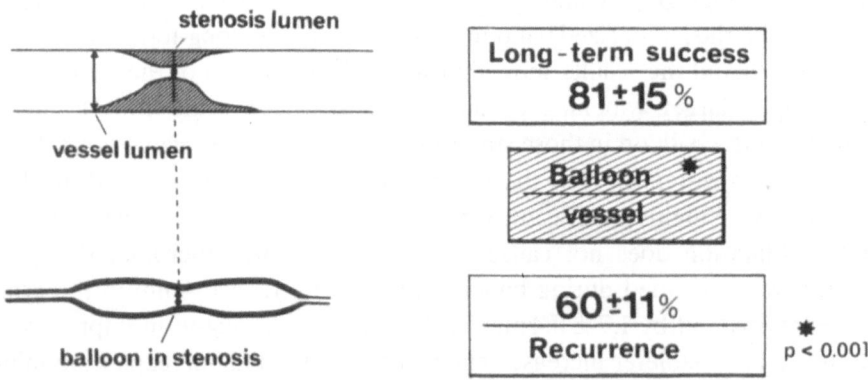

vessel diameter and $81 \pm 15\%$ in the group with long-term success (p<0.001), (Figures 2 and 3).

Thus these findings based on angiographic studies confirm the results from expermintal-anatomic investigations on the mechanism of angioplasty. Apparently, a certain degree of vessel dilatation is necessary for lasting success.

Conclusions

The long-term success rate of PTCA is mainly determined by the primary dilatation. It appears essential that an adequate degree of vessel dilatation is achieved. The actual balloon expansion in the stenosis in relation to the vessel diameter and stenosis lumen is of decisive importance.

Consequences for practical application

To chose the suitable balloon size it is wise to estimate the prestenotic vessel diameter directly before initiating PTCA (after administering vasodilative medication). This can be effected by simply tracing on the video screen the vessel contour and the catheter used for calibration. For a vessel lumen smaller than 3.2 mm we recommend to use a 3.0-mm balloon, and for diameters of 3.2 mm and larger the 3.7-mm balloon.

Since the balloon continues to expand during the course of inflation, (disappearance of the hourglass shape, decrease of impression), long periods of inflation appear to exert a favorable influence- also with regard to the physical aspect of stretching elastic structures. These times should be adapted to ischemia tolerance of the patient.

If a recurrent stenosis develops and dilatation is repeated, either a larger balloon should be chosen or inflation should be performed with higher pressures. Due to the flexibility of the balloon, enlargement can also be achieved by inflation with increased pressure.

The use of the 3.7-mm balloon did not lead to more complications than the 3.0-mm balloon. The risk of a dissection or of coronary occlusion appears to be more dependent on the vessel path (arcuation, tortuosity), stenosis shape (long, irregular), and the experience of the physician performing the PTCA.

References

1. Castaneda-Zuniga WR, Formanek A, Tadavarthy M, Vlodaver Z, Edwards JE, Zollikover C, Amplatz K (1980) The mechanism of balloon angioplasty. Radiology 135: 565
2. Dangoisse V, Val PG, David PR, Lesperance J, Crepean J, Dyrda I, Bourassa MG (1982)

Recurrence of stenosis after successful percutaneous transluminal coronary angioplasty (PTCA). Circulation 66 (Suppl. II): II-330

3. Faxon DP, Sanborn TA, Gottsmann SD, Haudenschild C, Ryan TJ (1983) The effect of aspirine and persantine on restenosis following experimental angioplasty. Circulation 68 (suppl. III): III-96

4. Gruentzig A, Senning A, Siegenthaler WE (1979) Nonoperative dilatation of coronary-artery stenosis. Percutaneous transluminal coronary angioplasty. N Engl J Med 301: 61

5. Hollmann J, Gruentzig A, Meier B, Bradford J, Galan K (1983) Factors affecting recurrence after successful coronary angioplasty. J Am Coll Cardiol I (2): 644

6. Holmes D, Vliestra R, Smith H, Kent K, Bentivoglio L, Block P, Dorros G, Gosselin A, Gruentzig A, Myler R, Simpson J, Stertzer S, Williams D, Bourassa M, Vetrovec G, Kelsey S, Detre K, Passamani E, Van Raden M, Mock M (1983) Restenosis following percutaneous transluminal coronary angioplasty (PTCA): a report from the NHLBI PTCA registry. Circulation 68 (Suppl. III) III-95

7. Leu HJ, Gruentzig A (1978) Histopathologic aspects of transluminal recanalization. In: Zeitler E, Gruentzig A, Schoop A (eds): Percutaneous vascular recanalisation, Springer Berlin 39

8. Levine S, Ewels CJ, Rosing DR, Kent KM (1983) Restenosis following transluminal coronary angioplasty (TCA). Circulation 68 (Suppl. III): III-96

9. Sanborn TA, Faxon DP, Haudenschild C, Gottsmann S, Ryan TJ (1983) The mechanism of transluminalangioplasty: evidence for formation of aneurysms in experimental atherosclerosis. Circulation 68 (5): 1136

10. Schmitz HJ, Meyer J, Kiesslich T, Effert S (1982) Greater initial dilatation gives better late angiographic results in percutaneous coronary angioplasty (PTCA). Circulation 66 (Suppl. II): II-123

Results of repetitive controls after successful transluminal coronary angioplasty

G. KOBER, C. VALLBRACHT and M. KALTENBACH

Introduction

Since its introduction as a therapy of coronary heart disease in 1977 transluminal coronary angioplasty (TCA) has been used for myocardial revascularization. Predominantly treated were patients with angina pectoris *and* ischemic findings at electrocardiographic and radionuclear investigations. Few patients had either anginal symptoms *or* ischemic reactions.

Since October 1977 983 transluminal coronary angioplasties have been performed in the Department of Cardiology of the University Hospital in Frankfurt. During the years the mean acute success rate increased from 52% to about 90%. The fatality rate is 2 patients with multivessel disease after myocardial infarction or 0.2%.

This is a report on follow-up studies after successful angioplasty in 2 non-selected subgroups of 90 and 84 different patients as well as on 439 routine follow-up angiograms. Especially the patients' case history, the exercise-ECG and the angiogram have proven to be suitable for the calculation of short and long-term success of the procedure. Follow-up was performed immediately, 3 months, and 12 months after TCA. So far a small part of the patients additionally had repeat follow-up several years after TCA.

Acute follow-up

By international definition successful angioplasty is defined as a reduction in diameter stenosis by 20% and more. Actually the reduction in stenosis is far higher. It ranges about 50%. Compared to the increase in diameter stenosis the increase in cross-sectional area is by far higher.

Among 90 consecutive patients meeting the criteria of successful angioplasty no patient had percentage stenosis of less than 50% before TCA, 84% had diameter stenoses higher than 75%. Fourty-nine percent of the patients had percentage stenosis of 90% and higher. After TCA percentage stenosis was less than 50% in 81% of the patients. In none of the patients it exceeded 75%.

In another group comprising 84 patients the TCA results were classified according to the degree of the previous stenosis. In the mean higher grades of

266

stenoses show a more extensive reduction. There was a mean reduction by 28% in obstructions ranging between 51 and 70%, whereas high-grade stenoses of 81 to 90% were reduced by 42% and those of 91 to 100% even by 56%. Thus the outcome is almost identical in all patients and nearly independent of percentage stenosis before dilatation (Figure 1).

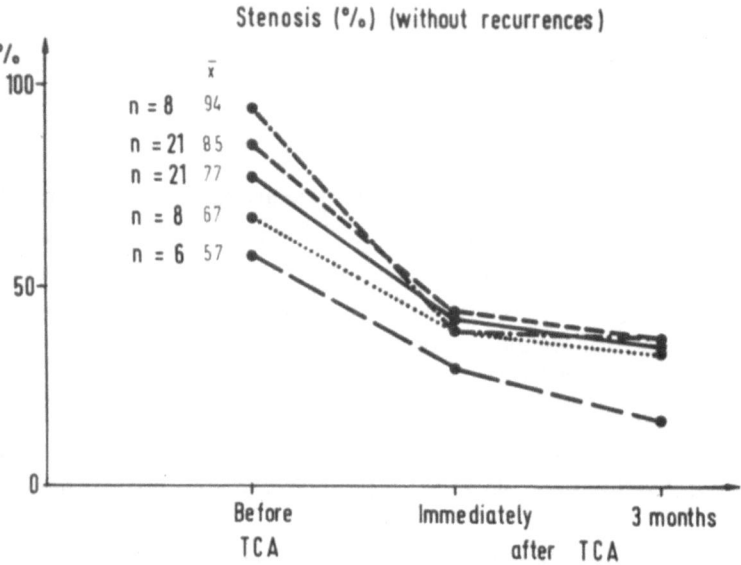

Figure 1. Reduction in stenosis dependent on pre-TCA percentage stenosis.

Among the 90 patients with successful TCA mentioned above 5 had no angina pectoris before TCA, 2 had uncharacteristic symptoms and 83 (92%) had angina pectoris of different severity. The day after TCA clinical symptoms of all symptomatic patients had improved by at least 1 class. Most of the patients were absolutely asymptomatic. The symptomatically unchanged patients were those without angina before TCA (Figure 2).

Before dilatation 87% of the patients had ischemic changes of different degrees at rest or in the exercise-ECG, 4 symptomatic patients had an exercise test only suspicious for ischemia. In most patients ischemic changes were no longer found the day after TCA even with higher and longer exercise-testing. In 15 patients (17%) there were still slight, yet mostly reduced ischemic reactions (Figure 3).

Thus there was a good coincidence between the acute angiographic improvement and the influence on symptoms and the exercise electrocardiogram.

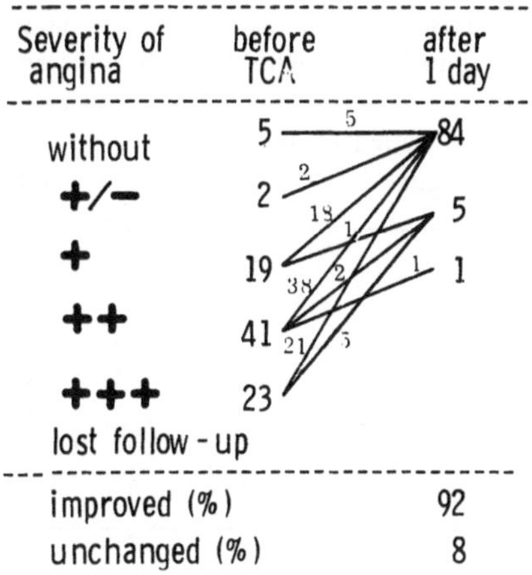

Severity of angina	before TCA	after 1 day
without	5	84
+/−	2	5
+	19	1
++	41	
+++	23	
lost follow-up		
improved (%)		92
unchanged (%)		8

Figure 2. Angina Pectoris in 90 patients with successful angioplasty.

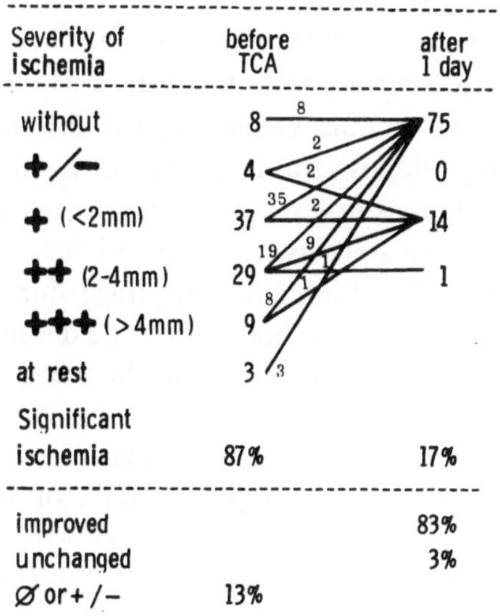

Severity of ischemia	before TCA	after 1 day
without	8	75
+/−	4	0
+ (<2mm)	37	14
++ (2-4mm)	29	1
+++ (>4mm)	9	
at rest	3	
Significant ischemia	87%	17%
improved		83%
unchanged		3%
Ø or +/−	13%	

Figure 3. Ischemic reaction in the exercise-ECG in 90 patients with successful TCA.

Follow-up 3 months after TCA

Of the 90 patients with successful TCA 86% reported to be still improved symptomatically after 3 months, 10% to have unchanged symptoms compared to the pre-TCA state or a recurrence of angina after an initial improvement. Informations were missing about 4 patients (Table 1). Among these 90 patients the exercise-ECG was still improved in 91%. In 5% of the patients there were signs of a recurrence. The angiograms showed restenoses of different severity in 13% of the patients. We took into account restenoses meeting the criteria of a loss

Table 1. Angina pectoris and exercise ischemia in comparison to the pre-TCA state and percentage stenosis during follow-up angiograms in 90 patients 3 months after successful TCA.

Compared to pre-TCA state	% Patients with		% Patients	Stenosis %
	angina	Ischema		
Improved	86	91	67	50
Unchanged	6	–	19	50–74
Reappearance	4	5	7 ⎫	75–89
			⎬13	
Unknown	4	4	6 ⎭	90
			2	no follow-up

of 50% of the dilatation-induced initial increase in lumen diameter or an increase in diameter stenosis by more than 30% compared to the acute TCA result (Table 1).

When comparing angiograms taken immediately after dilatation and those taken after 3 months 3 groups can be differentiated: The majority of 69% of the patients shows unchanged results with mean stenosis being 40% immediately after TCA and 37% after 3 months. Compared with the immediate result in 12% of the patients percentage stenosis was further improved during follow-up from a mean of 41% to 14% whereas in 19% of the patients restenosis occurred, thus increasing mean percentage stenosis from 32% to 60% (Table 2). Comparing restenosis rate 3 months after TCA and percentage stenosis (50 to 60%, 60 to 70%, 70 to 80%, 80 to 90%, >90%) before TCA no definite difference between the different groups of stenoses is discernible. The mean recurrence rate varied between 11 and 20%.

The low restenosis rate in our patients in comparison with other groups is also valid for bigger follow-up groups. Among a total of 311 routine follow-ups performed 1 to 5 months (mean 3 months) after TCA restenosis rate was 14%, among a total of 439 follow-ups performed 5.6 months (mean value) after TCA restenosis rate was 17%. Thus restenosis rate is about 50% of the values given in

Table 2. Caliper measurements in 84 stenoses before, immediately after and 3 months after successful TCA. Three groups with unchanged results, further improvement and restenoses compared to the acute TCA result can be differentiated.

TCA results at 3 months		Stenosis (mean %)		
		Before	Immed.	3 months
	n			
Constant (<20%)	58 (69%)	81	40	37
Improved (≥20%)	10 (12%)	73	41	14
Deteriorated (≥20%)	16 (19%)	77	32	60

the NIH-registry where they amount to nearly 34% within comparable follow-up intervals.

Follow-up 12 months after TCA

Here we refer again to the results of the above mentioned group of 90 patients who underwent acute successful TCA. A year after TCA the symptoms were still improved in most of the patients. When compared with their condition before TCA the number of patients whose symptoms were not altered or deteriorated after an initial improvement had remained unchanged. It is the same with the findings in the exercise-ECG. Among 81 of the 90 patients who had a repeat angiogram only 2 showed restenosis.

Follow-up 3 to 6 years after TCA

Three to 6 years (mean 3.8 years) after TCA questionnaires were sent to 61 patients who had had successful TCA in the period between 1977 and 1980. It was answered by 54 patients (88%) (Table 3). Nineteen of the patients stated to be absolutely free of symptoms, 32 to have still markedly improved symptoms compared to their condition before TCA. Only 2 patients reported that their condition had not changed and 1 patient that his symptoms had deteriorated after an initial improvement.

Of the 54 patients 23 consented to undergo repeat angiography. This showed good or unchanged regional long-term results in all patients. No change in the mean diameter of the dilated stenoses was found. Only 5 patients had remaining stenoses between 50 and below 75%. In no patient an increase in diameter stenosis of more than 10% had occurred compared to the study one year after TCA (Figure 4). In 5 patients, however, 4 with primary stenoses in the LAD, and 1 in the left circumflex artery (LCX), new hemodynamically effective stenoses developed, 4 in the right coronary artery and 1 in the LCX.

Table 3. Symptoms in 54 patients 3–6 years after TCA compared to the pre-TCA state.

Symptoms	Patients	
	n	%
None	19	35
Improved	32	59
No change	2	4
Reappearance	1	2

Repetitive Coronary Angiograms in 22 Patients

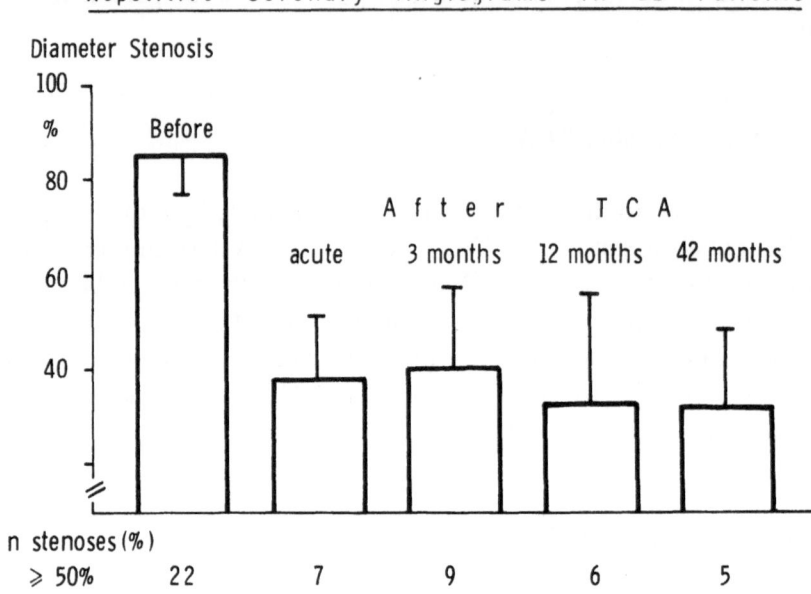

Figure 4. Mean stenosis in follow-up angiograms in 22 patients acutely after, 3 months, 12 months, and 42 months after successful TCA. Pre-TCA stenosis was more than 50% in all patients, more than 75% in 20 patients and 90% or more in 13 patients. During follow-ups, there were remaining stenoses in the dilated segments between 50% and less than 75% in only few patients.

Summary

TCA has proved to be a technique for myocardial revascularization showing not only acute or medium-term but also long-term success over a follow-up period of now up to 6 years.

Symptoms, ischaemic parameters especially in the exercise-ECG and angiographic findings are suited for follow-up investigations. In the period between the acute angiographic result and the follow-up angiogram after 3 months the majority of the patients showed stable angiographic results whereas in smaller patient groups further improvements or restenoses were observed. Regional restenoses were detected in 17% of the patients within the first year after TCA. Most often the restenoses are announced by a sudden recurrence of symptoms and by ischaemic changes in the exercise-ECG.

Long-term follow-up is characterised by permanent improvement of symptoms in most patients and the absence of regional restenosis if good success was confirmed after 12 months. But progression of the primary disease which was observed in 23% of the patients within 42 months at another location may be the reason for a recurrence of symptoms and the need for repeat revascularization.

Longterm results after angioplasty of stenosed coronary artery bypass grafts

MAMDOUH I. EL GAMAL, HANS R. BONNIER, HERMAN R. MICHELS, JAQUELINE M. HEYMAN and EDMOND G. STASSEN

Percutaneous transluminal angioplasty (PTA) of stenosed aorto-coronary bypass grafts is an alternative to re-operation in patients who develop recurrent angina pectoris following coronary bypass surgery [1, 2]. Although the procedure is easily performed with a high success rate and a low incidence of complications, there are only a few reports dealing with the long term follow up after an initial successful angioplasty [3, 4].

In the period between October 1980 and April 1982 we performed 26 successful PTA's in 16 patients: 20 first PTA, 4 second PTA, one third PTA and one fourth PTA. All patients were followed up to December 1983 (Table 1).

After a successful first PTA, angina and graft re-stenosis or occlusion occurred one to twelve months later in 9 out of the 16 patients (11 out of the 20 grafts). Angiography revealed restenosis in eight and total occlusion of three grafts. Three patients underwent elective coronary artery bypass grafting (CABG), two were treated conservatively and four patients (4 grafts) underwent a successful second PTA.

Two patients (2 grafts) remained clinically improved 28 and 29 months later. There were no angiographic sings of re-stenosis in the graft pertaining to the latter patient when restudied 23 months after PTA. The remaining two patients (2 grafts) developed recurrence of graft stenosis. One underwent CABG after 14 months, the other a third successful PTA after two months. The latter patient developed recurrence after 5 months. He underwent a fourth successful PTA, because satisfactory surgical revascularization was not possible. He remained clinically improved 18 months later. Seven out of sixteen patients remained asymptomatic 22 to 37 months after a first successful PTA (9 out of 20 grafts).

Five patients (6 grafts) consented to have repeat angiography that was performed 6 to 26 months after PTA. There was no recurrence of the stenosis in five grafts (3 to the left anterior descending and 2 to the circumflex artery). A single graft to the right coronary artery showed a 40% stenosis (prior to PTA 70%). We studied the relation between recurrence of stenosis and the initial site of the stenosed segment in the graft (Table 2). Vein grafts with multiple stenoses had the highest incidence of recurrence. Localised stenoses in the body of the vein had the lowest incidence of recurrence. As far as other sites were concerned, we were

Table 1. Longterm results after angioplasty of stenosed coronary artery bypass grafts.

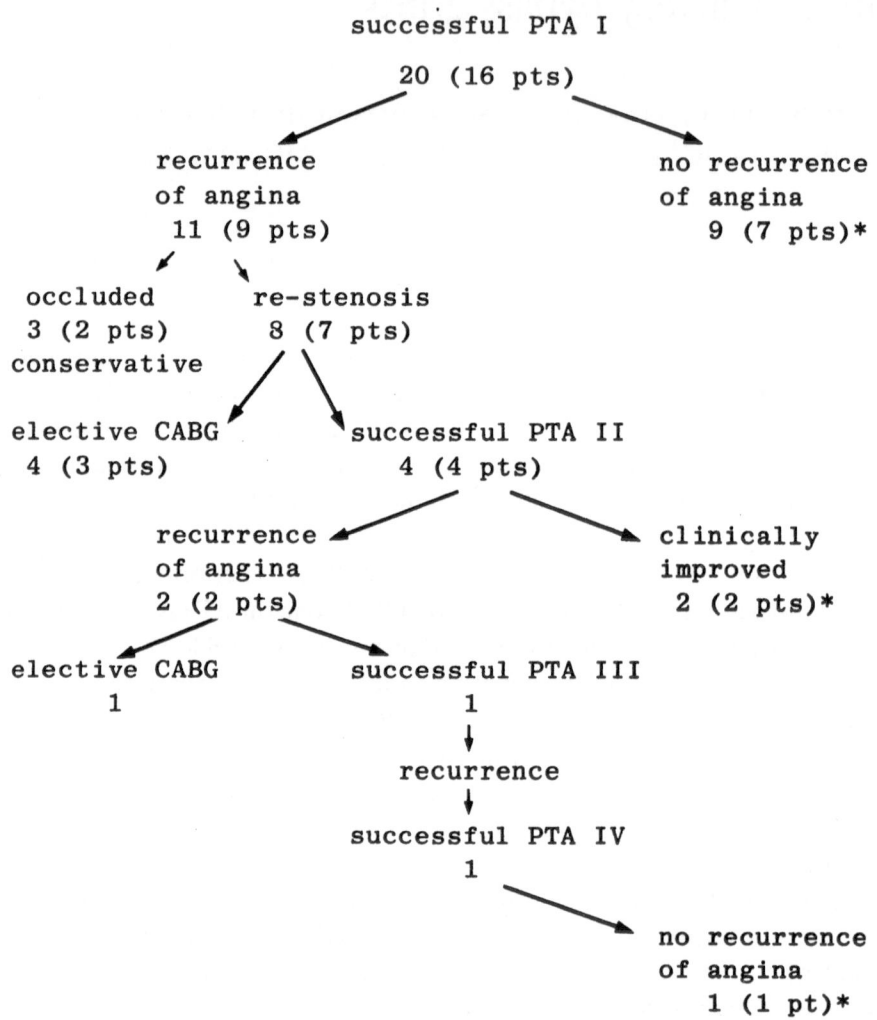

* Seven out of the ten patients had a repeat angiogram without signs of restenosis, three refused.

Table 2. Relation between recurrence and the initial site of the stenosed segment in the aorta-coronary bypass graft.

Site of stenosis	N	Recurrence
Ostium	2	1
Distal anastomosis	3	2
Body, localised	12	5
Body, multiple	3	3

unable to draw any conclusions because the numbers were to small. Recurrence of graft stenosis at a site that was not previously narrowed occurred twice.

The mean stenosis by angiography was 75% before and 31% after PTA in grafts that developed recurrence, while it was 76% before and 20% after in grafts that did not restenose. The difference is statistically significant ($p < 0.05$).

Thus in our series the total recurrence of graft stenosis after one or more PTA is 50%. Douglas et al. [3] reported a similar high recurrence rate (47%) for stenoses in the proximal anastomosis or body of the vein grafts, while Block et al. [4] reported a 38% recurrence.

In our series however 10 out of 16 patients (62%) remain clinically improved after a mean follow up of 26 months. In conclusion, PTA is useful in the long-term management of patients with stenoses of aorto-coronary bypass grafts and recurrent angina.

References

1. Ford WB, Wholey MH, Zikria EA (1981) Percutaneous transluminal dilatation of aorto-coronary saphenous vein bypass grafts. Chest 79: 529–535
2. Block PC, Palacios IF, Wholey MH (1981) Percutaneous transluminal angioplasty of stenotic coronary artery bypass grafts. Circulation 64-Supp IV: IV-109. (Abstr)
3. Douglas JS, Gruentzig AT, King SB (1982) Long-term results of percutaneous transluminal angioplasty for aorto-coronary saphenous vein graft stenosis. Circulation 66-Supp II: II-124 (Abstr)
4. Block PC, Cowley MJ, Kaltenbach M (1984) Percutaneous angioplasty of stenoses of bypass grafts or of bypass graft anastomotic sites. Am J Cardiol 53: 666–668

In vitro studies to investigate the possibility of protective intracoronary perfusion during percutaneous transluminal coronary angioplasty (PTCA)

F.M. McDONALD, M. FUCHS, J. KREUZER, A. HEINEN, H.W. HÖPP, Hj. HIRCHE, V. HOMBACH, V. HOSSMANN and H.H. HILGER

In order to investigate the possibility of providing a myocardial protective effect by intracoronary perfusion through the dilatation catheter during the phase of balloon inflation for PTCA, in vitro studies were performed to determine the relationship between proximal perfusion pressure and flow through the catheter. In addition, blood samples obtained proximal and distal to the catheter system were examined to establish whether a change in blood composition across the catheter occurs.

Initial studies were performed using the Grüntzig G-20-20 dilatation catheter (Schneider Medintag AG, Zurich), however we were unable to obtain flow rates of more than $10 \, ml.min^{-1}$ using this catheter (see Figure 1) and so all further experiments were carried out using the Grüntzig 'Steerable' 2.0 catheter from the same firm. The perfusates employed were heparinised pig blood (approx. 50 $IU.ml^{-1}$, giving TPT <10% and PTT >2 min) or pig blood diluted with 0.9% NaCl to a haematocrit of about 25%. Perfusion was performed at proximal pressures (P_{cath}) of 600, 900 and 1200 mmHg, both against atmospheric pressure and using a model coronary artery system [1] to provide a better approximation of in vivo conditions.

Figure 1 shows the relationship between P_{cath} and flow rate through the catheter when perfusion was performed against atmospheric pressure. Reduction of haematocrit to under 30% was associated with an increase in flow at all levels of Pcath, and flow rates in excess of $20 \, ml.min^{-1}$ were achieved at $P_{cath} = 1200$ mmHg. When perfusion was performed against a pressure of 40 mmHg in the model coronary artery system (this pressure was chosen as representing the intracoronary pressure in vivo after balloon inflation) there was again a marked increase in flow associated with the reduction in haematocrit (Table 1). The mean pressure distal to the catheter in the model system (P_c) approached values of 200 mmHg at a P_{cath} of 1200 mmHg.

Blood samples obtained proximal and distal to the catheter system showed no haemolysis or change in erythrocyte count, even at P_{cath} of 1200 mmHg, indicating that perfusion was not associated with mechanical damage to the erythrocytes. However, perfusion with whole blood (haematocrit ≥30%) led to a significant reduction in thrombocyte count across the catheter, independent of P_{cath} (proxi-

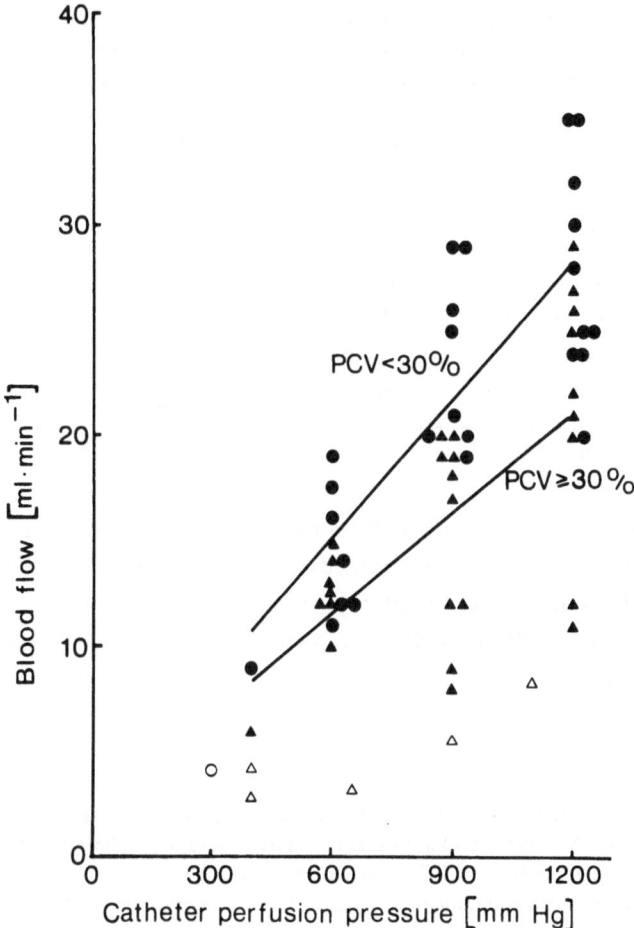

Figure 1. Relationship between catheter perfusion pressure and blood flow for the PTCA catheters Grüntzig G-20-20 (open symbols) and Grüntzig 'Steerable' 2.0 (filled symbols). Perfusion was performed against atmospheric pressure.
▲: Haematocrit (PCV) $\geqslant 30\%$, $y = 0.016x + 2.06$, $n = 27$, $r = 0.657$, $P<0.001$.
●: Haematocrit (PCV) $<30\%$, $y = 0.022x + 1.79$, $n = 26$, $r = 0.815$, $P<0.001$.

mal 388 ± 198 to distal $356 \pm 183 .10^3 . \mu l^{-1}$, $P<0.05$). When diluted blood was used, there was no significant change in thrombocyte count (proximal 279 ± 125 to distal $264 \pm 117 .10^3 . \mu l^{-1}$). Associated with this was the repeated finding during whole blood perfusion that the catheter lumen, particularly at the side-openings, became blocked by thrombus formation. The reason for this is presumably the greater lateral displacement of thrombocytes onto the catheter walls due to the higher erythrocyte number in whole blood [2].

In conclusion, the flow which can be obtained through the dilatation catheter should be sufficient to provide a protective effect, at least in cases where the coronary artery stenosis is not too proximal. Care should be exercised during in vivo perfusion, as these in vitro studies suggest that overperfusion may lead to the

Table 1. Relationship of proximal perfusion pressure (P_{prox}) and haematocrit (PCV) to flow through the dilatation catheter Grüntzig 'Steerable' 2.0 and the pressure measured distal to the catheter (P_c) during perfusion against A $\bar{P}_{myoc}$ of 40 mmHg.

P_{prox} mmHg	PCV %	Flow ml.min^{-1}	P_c mmHg	N
600	39 ± 8	9 ± 3	92 ± 21	7
	25 ± 2	13 ± 3	95 ± 27	6
900	35 ± 4	15 ± 4	141 ± 40	8
	24 ± 2	19 ± 3	152 ± 44	7
1200	35 ± 4	18 ± 3	180 ± 53	8
	23 ± 3	26 ± 4	198 ± 47	8

All values are mean ± S.D.

development of high intracoronary pressures. The use of diluted blood as the perfusate instead of whole blood reduces the risk of intracatheter thrombus formation, which would prevent further perfusion, and might lead to blockage in the vascular bed by thrombus fragments becoming detached from the catheter.

References

1. Fuchs M, McDonald FM, Kreuzer J, Höpp HW, Heinen A, Hossmann V, Heymans L, Arnold G, Hirche Hj, Hombach V (1984) Myokardprotektion durch Perfusion während perkutaner, transluminaler Koronarangioplastie (PTCA). Herz Kreislauf, in press
2. Baumgartner HR (1984) Blutstömung und Thrombogenese. Internist 25: 75–81

Haemodynamic and haemorheologic effects of intracoronary perfusion during percutaneous transluminal coronary angioplasty (PTCA)

M. FUCHS, F.M. McDONALD, H.W. HÖPP, A. HEINEN, J. KREUZER,
G. ARNOLD, L. HEYMANS, V. HOMBACH, Hj. HIRCHE,
V. HOSSMANN and H.H. HILGER

During PTCA, inflation of the catheter balloon to dilate the coronary stenosis produces complete coronary occlusion and results in myocardial ischaemia, thus limiting the duration of inflation. It was the aim of this study to determine if a protective effect can be obtained by blood perfusion through the dilatation catheter during the phase of balloon inflation, which might permit an increase in the duration of inflation. Such a protective effect would reduce the problems of repeated localisation of the catheter if the primary dilatation was unsuccessful, and if PTCA induced a critical phase for the patient requiring surgical intervention, this interval could be bridged by this new method of perfusion.

In 17 anaesthetised open-chest pigs, the catheter (Grüntzig 'Steerable' 2.0, Schneider Medintag, Zurich) was advanced via the right carotid artery into the left anterior descending coronary artery (LAD) until the balloon lay in the middle third of the LAD. The haemodynamic parameters (left ventricular systolic and end-diastolic pressure, LVdP/dtmax, mean arterial pressure, heart rate and local segment shortening proximal and distal to the balloon) were measured before and 1 min after balloon inflation. To determine the haemorheologic and haemostasiologic effects of inflation with and without perfusion (perfusate PCV $\geqslant 30\%$ or $<30\%$), blood samples were taken proximal and distal (coronary sinus) to the catheter.

Results: The catheter itself in the LAD prior to balloon inflation caused a significant deterioration of the haemodynamic parameters (Figure 1), accompanied by a slight increase in heart rate. This effect of the catheter is dependent on the relationship between catheter and coronary artery diameter: 0.6 mm to 0.92–2.18 mm (mean 1.33). In 5 experiments the catheter induced ventricular fibrillation, in these animals the mean LAD diameter was 1.18 mm compared to 1.43 mm in those which did not fibrillate. Balloon inflation for 1 min without perfusion caused further significant haemodynamic deterioration and induced a paradoxical systolic segment lengthening distal to the catheter. These haemodynamic changes could be prevented by simultaneous intracoronary perfusion during the 1 min inflation using whole blood (PCV $\geqslant 30\%$) or blood diluted with 0.9% NaCl (PCV $<30\%$) at a proximal perfusion pressure of 1200 mmHg, giving flow rates of 18 ± 3 and 22 ± 5 ml.min^{-1} respectively (Table 1). In relation to the weight of

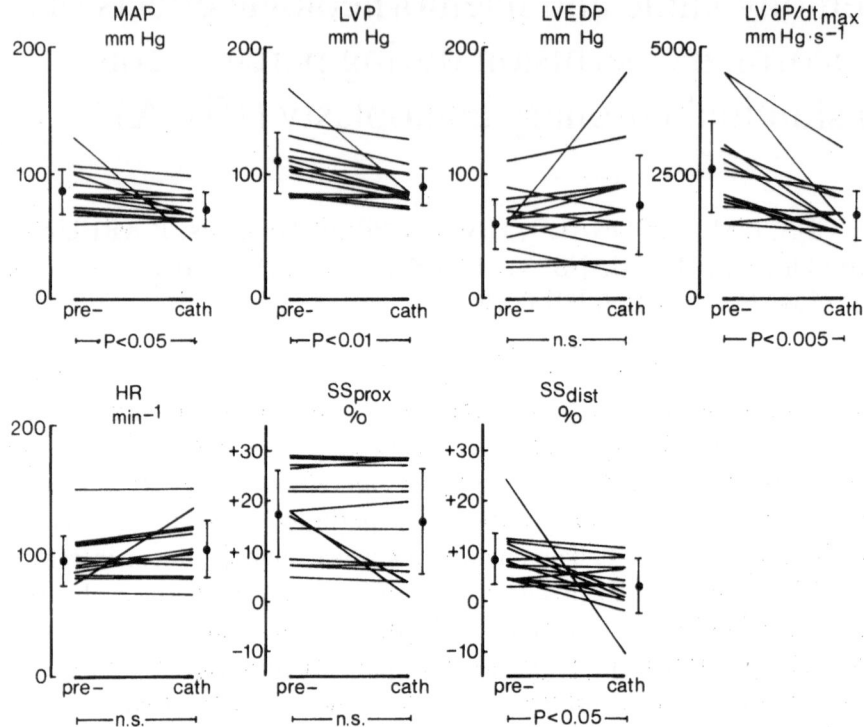

Figure 1. Haemodynamic changes caused by positioning the dilatation catheter in the LAD. The filled circles show the mean values ± s.d. when the catheter was in the aorta (pre-) and when the catheter was positioned with the balloon in the middle third of the LAD (cath).

tissue perfused, the estimated flow rate was 70–100 ml.100 g^{-1}.min^{-1}. In 8 other experiments, the proximal perfusion pressure was decreased to investigate the effect of perfusion at a lower flow rate (50–60 g^{-1}.min^{-1}). In these experiments a similar protective effect of perfusion during balloon inflation was seen. Coronary sinus blood samples obtained following inflation without perfusion showed an increased whole blood viscosity at low shear rates (0.03s^{-1}), this change was not observed following perfusion. Histological examination of myocardial samples obtained after inflation without perfusion (n = 9) showed the presence of fresh thrombi in the arteriolar segments on two occasions. After whole blood perfusion a thrombus was seen in one out of nine samples examined, and following perfusion with diluted blood none of the nine samples showed the presence of a fresh thrombus. In each experiment, the tip of the catheter had destroyed the endothelium in the middle third of the LAD, and in 3 hearts the intima was also injured.

In conclusion, the PTCA catheter positioned in the LAD caused sufficient myocardial ischaemia to influence the haemodynamic status. This effect was exacerbated by balloon inflation, and was accompanied by an increased structural viscosity in coronary sinus blood samples, suggesting an increased erythrocyte aggregation tendency, and possibly by an increased thrombus formation. Simultaneous perfusion during balloon inflation prevented the haemodynamic deterioration seen in the absence of perfusion and appears also to have a beneficial effect on the haemorheologic changes.

Improved tolerance of intracoronary balloon inflation with a modified Grüntzig balloon angioplasty catheter

ULRICH W. BUSCH, RAIMUND ERBEL, ULRICH PFEIFFER,
JÜRGEN MEYER, GÜNTHER BLÜMEL and HANS BLÖMER

Abstract

A modified Grüntzig coronary angioplasty catheter, designed to permit continuous antegrade perfusion during dilatation was evaluated. During in-vitro tests with blood, flow rates between 12 and 28 ml/min were measured at effective pressures between 50 and 100 mmHg. During in vivo tests in five dogs this catheter was compared with conventional catheter types which prevent antegrade flow during balloon inflation.

Time between balloon occlusion and appearance of the same degree of ischemia in the ECG ranged from 40 to 420 sec, mean 203 seconds, and 30 to 180 sec, mean 120 sec, for the modified and the conventional catheters, respectively. Prolongation of the intracoronary balloon inflation time may be valuable in selected patients.

Introduction

During coronary angioplasty, passage of a tight stenosis and balloon inflation often result in severe myocardial ischemia due to total interruption of antegrade flow, rendering prolonged balloon inflation intolerable and necessitating early balloon deflation or even catheter withdrawal. While pump perfusion via the regular dilatation catheter may help to prevent severe ischemia, this method requires an additional pump unit and is not without technical and biological problems [1–4]. To maintain antegrade flow in a different way the regular Grüntzig catheter was modified by creation of side holes proximal to the balloon and in communication with the distal orifice. This is a brief report of the results of our in-vitro and in-vivo tests of this catheter modification.

Methods

During in vitro tests, fully anticoagulated blood was allowed to enter the proximal holes of the distal catheter segment at a static pressure of 100, 75 and 50 mmHg. Flow rate was determined by timed collection of the blood leaving the distal

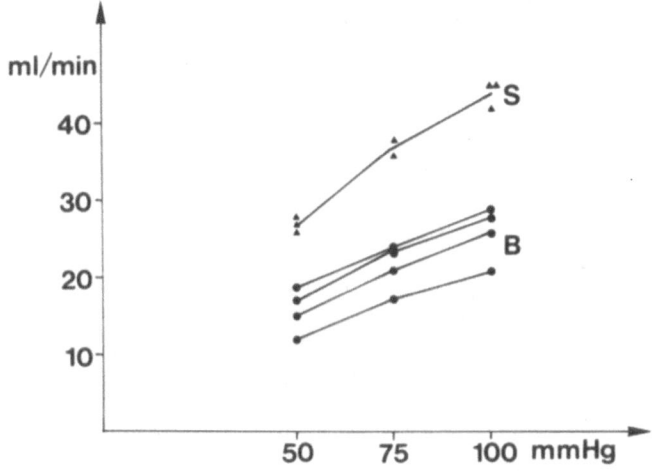

Figure 1. In vitro determined pressure/flow rate relation through the distal segment of the modified Grüntzig catheter. S = with saline, B = with blood.

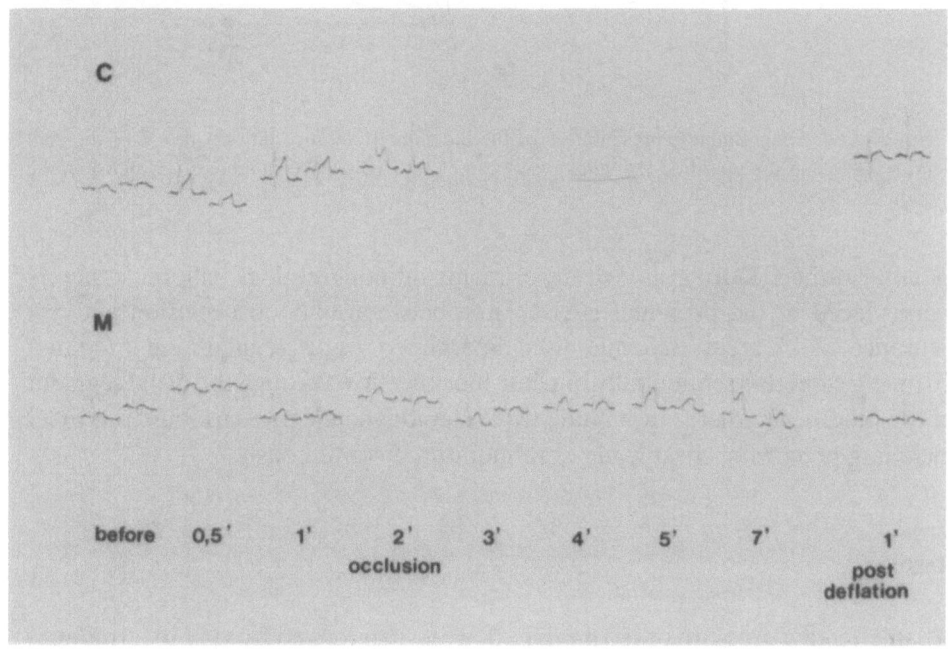

Figure 2. Time course of the electrocardiographic changes (V4 and V5) during balloon occlusion with the conventional (C) the modified (M) angioplasty catheter.

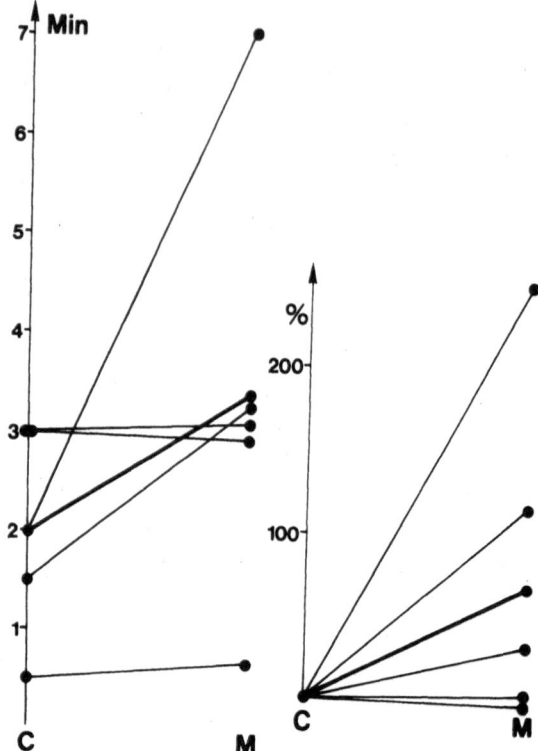

Figure 3. Left: Diagrammatic presentation of the individual tolerance times with use of the conventional (C) and the modified (M) angioplasty catheters. Right: Percent increase (with use of the modified catheter).

catheter orifice. During in vivo experiments in mongrel dogs balloon catheters were placed in the proximal LAD. Time between balloon occlusion and appearance of clearcut ischemia was determined using regular and modified Grüntzig catheters sequentially or while blocking flow through the distal segment of the modified catheter by a guide wire. Hemodynamic pressures and the ECG including precordial chest leads were monitored continuously.

Results

At an effective pressure of 100 mmHg, flow in vitro ranged from 21 to 28 ml/min, at 75 mmHg from 17 to 24 ml/min and at 50 mmHg from 12 to 19 ml/min. Pressure flow relation was slightly curvilinear, the increase in flow being less at higher pressures. Test blood hematocrit was in the normal range (39–45%). The higher flow rates obtained with saline (42 ml/min at 100 mmHg) reflect the influence of viscosity.

During in vivo tests in 5 dogs, time from balloon occlusion to manifest ischemia ranged from 30 to 180, mean 120 seconds using the regular catheters. With the modified catheters permitting residual antegrade flow, ischemia became manifest between 40 and 420, mean 203 seconds. The ECG changes were used as the most dependable and best comparable parameters for ischemia. In two of these five dogs, however, ischemia was not demonstrably delayed with the modified catheter by ECG criteria. Three other dogs could not be included in the study, one because of uncorrectable ventricular fibrillation shortly after the first balloon occlusion, a second because of absent ischemic changes after balloon occlusions and a third because of acute vessel occlusion from dissection and intramural hemorrhage after first balloon inflation (oversized balloon).

Comments

The modified Grüntzig catheter may allow a significant prolongation of the intracoronary balloon inflation time in dogs because the remaining antegrade flow through the catheter, though much reduced, delays the development of ischemia. It may, therefore, be useful in man when prolonged balloon occlusion during coronary angioplasty is a problem as in cases with proximal lesions of large, poorly collateralized vessels. Reasons for the failure to prolong inflation time in two dogs could be functional closure of the proximal or distal ostia through contact with the vessel wall or squeezing and kinking of the narrow segment inside the balloon. Therefore, further modification of the catheter (different location of the proximal ostia, reinforcement of the narrow segment) and in vivo testing is warranted. The inability to measure the transstenotic gradient with this catheter also should be mentioned.

References

1. Grüntzig A (1976) Perkutane Dilatation von Coronarstenosen-Beschreibung eines neuen Kathetersystems. Klin Wschr 54: 543–545
2. Meier B, Grüntzig AR, Brown JE (1984) Continuous distal perfusion of occluded coronary arteries with arterial blood through a percutaneous catheter (abstr.). Eur Heart J 5: 120
3. Busch U, Pfeiffer U, Baumann G, Sebening H, Blömer H (1984) Distal vessel perfusion via dilatation catheter after coronary artery occlusion (abstr.). Eur Heart J 5: 120
4. Spears JR, Serur J, Baim DS, Grossman W, Paulin S (1983) Myocardial protection with fluosol-DA during prolonged coronary balloon occlusion in the dog. Circulation 68/II: III-80

Pressure transmission characteristics of the Grüntzig superlow-profile catheter

ULRICH W. BUSCH, ROLAND HEINZE, HELMUT SEBENING
and HANS BLÖMER

Abstract

The pressure transmission characteristics of the recently introduced Grüntzig super-low-profile catheter were evaluated for comparison with those of other coronary angioplasty catheters in clinical use. After thorough elimination of air bubbles from the pressure transmitting system the frequency response was linear ($\pm 5\%$) up to 5 Hz and permitted recording of only minimally distorted arterial pressure tracings. With introduction of the 0.012″ guide wire arterial pressure tracings remained adequate as long as the narrow catheter segment beginning just proximally to the balloon was not entered. Passage of the wire through the narrow distal segment resulted in severe overdamping even below 0.5 Hz.

Introduction

Intracoronary pressure recordings provide important information during transluminal coronary angioplasty [1]. Frequently, however, they are markedly distorted due to overdamping, which usually is the result of minor air bubbles within the pressure transmitting system that includes the long and narrow lumen of the angioplasty catheter [2]. These catheter dimensions explain the much more devasting effect of even minute air bubbles on pressure recording quality as compared to conventional catheters. The recently introduced Grüntzig superlow-profile catheter is characterized by an even smaller lumen of the distal catheter segment. Therefore, we determined the pressure transmission characteristics of this catheter for comparison with other coronary dilatation catheters tested previously [2].

Methods

The tests were performed after complete elimination of even minute air bubbles from the pressure transmitting system. This was achieved by first replacing the room air inside the system by carbon dioxide and subsequent flushing with freshly boiled saline (contains less dissolved air). During initial flushing alcohol was added as a surfactant [2–4]. During measurements the catheter was immersed in a water bath of 37° C. Transmission of sine wave pressures (0.2–20 Hz) and of arterial pressure pulses reproduced from tape by use of a multifunction pressure generator was measured. Statham P23dB transducers, the Schneider Y connector, a NAMIC manifold and NAMIC adult pressure monitoring line were utilized. The catheter was kindly supplied by Schneider-Medintag AG, Zürich, Switzerland.

Results

The frequency response of the system was linear ($\pm 5\%$) up to 5 Hz (Figure 1). In the higher frequency range there was progressive reduction in amplitude. Arterial pressure tracings were transmitted with only minimal distortion (Figure 2). Flushing the catheter with diluted contrast medium resulted in additional damping of the frequency response.

Introduction of the 0.012″ guide wire into the larger lumen still yielded a satisfactory result in regard to the pressure curve contour as shown in Figure 2. Passage of the wire through the narrow distal segment, however, resulted in severe overdamping, even below 0.5 Hz, with gross distortion of the phasic arterial pressure curve.

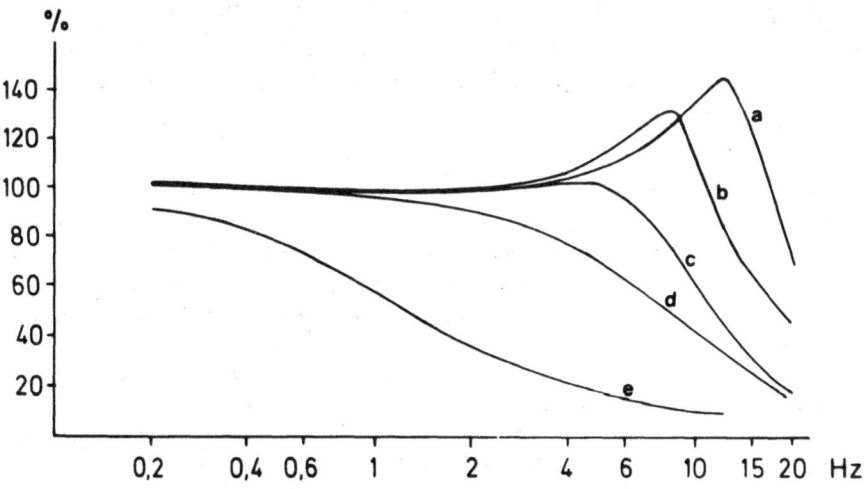

Figure 1. Frequency response curves of the Grüntzig super-low-profile catheter: a) connected to Statham P 23 dB via 60 cm pressure monitoring line; b) with additional manifold; c) as in b, with additional y connector; d) as in c, but filled with contrast medium instead of saline; e) with 0.012″ guide wire.

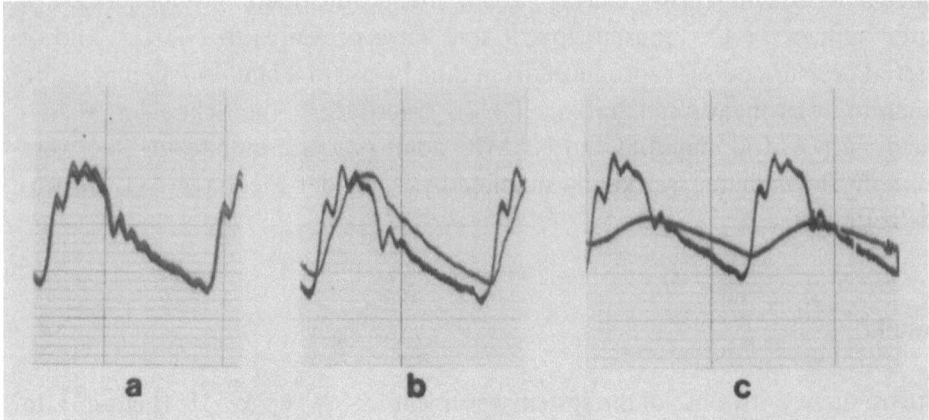

Figure 2. Examples of arterial pressure curves. Reference pressure and trans-catheter pressure recordings are shown superimposed: a) Without guide wire; b) With partially introduced guide wire; c) With guide wire passing through the distal narrow segment.

Comment

Despite its narrow distal segment, the frequency response of the Grüntzig super-low-profile catheter compares well with those of the regular size Grüntzig catheters and is still superior to the Simpson Robert catheter. All these catheter systems permit satisfactory phasic intravascular pressure measurements, provided the guide wire does not interfere with the narrow distal segment and the pressure transmitting system is optimally set up. This includes complete elimination of air bubbles as by the procedures mentioned above.

References

1. Meier B, Grüntzig AR, Senning A, Siegenthaler WE (1979) Nonoperative dilatation of coronary-artery stenosis: Percutaneous transluminal coronary angioplasty. N Engl J Med 301: 61–68
2. Busch UW, Sebening H, Beeretz R, Blömer H (1984) Zur Zuverlässigkeit der Druckregistrierung über Koronardilatationskatheter. Herz/Kreislauf 16: 304–308
3. Dear HD, Spear AF (1971) Accurate method for measuring dP/dt with cardiac catheters and external transducers. J Appl Physiol 30: 897–899
4. Yanof HM, Rosen AL, McDonald NM, McDonald DA (1963) A critical study of the response of manometers to forced oscillations. Phys Med Biol 8: 407–422

Increased hemolysis during coronary perfusion via angioplasty catheters as a result of side-hole jet effect

ULRICH W. BUSCH, ULRICH PFEIFFER, ULRICH KUSAWE,
HELMUT SEBENING, GÜNTHER BLÜMEL and HANS BLÖMER

Abstract

Hemolysis is one of the known possible problems that can occur with selective coronary perfusion through the dilatation catheter. In the present study we determined in vivo and in vitro the hemolysing effect of selective blood perfusion through different catheter types, using a specially designed perfusion pump. The in-vitro tests revealed that hemolysis was not directly determined by pump pressure, but by catheter design and flow rate. The side holes of the Grüntzig catheters were found to cause hemolysis, when blood was leaving through them in a jet like fashion.

The in vivo testing of the system in dogs revealed no clinically relevant hemolysis.

Introduction

Selective coronary artery perfusion may become a useful adjunct of coronary angioplasty. It may avoid severe schemia resulting from blockage of antegrade blood flow during passage of the catheter through a tight stenosis or during balloon inflation, as in cases with proximal lesions of large vessels in the absence of collaterals. It may also be beneficial in some cases of angioplasty-induced persistent coronary artery occlusion by providing flow to the jeopardized myocardium, until definitive surgical revascularization can be performed. One of the possible limitations of this method, however, may be the initiation of significant hemolysis and related problems [1–4]. In fact, severe hemolysis was observed by others with use of a roller pump at higher pump pressures as required for the Simpson-Robert catheter [3]. Because of somewhat different preliminary results from our own experiments [4] the present study was performed to further clarify the issue and to evaluate possible factors responsible for increased hemolysis.

Methods

A pressure and volume controlled perfusion pump was developed that is capable of producing the high pump pressures required for adequate perfusion rates through the catheter. During in vitro tests the pump pressure/flow rate relation for various angioplasty catheters as well as the degree of hemolysis were determined, using a recirculating blood pool of 100 ml. Tests were performed with both human and canine blood. Total plasma hemoglobin was used as an index of hemolysis and was determined with a benzidine reaction. In addition it was determined in vivo in dogs prior to and during prolonged selective coronary artery perfusion.

Results

With our pump model, continuous flow rates of up to 120 ml/min and a maximal pressure of 14 bar could be achieved. At flow rates of 60 ml/min, pressures ranged between 2.6 and 4.7 bar for the Grüntzig 'steerable', 5.4 and 7.2 for the Grüntzig super-low-profile and 7.8 and 13.7 for the Simpson Robert catheter, depending

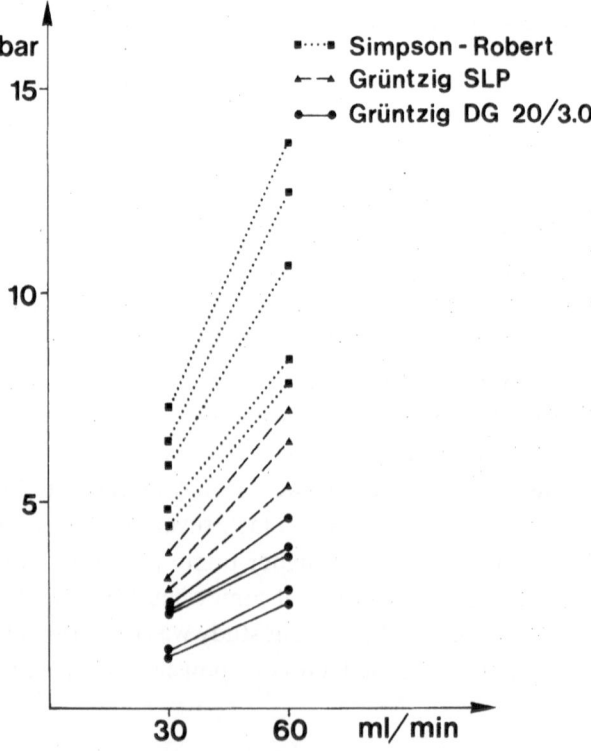

Figure 1. Pressure/flow diagram of various coronary angioplasty catheters.

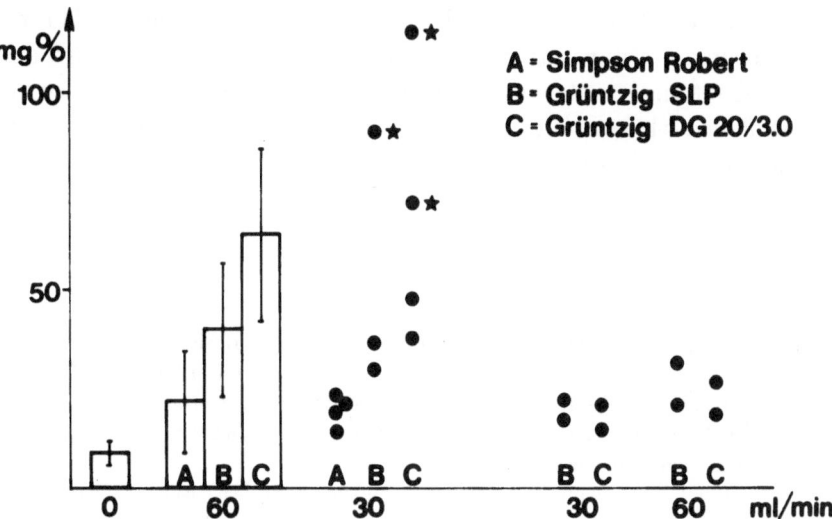

Figure 2. Change in plasma hemoglobin concentration during in-vitro testing with a recirculating blood pool of 100 ml. * denotes that the endhole was found occluded at the end of the test. The data to the right are obtained from catheters with cut-off tips (elimination of side holes).

upon blood viscosity. However, there was more hemolysis with the Grüntzig catheters. Plasma hemoglobin values after 15 minutes of in vitro testing were (mean + 2 SD): 0.22 ± 0.13, 0.40 ± 0.17 and 0.64 ± 0.22 g/l for the Simpson Robert, Grüntzig superlow profile and steerable, respectively. At the rate of 30 ml/min the difference was much less provided flow through the tip orifice was not inhibited. The increased hemolysis with the Grüntzig catheters was found the result mainly from blood leaving through the side holes near the catheter tip in a jet like fashion. The jet was always present with a flow rate of 60 ml/min. At 30 ml/min it was observed with clogging of the tip orifice. Avoiding this jet effect decreased hemolysis to values comparable with the Simpson Robert catheter. In dogs undergoing selective coronary hemoperfusion using catheters with tipholes only there was no clinically relevant rise in plasma hemoglobin after 2 hours of perfusion.

Comments

The data show that the degree of hemolysis is not directly related to the magnitude of the required pump pressure but is determined, at least in part, by differences in catheter design. For a given catheter, though, hemolysis increases with rising flow rate. The more severe hemolysis observed by others [3] with the Simpson Robert catheter in comparison with the Grüntzig catheters was not confirmed in this study and is not likely to result from higher shearing forces inside the catheter, the former having a smaller lumen and therefore a higher flow resistance than the latter. A possible explanation is that their roller pump becomes the site of erythrocyte destruction when working against a high output resistance even if this was shown to be negligible at zero output resistance. Since severe turbulence is known to cause hemolysis, its occurrence within the pathway of the blood used for perfusion should be reduced to a minimum.

References

1. Meier B, Gruentzig AR, Brown JE (1984) Continuous distal perfusion of occluded coronary arteries with arterial blood through a percutaneous catheter (abstr). Eur Heart J 5: 120
2. Spears JR, Serur J, Baim DS, Grossman W, Paulin S (1983) Myocardial protection with fluosol-DA during prolonged coronary balloon occlusion in the dog. Circulation 68/II: III-80
3. Meier P: personal communication
4. Busch U, Pfeiffer U, Baumann G, Sebening H, Blömer H (1984) Distal vessel perfusion via dilatation catheter after coronary artery occlusion (abstr). Eur Heart J 5: 120

Intraoperative angioplasty in the treatment of coronary artery disease

Introduction

Since Gruentzig's original description of the use of percutaneous transluminal coronary angioplasty in selected patients, there has been intense interest in extending the indications to include many subsets of patients with coronary artery disease [1]. One logical extension of this procedure is the use of angioplasty under direct vision in combination with coronary artery bypass. Intraoperative use of this technique has been described previously by others [2–6].

Whereas candidates for percutaneous coronary angioplasty usually have early symptoms of ischemia (a situation which maximizes chances of soft, easily compressible atheromatous lesions), patients for intraoperative angioplasty usually have well established multiple obstructions involving significant portions of the artery.

Indications

Theoretically, intraoperative angioplasty would have greatest appeal in patients with multiple segmental coronary artery lesions and when the obstructions are difficult to approach with normal bypass techniques. For anatomic locations in which the arterial obstructions are inaccessible (left anterior descending in the apical fat pad, distal right coronary at or near the interventricular-atrioventricular groove junction or proximal LAD adjacent to septal perforators), use of intraoperative angioplasty would have special significance. Obstructive lesions located in these areas are difficult to approach with usual coronary bypass techniques.

In addition to the treatment of multiple segmental or inaccessible obstructions, intraoperative angioplasty can occasionally be used to accomplish internally what would be difficult to accomplish externally. For example, heavily calcified or fibrotic arteries frequently cannot be safely entered for performance of either isolated or sequential bypass grafts. Surprisingly, in this situation intraoperative angioplasty has been successfully used to compress plaque of very diseased arteries far removed from the arteriotomy site.

Intraoperative angioplasty was begun at Emory University Hospital in September of 1981 and results reported herein extend through August 1984. During this period of time, 4,872 isolated coronary artery bypass operations have been performed and intraoperative angioplasty has been incorporated as an adjunctive procedure in 47 patients (1 percent). Intraoperative dilatations performed at our institution have primarily involved the anterior descending and posterior descending branches of the right coronary arteries. Arterial diameter down to 1.0 mm presents no unique limitation, and obstructions in the mid portion of the posterior descending branch of the right coronary artery have been dilated with satisfactory results. However, the mid and distal LAD arterial segments have been the most frequently dilated sites of obstruction (Figure 1). Primary sites for intraoperative dilatation include the left anterior descending at the apical fat pad, the distal right coronary artery at the interventricular-atrioventricular groove junction, and the proximal LAD at the site of the first septal perforator. However, the latter area has been considered somewhat dangerous because of the theoretical possibility of peripheral embolization of atherosclerotic plaque.

  Although intraoperative angioplasty appears to be a promising adjunctive procedure to the surgical treatment of coronary disease, angioplasty probably should not be employed whenever good sequential grafting is possible. Multiple obstructions of the proximal and mid anterior descending coronary artery which can be readily handled with sequential grafting should be treated with this technique until long term results of balloon angioplasty can be evaluated. Preliminary observations of percutaneous angioplasty at our institution suggest that the

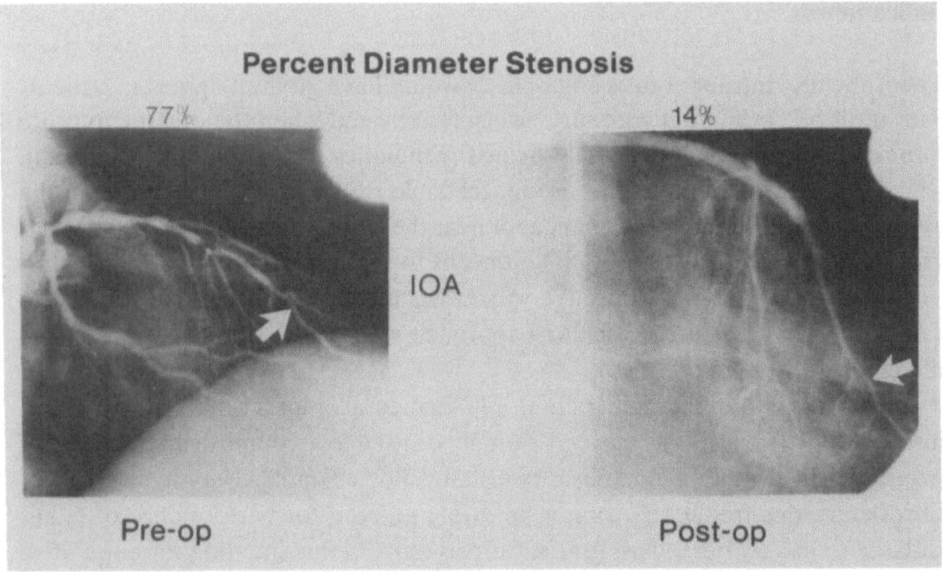

Figure 1. Site of intraoperative angioplasty in the distal left anterior descending coronary artery.

restenosis rate within the first six months is approximately 30 percent. Therefore, intraoperative angioplasty may be less satisfactory than additional grafting procedures when they can be applied. Stenoses located at the junction of the diagonal and anterior descending arteries should not be treated with intraoperative angioplasty since, as with the percutaneous approach, there is danger of compressing plaque into the diagonal branch.

Technique

The technique of intraoperative coronary angioplasty is simple and time to perform the procedure has averaged less than 10 minutes per obstruction dilated. Operative localization of the site of angioplasty can sometimes be difficult and is best done from a combination of the coronary arteriogram and external inspection or palpation. Obstructions in the apical fat pad or distal right coronary artery near the AV nodal artery can be identified by passing a small 1.0 mm metalic probe distal to the arteriotomy until the obstruction is encountered. This distance is carefully measured and a 2.0 or 3.0 mm balloon catheter is passed through the arteriotomy to the desired level. Regardless of which artery is dilated, the arteriotomy incision should not be placed close to the area for dilatation as a tear may occur into the arteriotomy site following balloon inflation.

The catheter is passed distally or proximally until the balloon bridges the obstruction (Figure 2). A hand-held saline-filled syringe is used to inflate the balloon to 4, 6, 8 and 10 atmospheres of pressure. Peak pressure at 10 atmospheres is held for 20 seconds. A total of 3 inflations is made over each obstruction. Once completed, the catheter is removed and the saphenous vein anastomosis performed in usual fashion. This technique does not allow for fluoroscopic visualization of the passage of the angioplasty catheter. This deficiency has concerned us but has not been a problem thus far, perhaps due to the lesions selected and the direct passage of the balloon catheter. Post dilatation arteriograms have not been employed to evaluate angioplasty results in the operating room because of the expensive equipment, danger of infection to the patient, and the added myocardial ischemic time necessary to evaluate results. The first 19 patients having operative angioplasty at our institution however, were recatheterized on the seventh day after surgery or just prior to hospital discharge.

Complications

Potential complications of intraoperative angioplasty are essentially those of sudden vessel closure due to dissection, spasm, or hemorrhage into the arterial wall. Late complications relate to recurrent stenosis.

We have noted no acute complications of the procedure and follow-up has not

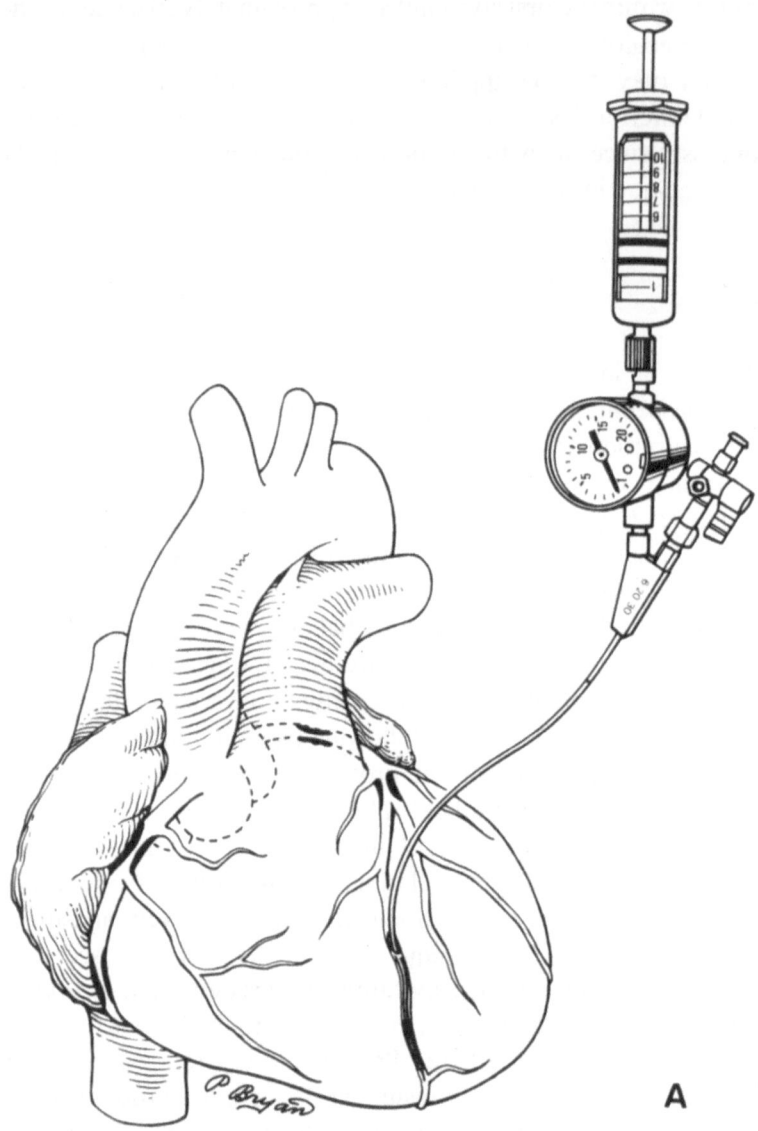

Figure 2. Technique of intraoperative angioplasty. A: Insertion of balloon catheter into distal left anterior descending artery through arteriotomy site. B: Inflation of balloon catheter to maximum of 10 atmospheres pressure after balloon bridges obstruction. C: Effect of transluminal angioplasty on atherosclerotic plaque. Specimen on left demonstrated persistent high grade obstruction adjacent to angioplasty site on right. Note compression of atheromatous material into wall of artery.

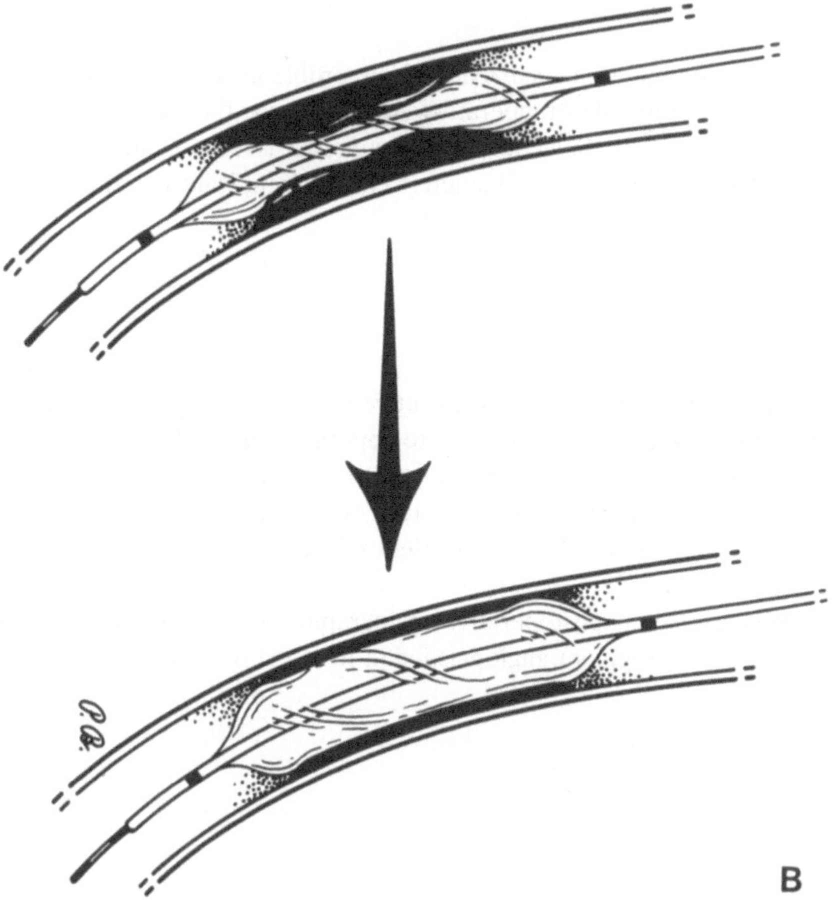

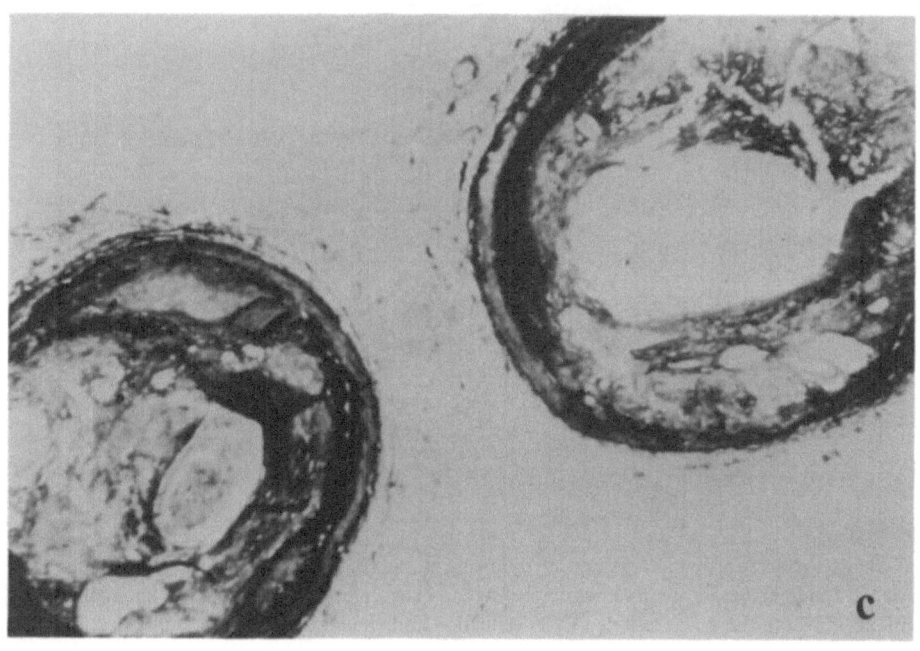

B

C

been sufficient to comment on occurrence of late problems. Initially, one of the primary reasons for failure of intraoperative angioplasty was the use of too small a balloon for the dilatation. Selection of balloon size is best made from the preoperative arteriogram as vessel diameters change significantly in the cooled anoxic heart.

Results

We now have complete data on 19 consecutive patients having intraoperative angioplasty for multisegmental or difficult to approach atherosclerotic coronary artery lesions. The most frequent site of intraoperative angioplasty has been the left anterior descending artery and accounted for 77 percent of all dilatations. There were no recognizable operative injuries or death and hospital mortality in the 4,872 patients was 1.5%.

Of the 19 patients having postoperative angiographic evaluation, the proximal or distal LAD was the segment angioplastied in 16 of the patients. The average

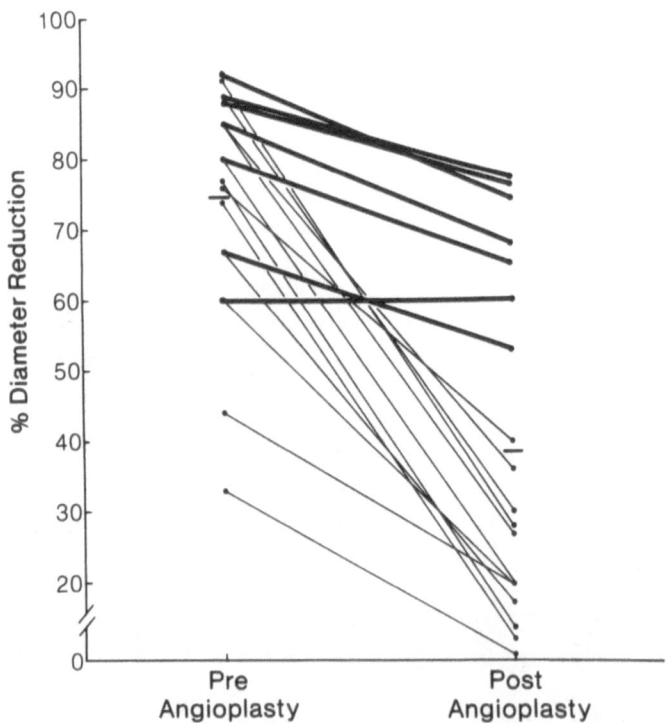

Figure 3. Changes in arterial diameter (stenosis) following intraoperative angioplasty. Heavy horizontal bars on left and right denote mean values before and after angioplasty. Heavy diagonal lines denote the 7 patients in whom there was less than 20% reduction in diameter stenosis after angioplasty.

preoperative diameter stenosis was 75% (range = 33 to 92%). The average diameter stenosis following intraoperative dilatation was 39% (range = 0 to 77%), a mean improvement in diameter stenosis of 36%. In 7 patients, improvement in diameter stenosis was less than 20% (Figure 3).

In the 47 patients undergoing intraoperative angioplasty, new Q wave formation occurred in one patient following the bypass procedure. There was loss of R wave voltage in two additional patients.

Discussion

In 1983, Mills and Ochsner [7] reported on intraoperative angioplasty in 93 atherosclerotic coronary artery obstructions at the time coronary bypass was performed. In their series of patients, the obstructions chosen for intraoperative angioplasty would not have otherwise been bypassed because of the small size of the arteries or inaccessibility. In one-half of the patients, the dilatations involved the distal left anterior descending coronary artery. In 19% of their patients, the obstructions could not be traversed, and of all lesions attempted only 57% were successfully dilated when recatheterized. In two of their patients the coronary artery was occluded distally at the time of recatheterization and this was attributed to dilatation of relatively normal intimal segments. Strong warnings were issued that balloon inflation should only occur in diseased segments of the arteries. The incidence of perioperative infarction in this series of patients was 2.4%, and they concluded that the length of the lesion rather than calcification determined success of the procedure. Roberts et al. in 1982 [8] reported on 21 dilated segments combined with coronary artery bypass. In 57% of their patients the lesions were unchanged at recatheterization and in 10% the obstructions were actually worse. In only 7 of the 21 dilated segments was there actual improvement and there was new intimal damage recorded in two of the patients.

Our experience substantiates the findings of these previous two series and 63% of all lesions dilated showed significant early improvement (greather than 20% reduction in diameter stenosis) at the time of recatheterization prior to hospital discharge. This would agree closely with the 57% reported by Mills and Ochsner [7].

Before using intraoperative angioplasty routinely, more extensive carefully controlled clinical trails should first be performed. Indiscriminate use of the procedure on all types and locations of obstructive lesions will probably yield uniformly poor results.

Intraoperative angioplasty can be performed very smoothly and rapidly, but in most situations probably offers no advantage over good multiple grafting procedures to the artery involved. The procedure has its greatest application in the treatment of obstructions which are inaccessible with normal grafting procedures or in arteries having multiple segmental lesions when balloon dilatation can be

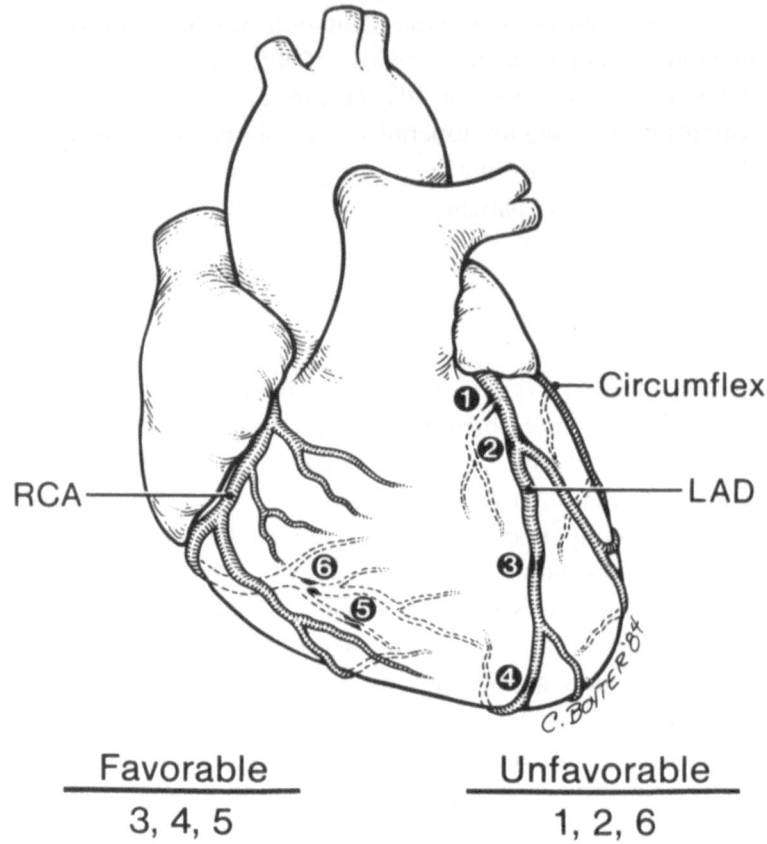

Favorable
3, 4, 5

Unfavorable
1, 2, 6

Figure 4. Favorable and unfavorable operative angioplasty sites.

used with multiple grafting techniques.

Intraoperative angioplasty may prove to be a substantial addition to the treatment of selected patients with diffused coronary disease. Favorable and unfavorable intraoperative angioplasty sites are depicted in Figure 4. Its ultimate value, however, will depend on the patency rate of the dilated arterial segments. Only further observation will decide whether the procedure will endure the test of time.

References

1. Gruentzig AR, Senning A, Siegenthaler WE (1979) Nonoperative dilatation of coronary artery stenosis: percutaneous transluminal coronary angioplasty. N Engl J Med 301: 61–8
2. Mills NL, Doyle DP (1982) Does operative transluminal angioplasty (OTA) extend the limits of coronary artery bypass surgery? Circulation 66 (suppl I)
3. Roberts AJ, Feldman RL, Conti CR, Selby JH, LaBrosse C, Knauf DG, Alexander JA, Watson

WD & Pepine CJ (1982) Preliminary experience with intraoperative transluminal balloon catheter dilation and coronary artery bypass grafting for the treatment of symptomatic diffuse coronary artery disease. Ann Thor Surg 32: 504

Fogarty TJ, Chin A, Sheon PM, Blair GL, Zimmerman JJ (1981) Adjunctive intraoperative arterial dilatation. Arch Surg 116: 1391

Wallsh E, Franzone AJ, Clauss RH, Bruno MS, Steichen F, Stertzer SH (1980) Transluminal coronary angioplasty during saphenous coronary bypass surgery. A preliminary report. Ann Surg 191 (2): 234

Wallsh E, Franzone AJ, Weinstein GS, Alcan K, Clavel A, Stertzer SH (1982) Use of operative transluminal coronary angioplasty as an adjunct to coronary artery bypass. J Thorac Cardiovasc Surg 84 (6): 843–848

Mills NL, Ochsner JL, Doyle DP, Kalchoff WP (1983) Technique and results of operative transluminal angioplasty in 81 consecutive patients. J Thorac Cardiovasc Surg 86: 689–696

Roberts AJ, Feldman RL, Conti CR, Selby JH, LaBrosse C, Kanuf DG, Alexander JA, Watson WD, Pepine CJ (1982) Preliminary experience with intraoperative transluminal balloon-catheter dilation and coronary artery bypass grafting for the treatment of symptomatic diffuse coronary artery disease. Ann Thor Surg 34: 5

Treatment of coronary artery stenosis by laser technique

JAMES J. LIVESAY, O.H. FRAZIER and DENTON A. COOLEY

Introduction

Current techniques of coronary bypass surgery have been effective in relieving stenosis, improving coronary perfusion, and prolonging life in numerous patients [1]. Atherosclerosis, however, involves the distal as well as the proximal coronary artery in 10 to 20% of patients and may either prevent successful revascularization initially or reduce the chance for long-term graft patency. Variations of distal atherosclerosis may be classified as tandem stenosis, discrete distal stenosis, multiple diffuse stenosis, or total coronary occlusion (Figure 1). Previously, manual endarterectomy and intraoperative angioplasty have been utilized for treating distal coronary disease. Both surgical techniques, however, have specific indications for use and limitations on their application [2, 3]. Consequently, alternate methods have been sought to deal with the problem of distal atherosclerotic disease.

Recent interest has focused on the use of high-intensity light energy to remove atherosclerotic plaques. Several investigators have described the capacity of laser radiation to vaporize plaques, relieve stenosis, and reopen occluded vessels [4–7]. The importance of a complete understanding of the biologic effects of laser radiation and the necessity for precise control of radiant energy was highlighted by reports of arterial wall injury, aneurysm formation, and perforation after laser angioplasty [8, 9]. Thermal damage to the arterial wall may lead to thrombosis of the vessel. Considering the small size of human coronary arteries with a wall thickness of only 0.1 to 0.5 mm and the heterogeneity of atherosclerotic plaque with lipid, fibrous, and calcific components, the difficulties of applying laser energy for this purpose are readily apparent. Nevertheless, experimental studies have demonstrated that arterial plaque can be removed successfully without injury to the arterial wall [10]. The exact parameters necessary for precise control of laser energy have been determined, and arterial healing after laser treatment has been observed in animals [11]. A prospective clinical trial has been initiated using laser endarterectomy as an adjunct to coronary bypass surgery.

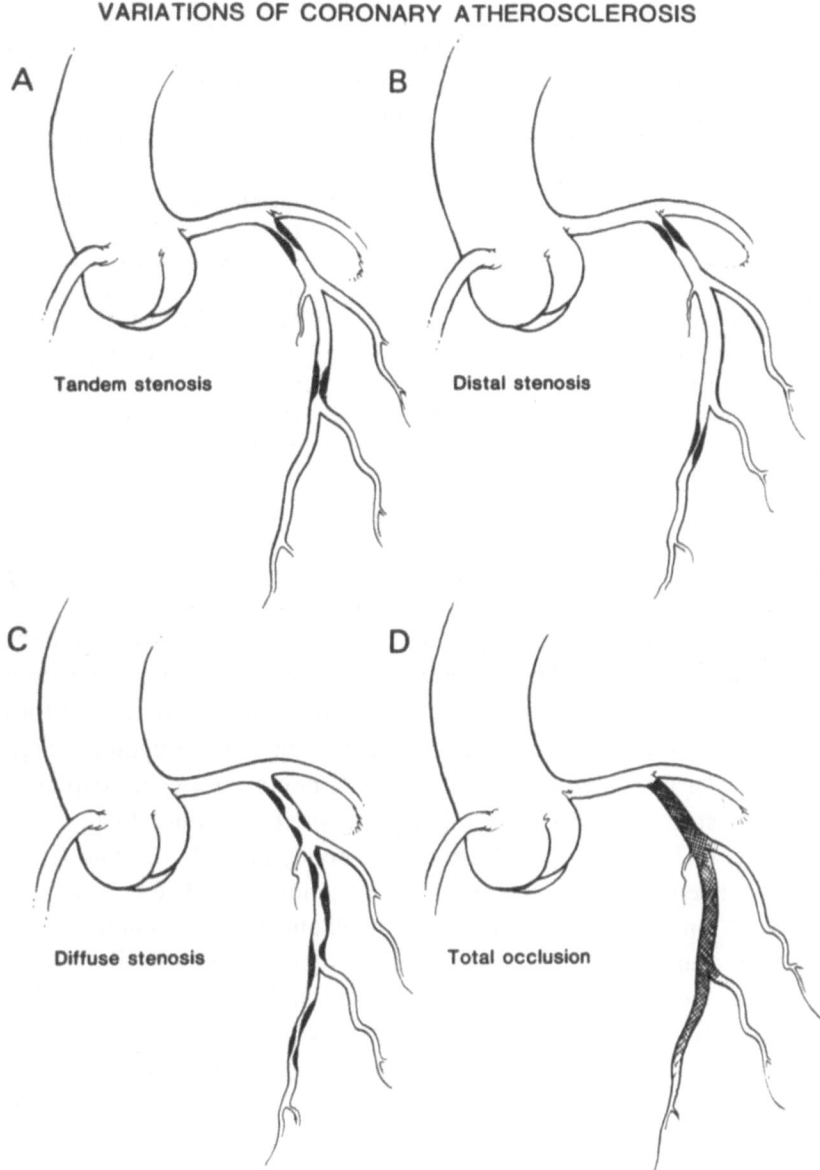

VARIATIONS OF CORONARY ATHEROSCLEROSIS

A

Tandem stenosis

B

Distal stenosis

C

Diffuse stenosis

D

Total occlusion

Figure 1. Variations of distal coronary atherosclerosis.

Medical laser systems

Knowledge of the physical properties of lasers is a prerequisite to successful use of laser technology for medical purposes [12]. A comparison of the characteristics of the four most commonly used lasers in medical treatment is provided in Table 1 (ruby, argon, neodymium-YAG, and carbon dioxide [CO_2]. Just as the wave-

Table 1. Comparison of Medical Laser Systems.

Laser	Wavelength (microns)	Transmission system	Tissue penetration	Tissue absorption	Medical applications
Ruby	Visible red (0.694)	Fiberoptic	High	Low	Blood flow sensors
Argon	Visible blue-green (0.488–0.515)	Fiberoptic	Intermediate	Intermediate (High-pigmented tissues)	Retinal detachment and hemorrhage Pigmented skin disorders
Neodymium-YAG	Invisible near-infrared (1.06)	Fiberoptic	High	Intermediate	GI bleeding GI, GU tumors
CO_2	Invisible far-infrared (10.6)	Articulated arm	Low	High (water and soft tissues)	'Ideal' surgical laser Eye, ENT, Neuro, GYN, Orthopedics & Vascular surgery

length of light varies from the visible red and green to the invisible, infrared range, so too does the interaction of light energy with body tissues, whether by penetrance or absorption. The biologic effects of laser radiation depend as much on the tissue absorption of a specific wavelength as the parameters set for laser energy (power [watts], power density [watts/cm^2], exposure time [sec], and energy [joules]). Consideration of these fundamental properties explains why one laser is best for cutting tissue and another for coagulating blood.

The effects of laser radiation from argon, neodymium-YAG, and CO_2 laser systems have been examined in atherosclerotic plaques [5]. The rapid absorption of CO_2 radiation results in vaporization of plaque at a low energy level (7.5 joules). Due to the lower tissue absorption at other wavelengths, the argon laser requires four times the amount of energy to vaporize the plaque, while the neodymium-YAG laser requires 20 times more energy for the same tissue effect. The absorption of CO_2 radiation is so high that 98% of the radiant energy is absorbed within 0.01 mm of tissue. Since soft tissues are composed of 70 to 90% water, CO_2 radiation is rapidly absorbed by body tissues, making it the ideal laser for surgical application.

The argon and neodymium-YAG lasers may be transmitted by small optical fibers, but a non-toxic fiber system is not presently available for the CO_2 laser. Instead, CO_2 radiation is transmitted through hollow cylinders by highly reflective mirrors in an articulated arm system. Previous CO_2 laser systems have been large, cumbersome devices which were overpowered (100 watts) for most surgical applications and lacked precise control mechanisms.

The recent development of a hand-held CO_2 laser has provided a conveniently-sized device for surgical application. The laser is compact and lightweight, measuring 30 cm in length by 3.2 cm in width and weighing 500 gms, which enables manual alignment.* Up to 15 watts of power can be delivered through a hollow metal waveguide, and variously sized arterial introducers are available for insertion into the coronary artery (outer diameter: 1.5, 2.0, 2.5 mm). A power meter is provided to measure the exact power setting (watts available). A laser controller determines the energy delivery and duration of radiant exposure by setting the pulse duration (1–50 msec) and the number of pulses (1–99). The laser is activated by a foot switch.

Experimental studies

Laser parameters and tissue effects

The parameters necessary for precise control of CO_2 laser energy were defined in studies using the normal canine aorta and the atherosclerotic aorta from a cadaver [10]. CO_2 laser radiation delivered at a low energy level vaporized a shallow intimal crater (0.9 mm diameter) in the arterial wall. Increasing laser energy (by raising power or exposure time) produced craters of greater depth without changing the width of the crater. If excessive laser energy was delivered, carbonization occurred on the walls of the crater.

The minimal energy necessary to penetrate the 1 mm arterial wall was determined in the canine aorta because of its uniform thickness. At 2 watts (power density 313 watts/cm²), the CO_2 laser produced only a shallow intimal crater, and penetration of the 1 mm wall was not accomplished despite 3.0 joules of energy. At 5 and 8 watts (power density 781 and 1250 watts/cm²), complete penetration of the 1 mm artery was consistently observed with 1.5 joules of energy. Minimal charring was present adjacent to the crater at low energy levels (1.5–4.0 joules), while moderate charring was seen at 4.5–7.0 joules, and more severe thermal effects were obvious at higher energy levels (7.5–12 joules). The minimal energy required to cut a 2 mm depth in the atherosclerotic human aorta was 2.5–5.0 joules due to the heterogeneity of plaque. To determine the influence of pulse duration on thermal effects, pulse duration was varied (31, 64, 97 msec) while laser power, beam size, and power density were kept constant. The number of laser pulses was increased so that thermal effects of equivalent energy levels could be compared. The results demonstrated that thermal effects and charring were diminished if pulse duration was limited to 30 msec or less.

Laser effects in human coronary arteries

The effects of CO_2 laser radiation on coronary stenosis were examined in 24

---

* Directed Energy, Inc., Irvine, California

human coronary arteries from 9 cadaver hearts [10]. Each artery was at least 1.5 mm in diameter and had a 50% or greater stenosis. The CO_2 laser parameters selected for laser endarterectomy were power, 10 watts; pulse width, 30 msec; and 5 pulses for a radiant energy of 1.5 joules. One to six applications were needed to relieve the stenosis completely in 19 arteries. In two arteries with complete occlusion, the laser recanalized segments from 2 to 4 cm in length without perforation. These arteries contained fibrous, lipid, and calcified atheromatous plaques. Two densely calcified plaques could not be vaporized despite repeated application of the laser. Higher levels of energy produced charring of the plaque without improvement in the stenosis. The laser was misaligned in one artery early in our experience, and perforation of the vessel occurred.

The histologic appearance of all laser-treated arteries was examined. In 21 arteries, the vessel diameter was increased 25 to 100% by laser vaporization of intimal plaque (Figure 2). A thin rim (7–30 microns) of charred material lined the crater. The surrounding architecture of the vessel wall was well preserved. There was no evidence of cellular swelling or disruption of the medial layer of the artery.

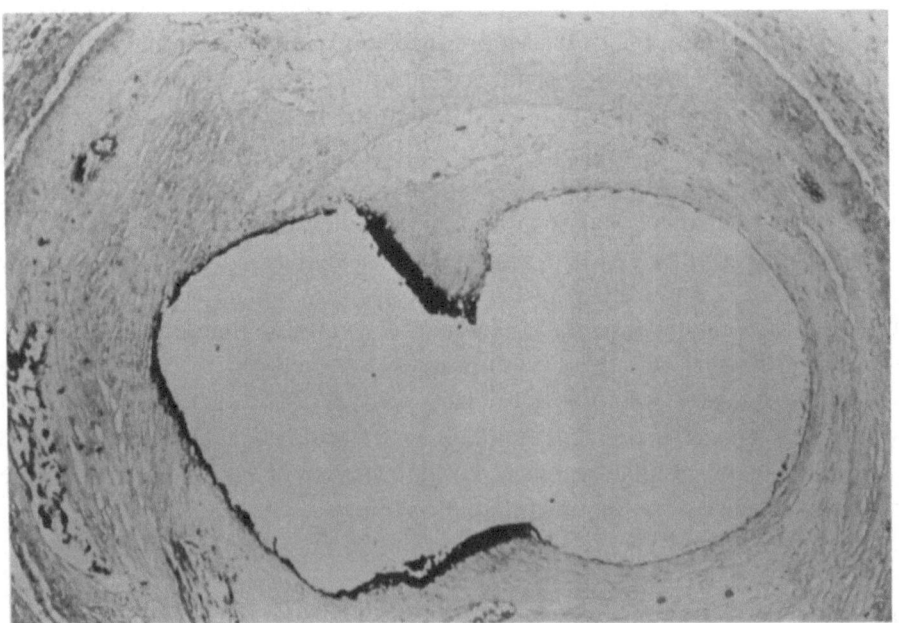

Figure 2. Effect of CO_2 laser radiation on atheromatous plaque of human (cadaver) coronary artery. Note the critical coronary stenosis has been relieved by laser endarterectomy. A thin rim of charring lines the laser crater, but no other thermal effect is observed in the arterial wall.

Proposed operative technique

Exposure of the heart is through a median sternotomy as in conventional revascularization (Figure 3). Normothermic cardiopulmonary bypass is established. After the aortic cross-clamp is applied, a cold cardioplegic solution is infused
into the ascending aorta to insure myocardial protection and to provide a motionless heart for surgical repair. A suitable site is selected for arteriotomy in the distal
coronary artery. A dry coronary field is achieved by gentle suction on the aortic

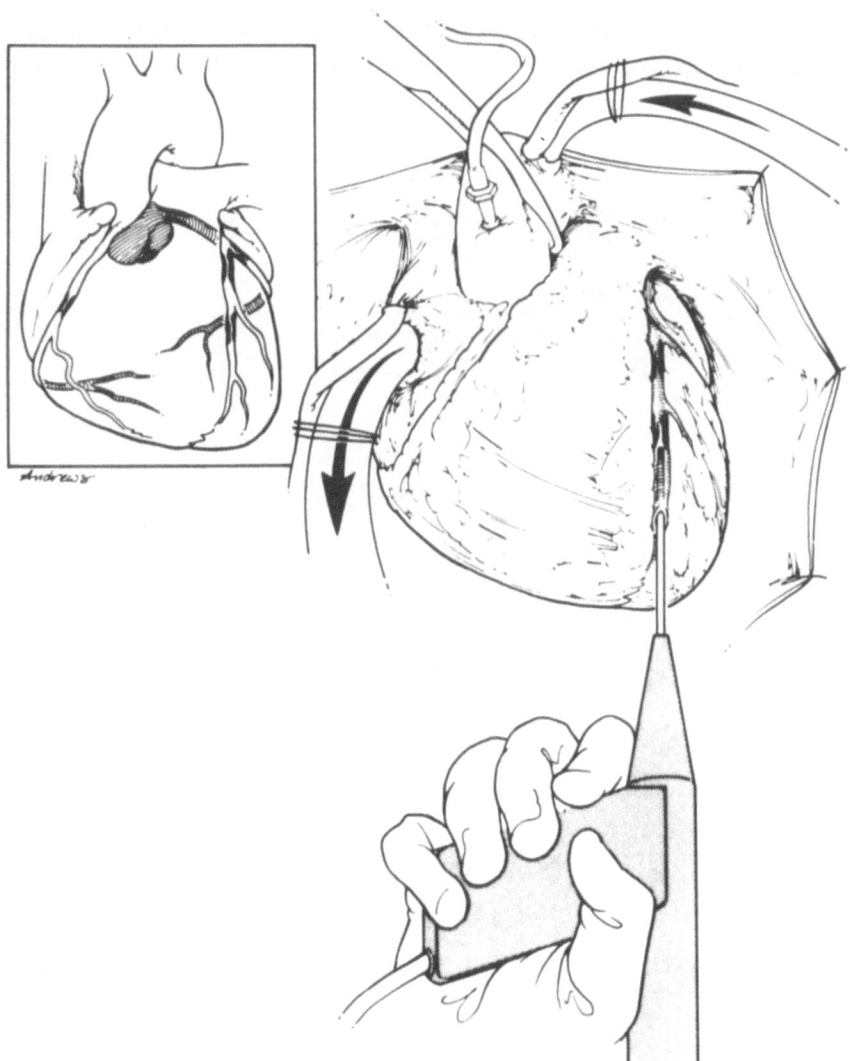

Figure 3. Proposed operative technique for laser coronary endarterectomy using a hand-held CO_2
laser for relief of distal atherosclerotic disease. Note cardiopulmonary bypass has been established
and cold cardioplegic arrest used to insure dry, motionless conditions.

306

vent. Flexible, calibrated coronary probes should be used to determine the location and severity of critical coronary stenoses. The laser coronary introducer is inserted through the distal arteriotomy and passed up to the level of the stenotic plaque. Once adjacent to the plaque, the instrument should be aligned to insure coaxial passage in the vessel. Each laser impulse cuts a shallow, cone-shaped wedge in the obstructing plaque (Figure 4). After a series of laser impulses, the stenosis is relieved and the coronary introducer advanced down the vessel. Smoke produced by laser vaporization of the plaque escapes through the distal arteriotomy or is aspirated by suction on the aortic vent. Particulate debris is flushed out the distal arteriotomy by reinfusion of cardioplegic solution.

Relief of coronary stenosis or recanalization of the vessel is confirmed by passage of calibrated coronary probes. The aortocoronary bypass, using saphe-

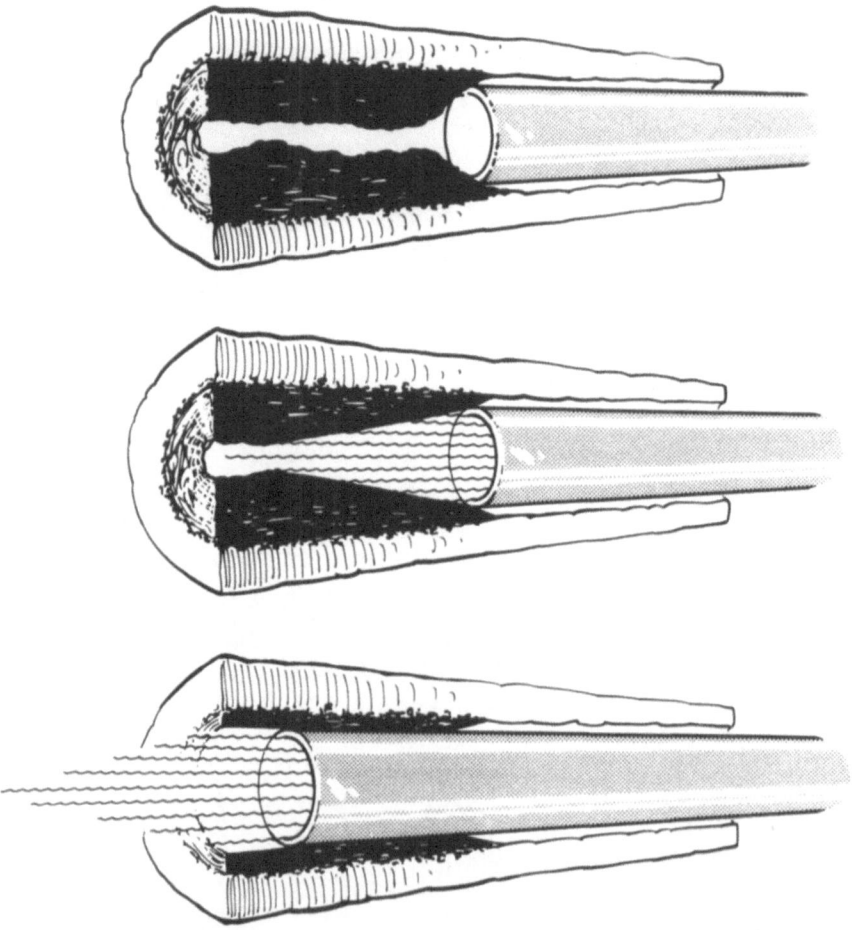

Figure 4. The coronary laser introducer is aligned for coaxial passage down the vessel. Each laser impulse cuts a conical path through the plaque. Multiple, short pulses of laser energy are desired to prevent thermal injury to the artery.

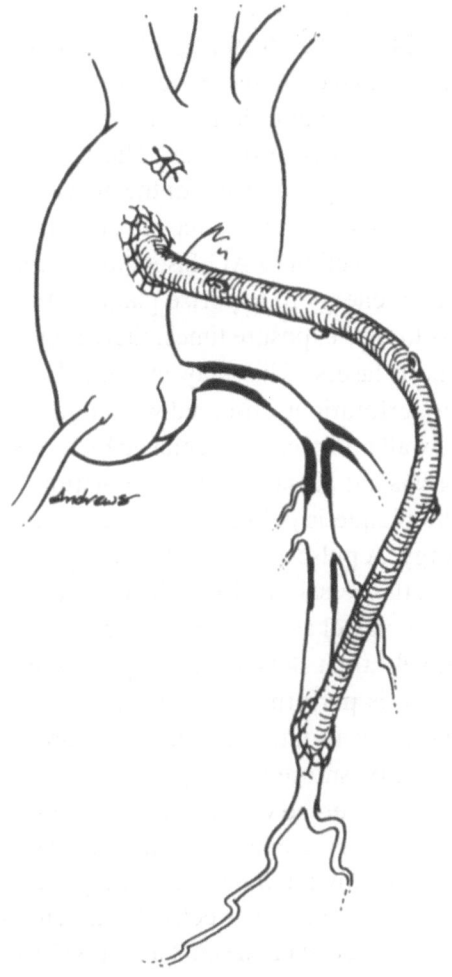

Figure 5. Coronary revascularization is accomplished by saphenous vein bypass to the distal coronary artery after laser endarterectomy has relieved intervening coronary stenosis and improved perfusion to additional tributaries.

nous vein graft or internal mammary artery pedicle, is completed by sutured anastomosis (Figure 5). After relief of intervening coronary stenosis by laser technique, blood flow from the graft fills the proximal and distal vessels. Improved coronary runoff is provided by opening additional tributaries.

Discussion

The use of laser energy to remove obstructing arterial plaques reveals a new horizon in the treatment of atherosclerotic cardiovascular disease. Prior investigations have demonstrated the capacity of lasers to relieve stenosis and to open totally occluded arteries [4–7]. An awareness of the physical properties of the particular laser used is necessary for successful application of the device. The relationship of power density and duration to cutting and coagulating effects are fundamental properties of each type of laser. The CO_2 laser has the optimal characteristics for vaporizing plaque because of the high energy absorption at this wavelength. There is minimal thermal effect on the adjacent arterial wall. In contrast, the argon and neodymium-YAG lasers are not absorbed as well and require greater amounts of energy to vaporize plaque. As a result of the excess energy delivered and prolonged exposure times, there is more thermal damage to the artery wall with these lasers. This may explain the reports of aneurysm formation and frequent perforations observed with argon laser systems [8, 9].

Prevention of arterial wall injury can be achieved by the use of an optimal laser system and by insuring coaxial passage of laser radiation. The minimal energy required to vaporize the plaque is delivered in small, graded amounts utilizing short pulses of laser energy. A pulse duration of 30 msec or less has been shown to reduce thermal effects on the vessel wall [10]. The rigid laser coronary introducer tends to straighten out the vessel as it passes through it and can be aimed more predictably intraoperatively than flexible catheter systems. Guidance is facilitated, since the procedure is performed under direct vision. In the controlled environment of the operating room, the risk of perforation is small, and the problem is easily remedied by suture techniques.

Arterial healing has been observed within two weeks after laser application [11, 13]. When exposed to blood elements, the intimal crater produced by laser vaporization of plaque is quickly lined by fibrin and platelets. Endothelial cells migrate to reline the crater within two weeks. Complete arterial healing with 100% patency has been observed even in small arteries (1.0 mm) exposed to CO_2 laser radiation [11]. The potential for thrombosis has been reported in arteries exposed to argon radiation and may in part be related to the magnitude of thermal injury [14]. Early occlusion in seven of nine human coronary arteries subjected to argon laser radiation at the time of coronary bypass was reported by Choy [15]. This may be related to thermal injury to the arterial wall, incomplete relief of stenosis, sluggish blood flow, or activation of platelet aggregation. The potential for thrombosis during laser endarterectomy suggests the need for antiplatelet therapy as recommended by Chesebro [16].

Experimental data from animal and cadaver studies suggest that laser endarterectomy can be applied safely in the controlled environment of the operating room. This new technique has promise as an adjunct to conventional coronary bypass procedures, especially in patients with advanced distal atherosclerosis. The principal indications are in patients with tandem coronary stenosis, discrete distal lesions, multiple or diffuse disease, total occlusion, and coronary artery dissection. A prospective clinical trial has been undertaken to establish the safety and efficacy of this new modality of treatment.

References

1. Cooley DA, Duncan JM (1983) Coronary bypass surgery: The total experience at the Texas Heart Institute. In Hurst J (ed): *Clinical Essays on the Heart,* Vol 2, New York, McGraw-Hill, pp 207–217

2. Miller DC, Stinson EB, Oyer PE, Reitz BA, Jamieson SW, Moreno-Cabral RJ, Shumway NE (1981) Long-term clinical assessment of the efficacy of adjunctive coronary endarterectomy. J Thorac Cardiovasc Surg 81: 21–29

3. Roberts AJ, Faro RS, Feldman RL, Conti CR, Knauf DG, Alexander JA, Pepine CJ (1983) Comparison of early and long-term results with intraoperative transluminal balloon catheter dilatation and coronary artery bypass grafting. J Thorac Cardiovasc Surg 86: 435–440

4. Choy DS, Stertzer SH, Rotterdam HZ, Bruno MS (1982) Laser coronary angioplasty: Experience with 9 cadaver hearts. Am J Cardiol 50: 1209–1211 ⋯-

5. Abela GS, Normann S, Cohen D, Feldman RL, Geiser EA, Conti CR (1982) Effects of carbon dioxide, ND-YAG, and argon laser radiation on coronary atheromatous plaques. Am J Cardiol 50: 1199–1205.

6. Lee G, Ikeda R, Herman I, Dwyer RM, Bass M, Hussein H, Kozina J, Mason DT (1983) The qualitative effects of laser irradiation on human arteriosclerotic disease. Am Heart J 105: 885–889

7. Livesay JJ, Johansen WE, Sutter LV, Cooley DA (1983) Can laser endarterectomy extend the effectiveness of coronary revascularization? Lasers in Surgery and Medicine 3: 173

8. Lee G, Ikeda RM, Theis JH, Chan M, Stobbe D, Ogata C, Kumagai A, Mason D (1984) Acute and chronic complications of laser angioplasty: Vascular wall damage and formation of aneurysms in the atherosclerotic rabbit. Am J Cardiol 53: 290–293

9. Sanborn TA, Faxon DP, Haudenschild CL, Gottsman SB, Ryan TJ (1983) Angiographic and histopathologic consequences of in vivo laser radiation of atherosclerotic lesions (Am Heart Monograph #101). Circulation 68 (4): Suppl II: 145

10. Livesay JJ, Johansen WE, Sutter LV, Klima T, Painvin GA, Follette DM (1984) Experimental technique of laser coronary endarterectomy and its immediate effects on atherosclerotic plaques in cadaver hearts. Texas Heart Institute Journal 11 (3), in press

11. Frazier OH, Painvin GA, Morris JR, Thomsen S, Neblett CR. Laser assisted microvascular anastomoses: Angiographic and anatomopathological studies on growing microvascular anastomoses. Surgery, in press.

12. Dixon JA (1983) *Surgical Application of Lasers.* Chicago, Year Book Medical Publishers, Inc., pp 11–28

13. Gerrity RG, Loop FD, Golding GAR, Ehrhart LA, Argeny ZB (1983) Arterial response to laser operation for removal of atherosclerotic plaques. J Thorac Cardiovasc Surg 85: 409–421

14. Treat MR, Weld FM, White JV, Forde KA, Feneglio JJ, L'Esperanza FA, Voorhees AB (1983) Effect of CO_2 laser on the luminal surface of blood vessels in vivo. Lasers in Surgery and Medicine 3 (3): 247–254

15. Choy DS, Stertzer SH, Myler RK, Marco J, Kaminow I, Fournial G (1984) Argon laser coronary angioplasty: Mass spectrometer evaluation, technetium 99 scintigraphy, human intraoperative evaluation. Report at American College of Cardiology, March.

16. Chesebro JH, Fuster V, Elveback LR, Clements IP, Smith HC, Holmes DR, Bardsley WT, Pluth JR, Wallace RB, Puga FJ, Orszulak TA, Piehler JM (1984) Effect of dipyridamole and aspirin on late vein-graft patency after coronary bypass operations. N Engl J Med 310: 209–214

Reoperative myocardial revascularization

DELOS M. COSGROVE and FLOYD D. LOOP

Recurrent angina after primary myocardial revascularization has resulted in an increasing number of patients undergoing a second revascularization procedure. At The Cleveland Clinic the number of these operations done in 1983 reached 276 cases which represents more than 11% of our total myocardial revascularization work.

Several factors influence the number of these operations which will be done. As the number of primary operations continues to increase, the pool of potential candidates has become huge with nearly one million procedures having been done in the United States. However, the percentage of these patients coming to reoperation is decreasing. More complete revascularization, improved patency rates, fewer single vessel disease cases and an increased age at primary operation tend to hold the number in check.

This decreasing proportion of patients who undergo reoperation is demonstrated when our results five years after primary revascularization are scrutinized. The percent of operated patients undergoing reoperation at five years has gradually decreased from 7% to 1.5% in 1977 suggesting that the primary operations have improved. Ten years postoperatively, 7% of the patients had undergone a second procedure.

Assuming that the number of primary revascularization operations will continue to increase to 200,000 cases per year by 1990 and that 7% of these patients will be candidates for reoperation ten years postoperatively, in 1990 there will be 14,000 coronary reoperations done per year in the United States.

The reported high morbidity and mortality rates associated with reoperation have made physicians reluctant to recommend reoperative surgery. With experience and refined surgical techniques, operative morbidity and mortality have been reduced and sicker patients are now considered to be candidates for reoperative myocardial revascularization. This is demonstrated by a review of the first 1000 patients [1].

The first 1000 patients undergoing a second myocardial revascularization procedure have been divided into four cohorts of 250 patients each. The nature of the primary operation has changed throughout this experience with half of the patients in the first cohort having had a Vineberg procedure done while in the final cohort only 10% had this operation as part of their primary operation.

Throughout this experience, angina was the principle indication for surgery with approximately 75% of the patients in each cohort being either Functional Class III or IV preoperatively.

The extent of coronary artery disease has increased slowly during our experience. In the last cohort, the incidence of left main coronary artery disease has increased to 18% while the incidence of triple vessel coronary artery disease has increased to 73% (Table 1).

Careful attention to perioperative detail is essential to achieve good results. This starts with careful review of the coronary angiogram. Angiographic assessment of potentially graftable vessels is the same as with primary revascularization and best results are achieved with large vessels with unobstructive run-off. Congestive failure is never an indication for reoperation. The angiographic indication for reoperative surgery may be divided into three catagories: graft closure, progression of atherosclerosis in previously ungrafted vessels, and a combination of graft closure and progressive atherosclerosis.

Initially, progressive atherosclerosis was the most common indication for reoperation, particularly during the period when single grafts and incomplete revascularization were common. Recently graft closure, particularly secondary to atherosclerosis, has become the most common angiographic indication for myocardial revascularization (Figure 1).

Salycilates, dipyridamole, antiinflammatory agents, anticoagulants, and antihistamines affect the hemostatic mechanism and should be eliminated at least one week preoperatively. It is important that propranolol, nitrates, calcium channel blockers and antihypertensives are continued through the day of surgery. This insures that the patient will arrive in the operating room in a nonischemic state.

Because of the relatively long period of anesthesia prior to beginning cardiopulmonary bypass, a Swan Ganz catheter is inserted in all patients prior to induction of anesthesia. Serial determinations of wedge pressure and cardiac

Table 1. Extent of coronary atherosclerosis (>50%).

Arteries	I	II	III	IV
One	23	18	10	7
	9.2%	7.2%	4.0%	2.8%
Two	84	62	56	60
	33.6%	24.8%	22.4%	24.0%
Three	143	170	184	183
	57.2%	68.0%	73.6%	73.2%
LMCA	27	36	48	45
	10.8%	14.4%	19.2%	18.0%

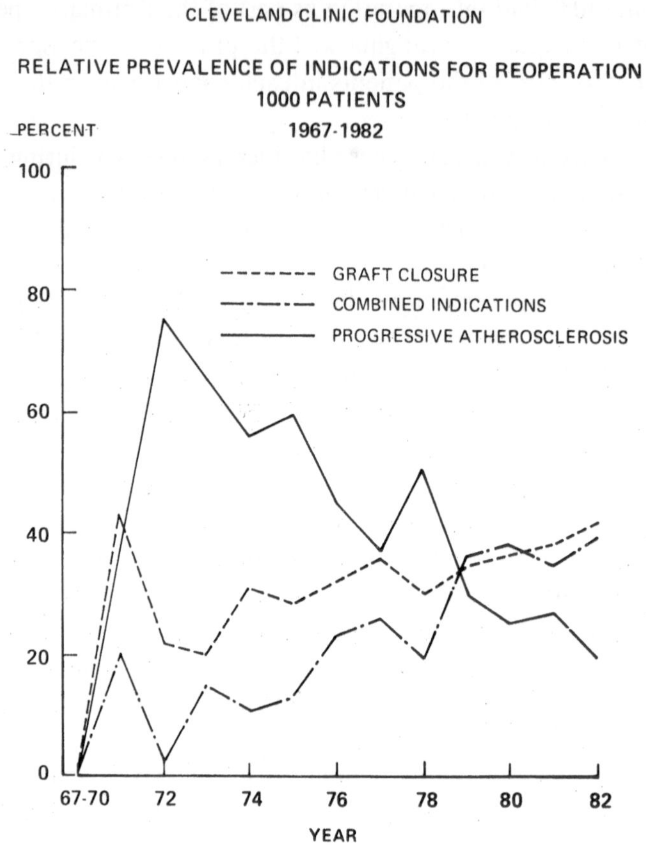

312

RELATIVE PREVALENCE OF INDICATIONS FOR REOPERATION
1000 PATIENTS
1967-1982

Figure 1. Graft closure has become the most common angiographic indication for reoperative surgery.

output are made. The EKG, including a V-5 lead, is carefully monitored to help detect ischemia while the heart is being exposed.

The safety of reentry has been greatly increased by the use of the oscillating saw which provides a more controlled sternotomy. The inner and outer tables of the sternum are carefully divided while the lungs are deflated, pulling mediastinal contents away from the sternum. The subxyphoid area is not probed as it is possible to damage the thin-walled right ventricle.

The posterior table of the sternum is dissected free from the mediastinal contents using electric cautery. Care is taken to stay as close as possible to the sternum. The internal mammary artery is dissected at this time.

Prior to heparinazation, dissection of the right heart is begun along the diaphragmatic surface. Dissection is generally easy in this location and vital cardiac structures are at a minimum.

Dissection is continued over the right atrium and aorta. The left ventricle is not dissected until the heart has been cannulated and cardiopulmonary bypass begun. A single venous cannula is used and the aorta vented through the cardioplegia cannula. These maneuvers help minimize dissection. Once the patient has been placed on cardiopulmonary bypass, the apex of the left ventricle can be dissected and the left ventricular surface exposed by cutting the pericardium along the anterior surface of the ventricle. This is easier than attempting to find the plane of fusion of the pericardium and ventricle anteriorly. Once target vessels have been identified and exposed, the aorta is cross clamped and cold cardioplegic solution injected into the aortic root.

Cardioplegia has been a major advance in reoperative surgery. Our series is evenly divided with half of the patients operated on since 1977 having had cardioplegia as a form of myocardial protection. Prior to 1977 patients had intermittent normothermic ischemic arrest. There has been a significant reduction in reoperative mortality and a trend towards lower perioperative infarction rate. At the same time, the patients have had a greater number of grafts performed and more complete myocardial revascularization has been achieved (Table 2.)

The mortality and morbidity associated with reoperative coronary artery surgery has been higher than with primary operations; however, it has gradually declined during the last decade. Operative mortality is now at 2%, perioperative infarction rate is 5.2%, reoperation for bleeding rate is 4%, neurologic deficit continues to run at approximately 2.5% with half of these being transient. Respiratory dysfunction, defined as patients requiring ventilatory support for more than 24 hours, is 0.4% and wound complications is 0.1%.

Table 2. Myocardial protection in reoperations.

Patients	530		470
Operative mortality	2.1%	p = 0.047	4.3%
Grafts per patient	2.2	p<0.01	1.5
Complete revascularization	64%	p<0.0001	39%
Perioperative myocardial infarction	5.1%	NS	7.7%

Table 3. Graft patency in reoperation patients 1967–1981.

	LAD	CX	RCA	Total
IMA	39/40	2/3	1/1	42/44
	97.5%	66.7%	100%	95.5%
SVG	49/59	53/67	53/73	155/199
	83.1%	79.1%	72.6%	77.9%
Total	88/99	55/70	54/74	197/243
	88.9%	78.6%	73.0%	81.1%

Patients Studied: 154. Mean Cath Interval: 29 months.

314

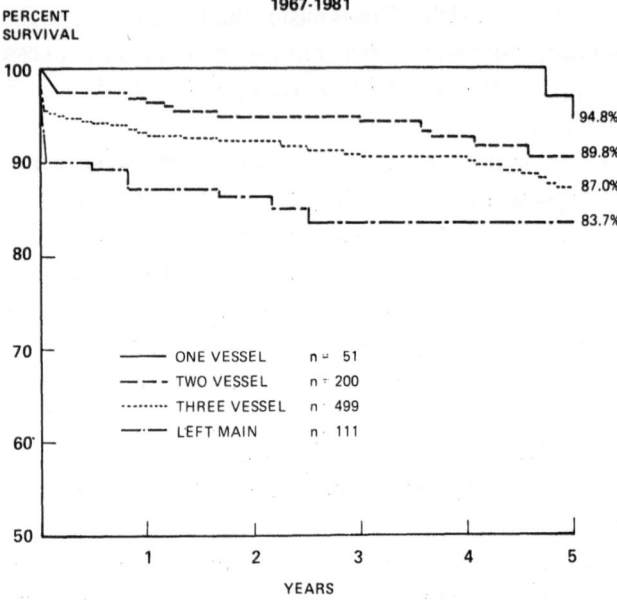

Figure 2. Five year survival was adversely influenced by increasing extent of disease.

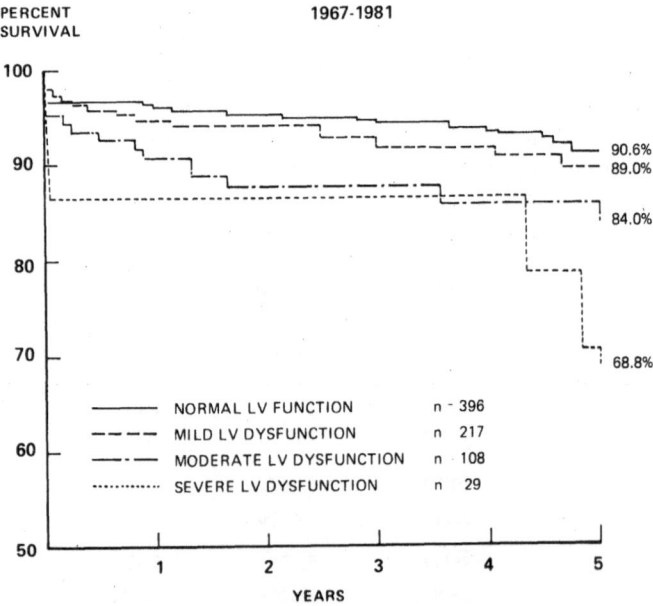

Figure 3. Five year survival was adversely influenced by deteriorating left ventricular function.

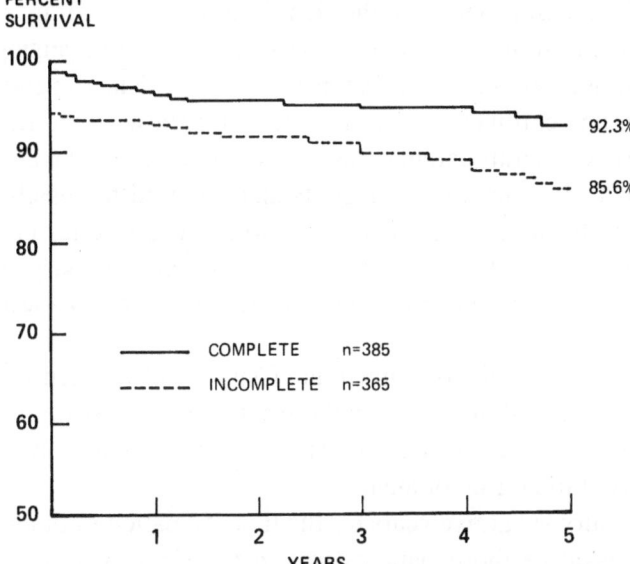

Figure 4. Patients who were completely revascularized had a greater five year mortality rate than incompletely revascularized patients.

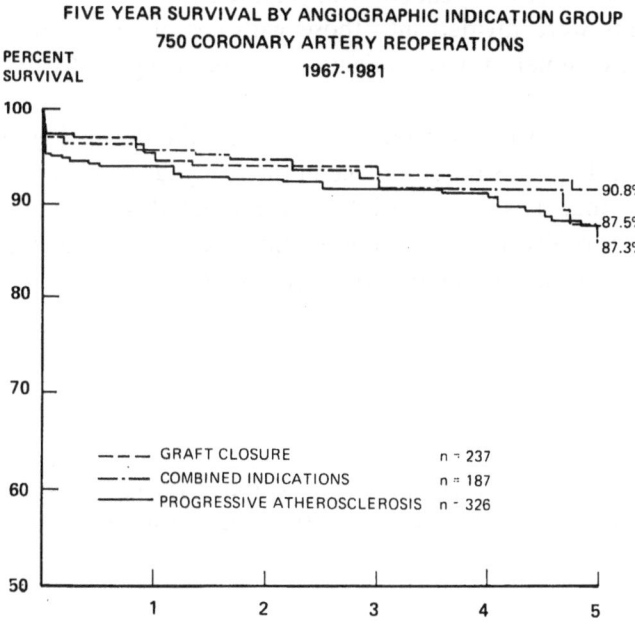

Figure 5. The five year survival was not influenced by angiographic indication for surgery.

Numerous preoperative and intraoperative descriptors were examined in an attempt to define those factors associated with high risks. Using a multivariate logistic regression analysis, it was demonstrated that incomplete revascularization at reoperation, left main trunk stenosis, incomplete revascularization at first operation, and increasing age were the significant predictors of mortality.

One hundred fifty-four patients underwent postoperative angiography at a mean of 29 months postoperatively. Patency rates were highest in grafts to the left anterior descending coronary artery and lowest for those to the right coronary artery (Table 3). Vein graft patency was 78% where as internal mammary artery patency was 96%. Patency rates for grafts anastomosed to vessels, previously involved with graft failure, were compared with those arteries previously not grafted. Patency rate for both vein grafts and internal mammary arteries were similar, suggesting failure of a graft is not a contraindication to a second surgical attempt.

New York Heart Association Functional Class for 659 patients with a mean follow-up of 57 months, showed 52% of these patients to be asymptomatic. This is lower than with primary revascularization patients at five years, 70% of whom are generally reported to be free of angina.

The actuarial survival at five years for the first 750 patients demonstrated that the highest survival of those patients was in the single vessel disease group followed by two vessels, three vessels, and left main trunk disease (Figure 2).

Left ventricular function was divided into groups with normal, mild, moderate, and severe left ventricular dysfunction. Patients with the worst left ventricular function have the worst five year survival (Figure 3).

When patients were divided into those with complete and incomplete revascularization, complete revascularization carried a higher five year survival (Figure 4).

When actuarial survival was examined with respect to the angiographic indication for surgery, there was no difference in the five year survival (Figure 5).

We conclude that it is now possible to carry out this operation with little morbidity and mortality and that patients who have recurrent angina should be considered for repeat angiography and are potentially candidates for reoperative surgery.

References

1. Loop FD, Lytle BW, Gill CC, Golding LAR, Cosgrove DM, Taylor PC (1983) Trends in selection and results of coronary artery reoperations. Ann Thor Surg 36: 380–388

Aortocoronary polygrafting and coronary endarterectomy in diffuse cad

H.H. SCHELD, M. GOTTWIK, G. GÖRLACH, U. BAUER, J. MULCH,
R. HÖGE, D. KLING and F.W. HEHRLEIN

Introduction

In coronary surgery the best results can only be achieved if complete revascularization is done [1, 2]. Patients with diffuse coronary disease can only completely revascularizised by performing multiple coronary bypass and coronary endarterectomy. But the performance of complete revascularization in diffuse coronary disease is still a matter of discussion [3]. Some propose to bypass only the great coronary arteries. They argue that bypass to small vessels will fail [4, 5]. The purpose of our study was to demonstrate that coronary endarterectomy and multiple bypass even to small vessels can be successfully performed.

Clinical data

Between 1980 and 1984 we did coronary surgery in 1873 patients. In 44 of these patients we performed multiple bypass grafting. The average age of these patients was 58 years. Forty-two patients were men and 2 were women. All had diffuse coronary three vessel disease. Percent 63,5 had myocardial infarction prior to surgery. Left ventricular ejection fraction was in 16% below 30%, in 43% between 31 and 60% and in 21% greater than 61%. In 48% left ventricular wall motion was normal, in 29% abnormal motion of one wall and in 23% of two or more walls existed.

All distal anastomoses were performed during one cross-clamping period. In all cases BRETSCHNEIDER HTP* cardioplegia was used for myocardial protection. After an initial infusion of 2 litres of cardioplegia we administered additional cardioplegia after performance of each distal anastomosis. For intermittent infusion of cardioplegia we used the already anastomosed coronary vein grafts. During heart arrest the body temperature was reduced to 28° C and the myocardial temperature was adjusted below 15° C.

We did from 6–12 distal anastomoses. The mean number of distal anastomoses was 7,48. In 32 arteries we also performed coronary endarterectomy and in 6

---

* Köhler Chemie, Alsbach

vessels intraoperative angioplasty was done. The mean cross-clamping period was $92 \pm 7,4$ minutes and the average duration of cardiopulmonary bypass was $162,2 \pm 12,1$ minutes.

Results

The mortality was 2% during the first 30 days after surgery. Perioperative infarction rate measured 2%. One patient died during the observation period ranging from 6–42 months (mean 25 months) after surgery. None of the patients showed disturbances of rhythm during the observation period. The patency rate of all bypass was 87,4% (Figure 1). There was a difference of the patency rate depending on the size of the coronary arteries. The pactency rate of vessels with a diameter greater than 2 mm was 90,7% and the patency rate measured 86,9% in vessels with a diameter of 1,5 mm while it measured 78,2% in vessels with a diameter of smaller than 1 mm (Table 1).

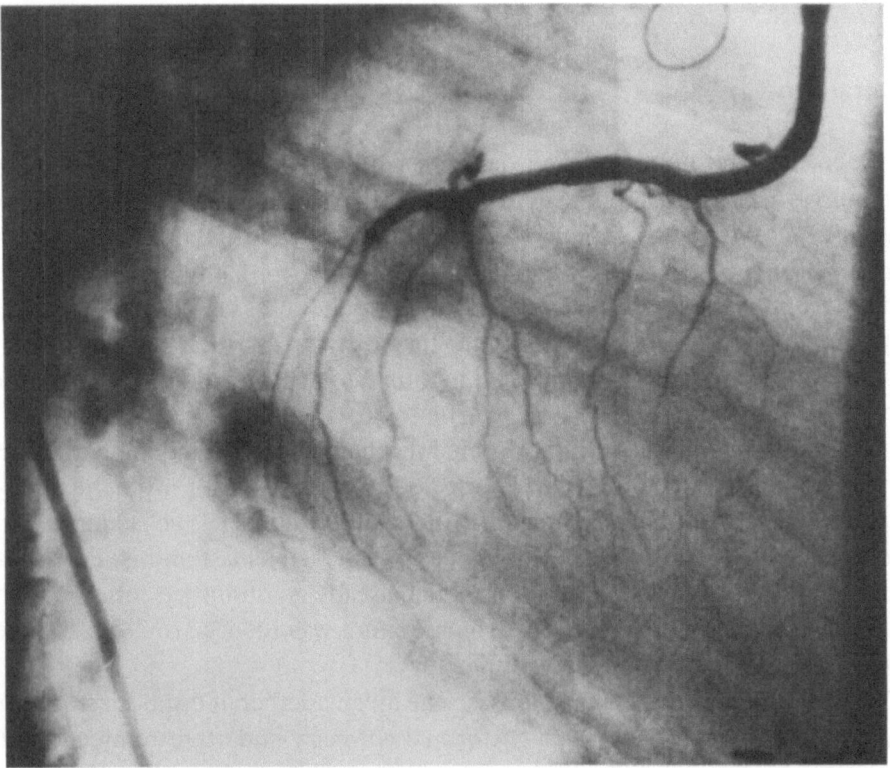

Figure 1. Postoperative angiography showing 6 coronary anastomoses done by one graft.

Table 1. Patency rate and coronary artery size in CAB-Polygrafting.

Size of grafted coronary artery	<1,0 mm	1,5 mm	>2,0 mm	Total
Number of restudied anastomoses	23	137	86	246
Patent grafts	18	119	78	215
Patency rate	78,2%	86,9%	90,7%	87,4%

Conclusions

Even in diffuse coronary disease complete revascularization is possible, if bypass to all diseased arteries are performed. If at the most distal point of an artery where an anastomosis can be done the artery is obstructed an endarterectomy often can be successfully performed or intraoperative angioplasty can be done. By these methods run off, which is an important factor for patency increases. According to a clinical study incomplete revascularization appeared to be a risk in coronary surgery. Life expectancy of patients with coronary disease is comparable to the normal population after complete revascularization, which is the basis for being free of angina pectoris [6]. As a consequence complete revascularization always has to be the goal of coronary surgery. Our results demonstrate, that the performance of multiple bypass even to small vessels must not be connected with a reduced patency rate. Therefore revascularization of only the great coronary arteries in diffuse coronary disease limits the success of surgical therapy in coronary surgery and can not be justified by the argument that bypass to small vessels will fail.

References

1. Meisner H, Schmidt-Habelmann P, Struck E, Sebening F (1983) Coronarchirurgie – Behandlung, Verfahrenswahl und Ergebnisse, Chirurg 54: 715–721
2. Buda AJL, McDonald L, Anderson MJ, Strauss MD, David TE, Berman ND (1981) Long-term results following coronary bypass operations. J Thorac Cardiovasc Surg 82: 383–388
3. Johnson LWD (1982) Diffuse Coronary Artery Disease; Is it a Contraindication for Surgery, in: Coronary Heart Surgery, Springer Verlag, Berlin, pp 80–84
4. Schmuziger M, Roskamm H, Stürzenhofecker P, Hahn Ch, Stolte M (1979) Is Revascularization Limited to Good Quality and High Caliber Vessels? In: Coronary Heart Surgery, Springer Verlag, Berlin, pp 73–79
5. Effler DB (1976) Revascularization with Little Coronary Arteries, Ann Thorac Surg 21: 83–89
6. Roskamm H (1982) Kurz- und Langzeitergebnisse der aortokoronaren Bypass-Operation, in: Operative Therapie der koronaren Herzkrankheit, perimed-Verlag, Erlangen, 127–136

Coronary artery bypass in the elderly

MacARTHUR A. ELAYDA, ROBERT J. HALL,
VIRENDRA S. MATHUR, GRADY L. HALLMAN,
ALBERT G. GRAY and DENTON A. COOLEY

Introduction

Coronary artery bypass is being performed with increasing frequency in various subsets of patients who appear to be at an increased native risk from their disease. The elderly patient who has coronary artery disease is one of the subsets which appears to carry an increased operative risk. Our institution's interest in elderly surgical patients span for more than two decades as evidenced by earlier reports [1–3]. Several recent studies have shown that the advances in all phases of coronary care contribute immensely to the application of coronary bypass in the elderly with gratifying surgical results [4–13]. This study presents our experience with consecutive elderly patients who underwent coronary artery bypass alone from 1970 to 1983.

Materials and methods

From January 1971 to December 1983, 28,130 patients underwent coronary artery bypass alone at the Texas Heart Institute-St. Luke's Episcopal Hospital. Of these, 1,972 (7.0%) were 70 years of age or older. There were 1,431 males and 541 females. Patients who had concomittant or other cardiac operations were excluded from this study. The primary indication for surgery was the persistence of incapacitating symptoms in spite of intensive medical therapy. According to the New York Heart Association functional classification, 8% were in class II, 68% in class III and 24% in class IV. In this same period, a total of 26,158 younger patients (69 years and younger) underwent coronary artery bypass in our institution. Table 1 shows the annual distribution of elderly patients. Figure 1 further demonstrates the progressive increase in the number of elderly patients operated on in our institution through the years.

Catheterization data

Selective coronary arteriography was performed in all patients and revealed single vessel disease in 178 patients (9%), double vessel disease in 237 (12%) and

Table 1. Patients who underwent isolated coronary artery bypass between 1971 and 1983.

Year	Overall no. of patients	Elderly	
		No.	%
1971	737	15	2.04
1972	787	14	1.8
1973	1025	23	2.2
1974	1294	44	3.4
1975	1806	62	3.4
1976	2402	112	4.7
1977	2499	136	5.4
1978	2722	173	6.4
1979	2881	203	7.0
1980	2987	270	9.0
1981	3157	267	8.5
1982	3041	302	9.9
1983	2792	351	12.6
Total	28130	1972	7.0

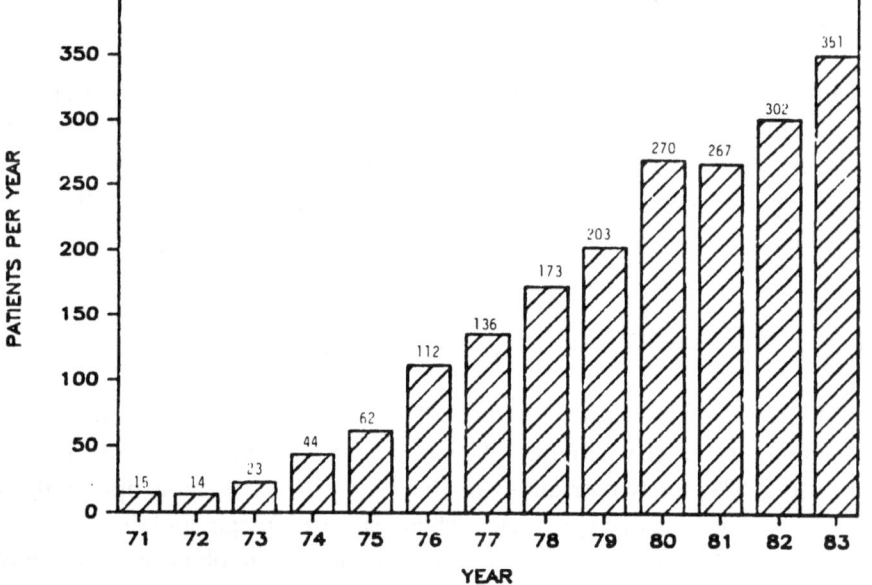

Figure 1. Number of elderly patients who underwent isolated coronary artery bypass from 1971 to 1983.

triple vessel disease in 1,557 patients (79%). Of the total elderly population, 1,577 patients (80%) had left ventriculographic study; 158 patients (10%) had evidence of aneurysm, 551 (35%) had a pronounced hypokinetic or akinetic area of the left ventricular wall, 726 (46%) had hypokinesia and 142 (9%) had normal ventricular wall motion. In the same time period, a total of 1,973 patients underwent combined coronary artery bypass and left ventricular aneurysmectomy, 119 of these were elderly patients with an early mortality of 14.3% (17 patients).

Coronary bypass surgery

Myocardial revascularization was accomplished with the use of reversed saphenous vein graft with hemodilution techniques. The operative technique, which was described in an earlier report, was the same for all patients [14]. The use of hypothermic chemical cardioplegia for myocardial preservation was introduced in our institution in 1976 and became routine in January 1977 and thereafter [15].

The results of surgery were examined with focus on the role of hypothermic chemical cardioplegia. For a better comparison of results, we divided our study period into two groups. Group I included 270 patients who were operated on from 1970 to 1976 prior to the use of hypothermic chemical cardioplegia while group II included 1,702 patients operated on from 1977 to 1983 with the routine use of hypothermic chemical cardioplegia.

Follow-up

Follow-up information was gathered by means of direct contact with patients at the outpatient clinic of our institution, interviews with the patient or his personal physician or through responses to questionnaires sent at 3 and 6 month intervals. Cummulative survival was calculated by the actuarial method of Cutler and Ederer [16].

Results

A total of 121 patients died within 30 days after surgery for an early mortality rate of 6.1% among the elderly patients. The early mortality for patients 69 years and younger was 2.5%. Early mortality was 10.7% in group I patients operated on prior to the routine use of hypothermic chemical cardioplegia and decreased to 5.4% in group II patients when hypothermic chemical cardioplegia was routinely used in coronary bypass procedures. The decrease in early mortality observed in elderly men and women in both groups was also reflected in patients 69 years and younger (Table 2). Death was attributed to cardiac causes (MI, arrhythmia,

Table 2. Early Surgical Mortality by Group and Age.

Patients	No. of Patients	Early mortality (%)
A. Patients 70 years and older		
1971 to 1983	1,972	6.1
Male	1,431	5.5
Female	541	7.9
Group I: 1971–76	270	10.7
Male	206	9.2
Female	64	15.6
Group II: 1977–83	1,702	5.4
Male	1,225	4.8
Female	477	6.9
B. Patients 69 years and younger		
1971 to 1983	26,158	2.5
Male	22,699	2.2
Female	3,459	4.9
Group I: 1971–76	7,781	3.8
Male	6.752	3.4
Female	1,029	6.5
Group II: 1977–83	18,377	2.0
Male	15,952	1.7
Female	2,435	3.9

pump failure and sudden death) in 77% of the 121 early deaths. The other causes of early deaths are shown in Table 3.

Number of bypasses

The number of bypasses performed in the elderly patient as well as the respective early mortality rates is shown in Table 4. The overall average number of bypasses implanted was 3.2 grafts per patient. It averaged 2.7 and 3.3 grafts per patient in group I and group II patients, respectively. Sequential grafting was performed in 4.4% of group I patients (all in 1976) and in 39.3% of group II patients. Eighty-six percent of group I patients had 1 to 3 bypass grafts while 81% of group II had 2 to 5 bypass grafts. The difference was mostly due to the 48% decrease in the number of patients with 2 bypass grafts from group I to group II while a 54% increase was observed in patients having four bypass grafts from group I to group II. Endarterectomy, mostly involving the right coronary artery, was performed in 20%.

324

Table 3. Causes of early death.

	Number of Patients
MI/Arrhythmia	63
Pump failure	25
Sudden death	5
Pulmonary complications	9
CVA	7
Renal failure	4
Infection	2
Other	6
Total	121

Table 4. Number of bypasses performed on 1972 patients.

Bypasses no.	Patients		Early mortality %
	No.	%	
1	88	4.5	7.9
2	330	16.7	5.2
3	818	41.5	7.2
4	576	29.2	4.9
5	146	7.4	6.2
6+	14	0.7	7.1

Follow-up period

Continued follow-up of the survivors is being carried out. They have been followed for a period ranging from 3 to 157 months (mean of 59.8 months). Seventy-two percent of the patients were free of angina, 17% had fewer anginal episodes compared to their preoperative status, 2% the same as preoperatively, 6% who were initially asymptomatic had recurrence of angina and 3% claimed worsening of angina after surgery. On an actuarial basis, 67% of the survivors of surgery continued to be free of angina for 3 years, 53% for 5 years and 34% for 10 years (Figure 2). No significant difference was discerned on anginal relief between group I and group II patients. After a mean follow-up of 59.8 months 169 late deaths occurred (9.1%). The actuarial survival for the entire series was 90% in the first year, 86% in the third year, 79% in the fifth year and 52% in the tenth year (Figure 3). Comparison of the survival pattern in group I and group II is shown in Figure 4). The late survival in group II patients improved over that in group I because of improved early mortality. Figure 5 shows the comparative survival rates in the elderly and the younger patients.

325

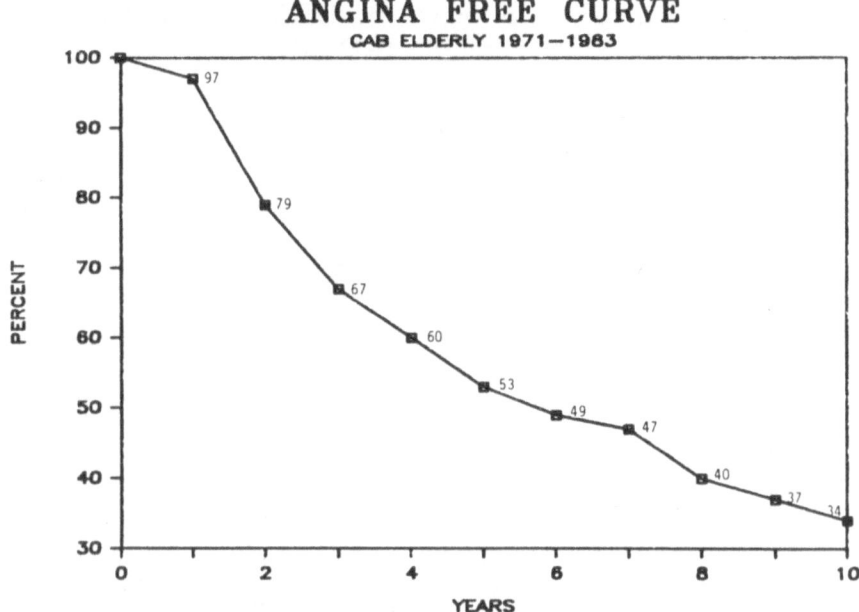

Figure 2. Angina-free curve of the survivors of surgery among the 1,972 elderly patients who underwent coronary artery bypass.

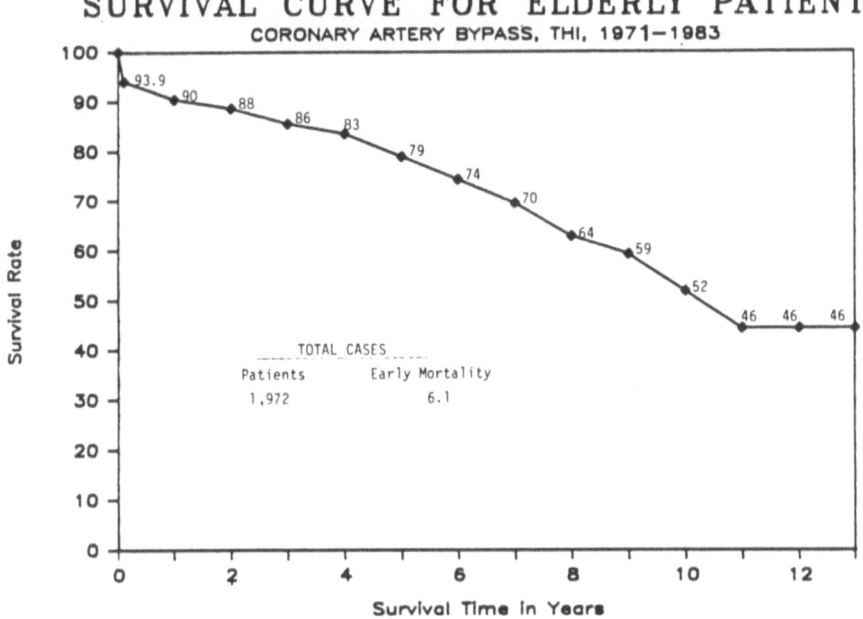

Figure 3. Life survival curves for all 1,972 elderly patients who underwent isolated coronary artery bypass.

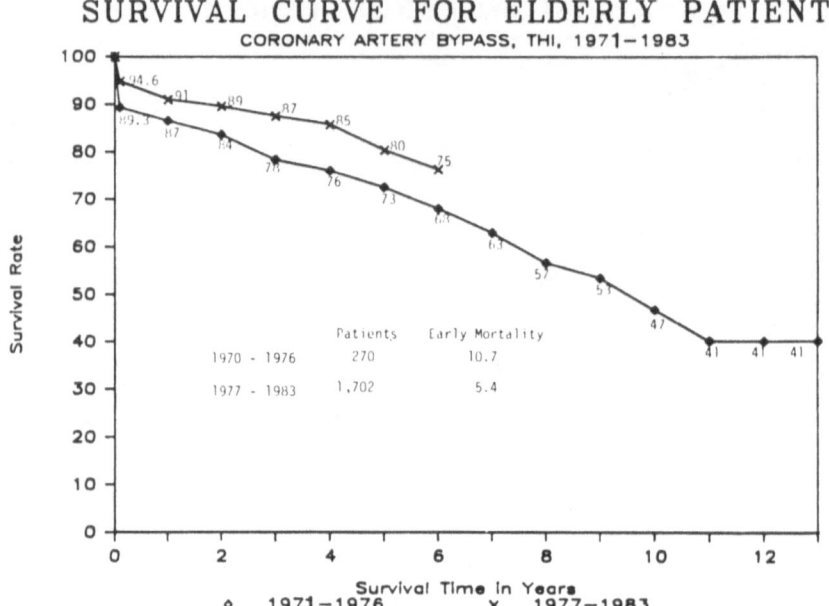

Figure 4. Life survival curve of patients in group I, 1971 to 1976, compared with patients in group II, 1977 to 1982.

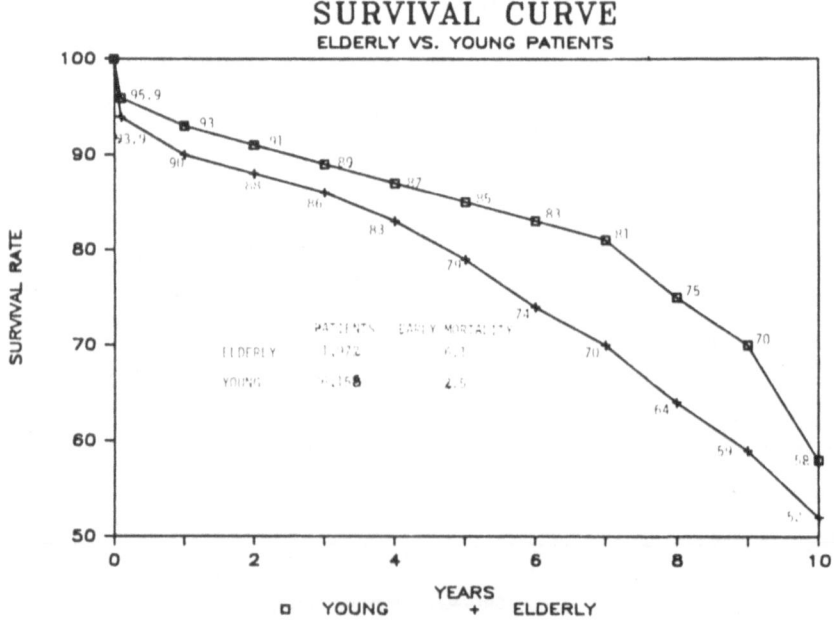

Figure 5. Life survival curves of 1,972 elderly patients compared with 26,158 younger patients who underwent isolated coronary artery bypass from 1971 to 1983.

Discussion

In recent years an increasing number of elderly patients have undergone coronary artery bypass in our institution as palliative treatment of coronary artery disease. This may be attributed to the wider acceptance of coronary bypass in the elderly as documented by reports, during the last 15 years, of decreasing operative mortality and morbidity [4–13] and good long-term surgical results [4–11, 12–13]. Moreover, the number of elderly individuals in our population is increasing. The observed decrease in early mortality in our series (5.4% in group II vs. 10.7% in group I) (p<.05) may be related to improved myocardial preservation, as well as technical advances in coronary care and surgery and improved angiographic techniques. Quite importantly are the increased incidence of serious, fatal and non-fatal complications and prolonged recovery time in the elderly compared to the younger patients [4–13]. The reason has been given as the higher prevalence of advanced coronary artery disease and other medical problems in the elderly.

Palliation from anginal symptoms was obtained in 89% of our patients. A similar report on decrease in anginal symtoms has been reported from other studies [5–13] as well as from initial experience in our institution in 95 elderly patients [10]. Long-term survival of our patients shows prolongation of life and can be favorable compared with the various groups of patients undergoing coronary artery bypass alone in our institution [17].

The therapeutic implications gained from our series are: a) the use of hypothermic chemical cardioplegia has reduced early mortality; b) the improvement in all phases of cardiovascular technology has reduced risk and improved the predictability of good surgical outcome; c) our results and those of others showed that elderly patients who are well preserved physiologically and mentally and with good motivation for improved life-style can undergo palliative therapy for disabling angina pectoris with an operative risk that is modestly higher than that observed in middle-aged patients. Therefore, advanced age, *per se,* should not deter or exclude a patient for consideration for surgery.

References

1. Bowles LT, Hallman GL, Cooley DA (1966) Open-heart surgery in the elderly: Results in 54 patients over age sixty. Circulation 33: 540–544
2. Bowles LT, Hallman GL, Cooley DA (1969) Open-heart surgery in patients over sixty years of age. J Amer Geriatrics Soc 17: 817–821
3. Messmer BJ, Hallman GL, Cooley DA (1970) Geriatric open heart-surgery: Experience with 292 patients over 60 years of age. J Cardiovasc Surg 11 (Suppl to No 3): 29–34
4. Berry BE, Acree PW, Davis DT, Sheely CH, Calvin S (1981) Coronary artery bypass operation in septuagenarians. Ann Thorac Surg 31: 310–313
5. Gann D, Colin C, Hildner FJ, Samet P, Yahr WZ, Greenberg JJ (1977) Coronary artery bypass surgery in patients seventy years of age and older. J Thorac Cardiovasc Surg 73: 237–241

6. Knapp WS, Douglas JS Jr, Craver JM (1981) Efficacy of coronary artery bypass grafting in elderly patients with coronary artery disease. Am J Cardiol 47: 923–930

7. Tucker BL, Lindesmith GG, Stiles QR, Hughes RK, Meyer BN (1977) Myocardial revascularization in patients 70 years of age and older. West J Med 1126: 179–183

8. DuCailar C, Chaitman BR, Castonguay Y (1980) Risk and benefits of aortocoronary bypass surgery in patients aged 65 years or more. Can Med Assoc J 122: 771–774

9. Smith JM, Lindsay WG, Lillehei RC, Nicoloff DM (1976) Cardiac surgery in geriatric patients. Surgery 80: 443–448

10. Meyer J, Wukasch DC, Seybold-Epting W, Chiariello L, Reul GJ Jr, Sandiford FM, Hallman GL, Cooley DA (1975) Coronary artery bypass in patients over 70 years of age: Indications and results. Am J Cardiol 36: 342–345

11. Gooch JB, Garrett HE, Davis JT Jr, Richardson RL June 1983. Coronary artery bypass surgery in the septuagenarian. Texas Heart Institute Journal 10 (2): 137–141

12. LaFollette L, Jacobson LB, Hill JD (1980) Isolated aortocoronary bypass operations in patients over 70 years of age. West J Med 133: 15–18

13. Ashor GW, Meyer BW, Lindesmith GG (1973) Coronary artery disease: Surgery in 100 patients 65 years of age and older. Arch Surg 107: 30–33

14. Cooley DA, Norman JC (1975) Techniques in Cardiac Surgery. Houston, Texas Medical Press, pp 153–156

15. Wukasch DC, Cooley DA, Halla RJ, Reul GJ, Sandiford FM, Zilgitts SL (1979) Surgical vs. medical treatment of coronary artery disease: Nine year follow-up of 9,061 patients. Am J Surg 137: 201–208

16. Cutler SH, Ederer F (1968) Maximum utilization of the life tables method in analyzing survival. J Chronic Dis 8: 699–712

17. Hall RJ, Elayda MD, Gray AG (1983) Coronary artery bypass: Long-term follow-up of 22,284 consecutive patients. Circulation 68 (Suppl) II: 20–26

Combination of valve replacement and coronary bypass

CARMINE MINALE and BRUNO J. MESSMER

Introduction

The combination of valve disease and coronary artery disease (CAD) has been reported to be as high as 64% [1–5]. In 28% of these cases, CAD can be completely asymptomatic [6]. The association of the two conditions has been blamed for increased morbidity and mortality after surgical correction of valve disease [2, 3].

Linhart and coworkers [1, 2] found that in patients (pts) with impaired left ventricular function following valve replacement, the most frequent associated condition was CAD.

Unfortunately, most symptoms and ECG patterns of combined valve and coronary artery disease are similar to those of isolated valve disease. Angina i.e. is a common symptom, particularly of aortic stenosis, but in 25% to 33% of such cases an additional significant LAD stenosis is revealed by angiography. On the other hand, angina is relatively uncommon in mitral disease because dispnea generally appears before the patient has sustained an effort great enough to cause angina. Moreover, ECG patterns of ventricular hypertrophy with strain cannot be exactly differentiated from those of ischemia due to coronary heart disease. With introduction of coronariography in the routine hemodynamic and angiographic investigations it was possible to discover concomitant lesions of the coronary arteries.

Since 1971 [7, 8], combined correction of coronary artery and valve disease is done routinely in many centers. Early experience was somewhat disappointing because overall hospital mortality averaged 16% [9, 10]. It was 12% for aortic pts [5, 11–16], 23% for pts with rheumatic mitral disease [16, 18], and for pts with ischemic mitral regurgitation even as high as 60% [18, 19]. The combined approach of valve repair and aortocoronary bypass graft (CABG) carried a significantly higher risk than for valve replacement alone. Perioperative myocardial infarction rates up to 21% were not infrequent in the literature [20].

The time-frame of operation, however, is significant since, with introduction of cold cardioplegic myocardial protection, with improvement of operative techniques and with use of inothropic and mechanical support of the heart during the postoperative period, hospital mortality and morbidity has decreased to rates that superimpose those of valve surgery alone [5, 21, 22].

This report evaluates our experience with the combined operative treatment of valvular and obstructive coronary artery disease since 1977.

Clinical material and methods

Between February 1977 and August 1984, 194 patients with combined significant valvular and coronary artery disease (Table 1) were operated on at our institution.

Onehundred-twentyseven patients underwent aortic valve replacement and 63 pts underwent mitral valve operation of either repair or replacement. Of these latter groups, 42 pts had mitral disease of rheumatic or degenerative origin and 21 of ischemic origin. Three patients had combined mitral and aortic disease, and 1 patient had tricuspid valve incompetence.

The left anterior descending artery (LAD) was the most frequently obstructed vessel, as well with aortic as with mitral valve disease (Table 2). No significative difference in distribution of coronary disease could be found among the three groups of patients.

One vessel disease was present in about the half of patients (Table 3), whereas 2 and 3 vessel disease accounted each for about $\frac{1}{4}$ of the patient's out. Left main stem stenosis was seen in 2.6% of the cases.

Of particular interest is the pathology of the so called 'ischemic mitral disease', where the mitral valve disfunction is not associated but due to CAD. We

Table 1. Valve replacement and bypass surgery (Feb. 1977–Aug. 1984).

No. of patients		194
137 Men	age 57 ± 7.5	(36–74)
57 Women	age 61 ± 6.3	(41–74)

Table 2. Aortic valve and CABG, n. = 127

	103	(81%)
LAD	103	(81%)
RCA	63	(49%)
CX	52	(41%)

Mitral valve and CABG, n. = 63

	non ischemic	ischemic
LAD	33 (78%)	19 (90%)
CX	20 (47%)	10 (47%)
RCA	17 (40%)	10 (47%)

Table 3. Coronary disease. n. = 194.

1 Vessel disease	93 (48%)
2 Vessel disease	55 (28%) *1
3 Vessel disease	46 (24%) *4

* Left stem st.	5 (2.6%)

encountered 16 prolapsing mitral valves due to hypo- to akinesia of the posterior wall following posterior myocardial infarct, 2 cases of papillary muscle disruption, and 3 cases of posterior wall aneurysm with mitral regurgitation.

Preoperative functional status of the 3 groups of patients is represented in Table 4. The NYHA classification has been used because it is more pertinent for primarily valve patients, even though it does not necessarily reflect the severity of CAD. More than 90% of the patients belong to the class III or IV.

All operations were done using standard cardiopulmonary bypass techniques, moderate systemic hypothermia and cold cardioplegic cardiac arrest with Kirsch cardioplegia [23]. Generally it was tried to avoid cross clamp times of more than 90−, either by adopting an operative strategy for the individual patient or by using a double cross-clamp. Technical details of surgery have already been described elsewhere [24, 25].

The aortic valve was replaced in all instances whereas the mitral valve was repaired, especially in younger people, by means of a Carpentier ring or by Kay-Wooler plastic, whenever possible. If not, it was replaced. With few exception mechanical valves were preferred for aortic valve replacement to avoid reoperation in patients with CABG anastomoses on the ascending aorta.

For mitral valve replacement we gave our preference to bioprosthesis, since in our opinion the risk of thromboembolism overwelms the risk of reoperation [24].

The aortic valve group became an average of 2.0 ± 1.2 CABG and the two mitral valve groups 1.9 ± 1.7 CABG pro patient with a range from 1 to 5 CABG.

Before discontinuing cardiopulmonary bypass, all patients became an inothropic support of 5 μg Dopamine/Kg.b.w. and if the cardiac output was not considered satisfactory, Suprarenin 0.01 to 0.15 μg/Kg.bw was combined to Dopamine.

Table 4. Preoperative functional status.

Nyha	Aorta	Mitral non isch.	Mitral isch.
	n = 127	n = 42	n = 21
I–II	2.5%	2.5%	
III	85.0%	85.5%	76.0%
IV	12.5%	12.0%	24.0%

332

Postoperatively all patients received warfarin for a minimum of three months. Long term anticoagulation was prescribed for patients with mechanical prostheses, with atrial fibrillation, for patients who had previous history of thromboembolism and/or atrial thrombi at operation.

Follow-up

Follow-up information has been obtained mainly by interviewing the patients in our outpatient clinic at regular intervals. For pts living at a far distance, a questionnaire was send to the patient and to the referring physician.

All deaths of unclear origin were attributed to cardiac related cause. Thromboembolic complications include peripheral arterial emboli as well as all new focal neurologic defect, either transient or permanent, unless they were proved to be of other origins.

Statistics

Continuous variables are presented with ± 1 standard deviation of the mean. Late mortality and morbidity are presented as linearized (% per patient-year) occurence rate.

Results

Overall average hospital (30 days) mortality was 2.6% with 5 deaths among 194 cases (Table 5). The specific mortality was lower in the aortic valve group (1.6%), somewhat higher in the non ischemic mitral group (3.3%) and definitively higher (9.5%) in the 'ischemic' mitral group. A significative difference, however, could not be demonstrated mainly because the samples of subjects at risk were relatively small. None of the few patients with isolated tricuspid or double valve replacement died.

Major causes of hospital mortality and morbidity are shown in Table 6.

Table 5. Hospital mortality.

Aorta	Mitral non isch.	Mitral isch.	AO & MI	Tricusp.
n = 127	n = 42	n = 21	n = 3	n = 1
2 (1.6%)	1 (2.3%)	2 (9.5%)	0	0

Average mortality: 2.6% (5/194)

Table 6. Major causes of hospital morbidity.

	Aorta n = 127		Mitral non isch. n = 42		Mitral isch. n = 21	
	n.	(%)	n.	(%)	n.	(%)
Ventr. fibrillation	24	19.0	2	5.0	5	23.0
Low cardiac output	11	9.0*	2	5.0	1	4.8*
Cardiac infarct					1	4.8*
Multiple organs failure	1	0.8*			1	4.8
Thromboembolism	1	0.8			1	4.8*

Each * = 1 fatal outcome.

Cardiogenic shock was the most determinant factor of fatal outcomes, followed by multiorgan failure, including gastrointestinal bleeding. There was only one, but fatal postoperative infarct in the ischemic mitral group. Also interesting is the higher rate of postoperative ventricular fibrillation in the aortic group versus the other two groups.

In 6.7% of the cases, intraortic balloon counterpulsation was necessary, mainly because of low cardiac output unresponsive to cathecholamines, and in 3 cases after high dosage of β-blockers because of serious rhythm instability (Table 7).

Survivors were followed-up to a total of 363 patient-years with a mean of 2.7 years and range between 5 months and 7 years (Table 8).

Average late cardiac related mortality was 2.5% per patient-year (Table 9). In this rate are also included all sudden deaths and all deaths of unknown nature.

Table 7. Intraortic counterpulsation.

Indications	Aorta n = 127	Mitral non isch. n = 42	Mitral isch. n = 21
Low cardiac output	8	1	1
Rhythm Instability	0	2	1

Average 6.7% (13/194)

Table 8. Follow-up.

No. of survivors	189
No. of pts. followed-up	134 (71%)
Follow-up duration (yrs)	363
mean	2.7 ± 1.7
range	(0.4–7)

Common causes of late morbidity were anticaogulation bleedings and thromboembolism (Table 10), boths generally presumed to be related to CAD and/or valve prostheses.

Incidence of late myocardial infarction was relatively low (average 1.7%) and no recurrence in the ischemic mitral group was observed. The differences are, however, not significant.

Late functional status (Table 11) shows a tremendous change in all patients groups. More than 80% of patients are asymptomatic or have minimal symptoms.

Table 9. Late mortality.

	Aorta n = 91		Mitral non isch. n = 28		Mitral isch. n = 15		Average n = 134	
	n.	(%)	n.	(%)	n.	(%)	n.	(%)
Cardiac related (incl. sudden death)	5	2.0	2	2.6	2	4.8	9	2.5
Non cardiac related	1	0.4					1	0.4

All percentage are expressed as % per patient-year.

Table 10. Late morbidity.

	Aorta n = 91		Mitral non isch. n = 28		Mitral isch. n = 15		Average n = 134	
	n.	(%)	n.	(%)	n.	(%)	n.	(%)
Minor bleedings	12	4.8	5	6.7	1	6.6	18	5.5
Major bleedings	1	0.4*	1	1.3			2	0.5
Thromboembolism	6	2.4*	2	2.6*	2	13.0	10	2.8
Myocardial infarct	5	2.0	1	1.3			6	1.7
Endocarditis	1	0.4					1	0.4

Each * = one fatal outcome.
All percentage are expressed as % per patient-year.

Table 11. Late functional status.

Nyha	Aorta n = 89	Mitral non isch. n = 28	Mitral isch. n = 16
I–II	94.4%	79.0%	100%
III	5.6%	10.5%	
IV		10.5%	
		p = 0.02	

Table 12. Degree of improvement.

Nyha	Aorta n = 89	Mitral non isch. n = 28	Mitral isch. n = 16
+1 Cl.	60.0%	68.0%	50.0%
+2 Cl.	36.0%	18.0%	44.0%
+3 Cl.	3.0%	7.0%	6.0%
−1 Cl.	1.0%	7.0%	
mean	1.4 ± 0.6	1.3 ± 0.7	1.6 ± 0.6

A slight significant difference was noted between improvement of the aortic valve and the mitral valve group. It is a common observation that the benefit of the operation in more evident in the aortic disease than in the mitral disease, since in the latter group a chronic myocarditis component is often present. All survivors of the ischemic mitral group are doing well. This is probably due to the fact that in many cases, the ventricular wall motion can restore after myocardial revascularization and the symptoms disappear drammatically.

The degree of improvement is shown in Table 12. Formally there is no significant difference among the three groups and the majority of patients improved at least 1.5 functional classes.

Finally, actuarial survival and complication-free actuarial survival are graphically represented in Figure 1. These curves can be considered significant up to 5–6 years. The overall survival is 85% and the complication-free survival 50%. This low complication-free survival rate is due to the fact that all minor and irrelevant episodes have been included.

The specific survival diagram (Figure 2) shows no significant difference be-

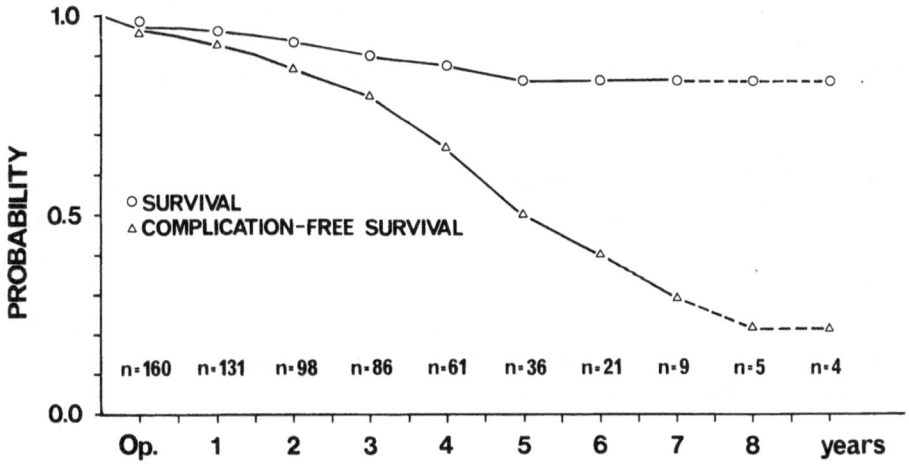

Figure 1. Valve replacement and CABG. Overall actuarial survival.

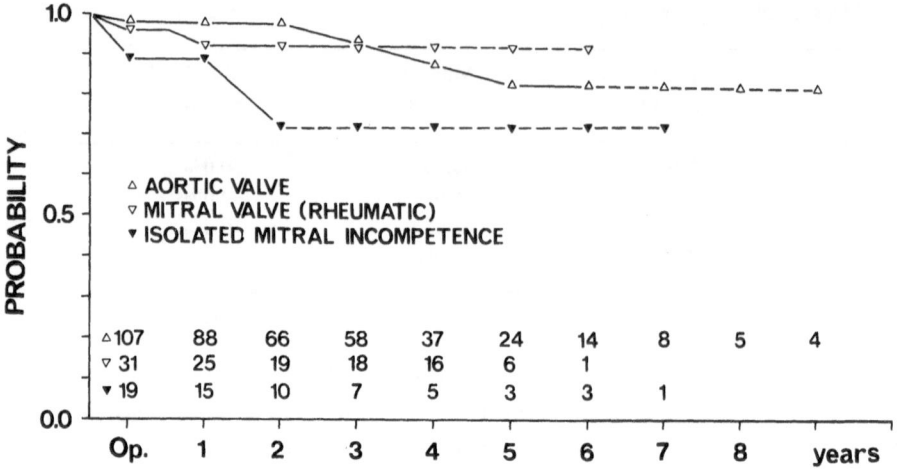

Figure 2. Valve replacement and CABG. Specific actuarial survival.

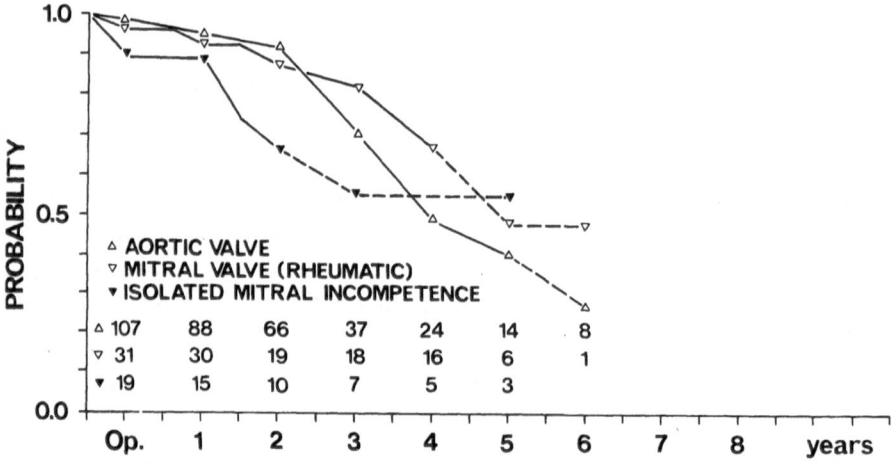

Figure 3. Valve replacement and CABG. Specific complication-free actuarial survival.

tween the three groups of patients. Of some concern may be, however, the ischemic mitral group whose survival curve drops more rapidly than the other two ones. The sample of subjects at risk is, however, too small to get statistical significance.

The same can be said of the complications-free intervals curves (Figure 3), where the ischemic mitral group has the higher incidence of complications, mainly thromboembolic complications.

Concluding remarks

Coronary artery disease can always be possible in adult patients with valvular disease over age 40 [1]. For this reason coronariography prior to operation is mandatory not only in patients with aortic or ischemic mitral valve disease but also in patients with rheumatic or degenerative mitral valve disease as well as in patients with isolated aortic insufficiency.

Earlier studies of simultaneous valve replacement and coronary bypass operation demonstrated a higher risk for the combined procedure [5, 7, 8, 11, 26–28] but more recent experience has shown an improved survival which approaches that of valve repair alone [15, 16, 18].

The correction of two pathological processes during the same procedure is indeed extremely important because omitted correction of a secondary condition could have detrimental effect on the outcome of repair for the primary condition. The rate of postoperative myocardial infarction after valve operation alone can be as high as 36.5% [29]. For combined valve repair and coronary revascularization it varies between 3 to 17% [30, 31]. In the present series it occurred only in one patient of the ischemic mitral group (Table 6), which amounts to 0.5% for the total group of 197 patients.

Some degree of scepticism concerns surgical treatment of the ischemic mitral valve disease. Early and late results are often unsatisfactory [18, 19, 32]. Our results are, however, encouraging as hospital mortality was 9.5% and late mortality 4.8% per patient-year, in spite of the fact that 9 of these patients had a proved myocardial infarct preoperatively. Baudet [33] reported recently of 9 patients without operative and postoperative mortality at an average follow-up of 21 months.

Complete rupture of a papillary muscle occurs infrequently after myocardial infarction, but it is typically associated with acute left ventricular failure, pulmonary edema and rapid clinical deterioration. Early mortality after such an event, if untreated, is approximatively 80%–90% [34]. The operation in these cases carries a high risk [35], but must be considered as a life-saving emergency.

Some authors concluded that severe coronary arteriosclerosis may adversely affect longevity, despite bypass grafting [5]. More recently, other authors have presented data suggesting that the overall survival rate of patients undergoing combined valve repair and CABG does not differ from the results obtained with valve repair alone in absence of coronary disease [21, 36]. The present results support this contention and we even can conclude that survival curves approximate those of matched normal population.

Summary

Between February 1977 and August 1984, a total of 194 patients (Pts) underwent combined coronary artery and valvular operation. One hundred-twentyseven Pts had combined coronary artery bypass grafting (CABG) and aortic valve replacement (AVR), 63 Pts had CABG with mitral valve operation (MVO), 1 Pt with AVR & MVO, and 1 with tricuspid valve replacement. There were 137 men and 57 women, whose age averaged 57 ± 7.5 (36–74) and 61 ± 6.3 (41–74) years respectively. One vessel disease was present in 48%, 2 vessel in 28%, and 3 vessel disease in 24% of the cases. Left main stem stenosis was present in 2.6% of Pts. Among Pts with MVO, 21 had isolated mitral incompetence (MI) of ischemic origin and 42 had a combined rheumatic mitral valve disease (MSI). An average of 2 [1–5] bypasses was done in the AVR group and 1.9 [1–5] in the MVO group. Mitral valve was replaced in all but one instances of MSI and in 15 cases of MI. In 6 patients the mitral valve was repaired by Kay-Wooler or ring plastic. Overall early mortality was 2.6% (5 cases) while specific mortality was 1.6% for AVR, 2.3% for MSI, 9.5% for MI. Postoperatively intraortic balloon pump support was needed in 13 cases (6.7%). One patient with MI sustained a fatal myocardial infarct postoperatively. One-hundred thirty-four Pts could be followed for a total of 363 patients-years (average 2.7 ± 1.7), range 0.4–7 years. Overall late mortality was 2.9% per Pt-year and presumed cardiac related mortality 2.5% per Pt-year. Late morbidity includes minor bleeding, 5.5% per Pt-yr; major bleeding, 0.5% per Pt-yr; thromboembolism, 2.8% per Pt-yr; myocardial infarct, 1.7% per Pt-yr; and infective endocarditis, 0.4% per Pt-yr. Functional improvement of at least 1–2 classes was observed in about 90% of Pts and there was no significant difference among the 3 groups. Six year actuarial survival was 0.83 for AVR, 0.92 for MSI and 0.72 for MI.

The small increase in risk compared to the significant improvement from the combined approach has led to the following conclusions: (1) coronary arteriography is mandatory on all adult patients requiring valvular operations, (2) bypass of all significant coronary lesions and (3) restoration of valvular function and hemodynamics must be performed.

References

1. Linhart JW, Wheat MW (1967) Myocardial dysfunction following aortic valve replacement. The significance of coronary artery disease. J Thorac Cardiovasc Surg 54: 259
2. Linhart JW, De La Torre A, Ramsley HW, Wheat MW (1968) The significance of coronary artery disease in aortic valve replacement. J Thorac Cardiovasc Surg 55: 811
3. Coleman EH, Soloff LA (1970) Incidence of significant coronary artery disease in rheumatic valvular heart disease. Am J Cardiol 25: 401
4. Lacy J, Goodin R, McMartin D, Masolen R, Flowers N (1977) Coronary atherosclerosis in valvular heart disease. Ann Thorac Surg 23: 429

5. Loop FD, Phillips DF, Roy M, Taylor PC, Groves LK, Effler DB (1977) Aortic valve replacement combined with myocardial revascularization. Late clinical results and survival of surgically-treated aortic valve patients with and without coronary artery disease. Circulation 55: 169

6. Loop FD, Favaloro RG, Shirey EK, Groves LK, Effler DB (1972) Surgery for combined valvular and coronary heart disease. JAMA 220: 372

7. Di Matteo J, Vacheron A, Cacherà JP, Heulin A, Lafont H (1971) Pontage aorto-coronarien avec replacement valvulaire aortique et commissurotomie mitrale. Ann Med Interne (Paris) 122: 867

8. Diethrich EB (1971) Technical considerations in combined valvular replacement and coronary artery bypass operations. Surg Gynecol Obstet 133: 1015

9. Callard GM, Flege JB, Todd JC (1976) Combined valvular and coronary surgery. Amer J Thorac Surg 22: 338

10. Cacherà JP, Vouhe P, Loisance D, Poulain H, Galey JJ (1977) La chirurgie combineé des lesions valvulaires et coronariennes. Coeur et Medicine interne 16: 259

11. Berndt ThB, Hancock EW, Shumway NE, Harrison DC (1974) Aortic valve replacement with and without coronary artery bypass surgery. Circulation 50: 967

12. Macmanus Q, Grunkemeier G, Lambert L, Dietl C, Starr A (1978) Aortic valve replacement and aorta-coronary bypass surgery. Results with perfusion of proximal and distal coronary arteries. J Thorac Cardiovasc Surg 75: 865

13. Thompson R, Ahmed M, Ilsley C, Seabra-Gomes R, Rickards A, Yakoub M (1979) Evaluation of combined homograft replacement of aortic valve and coronary bypass grafting in patients with aortic stenosis. Brit Heart J 42: 447

14. Luxereau Ph, Heulin A, Verdier-Taillefer MH, Cabrol C, Cacherà JP, Marchand M, Milon H, Cassagnes J, Acar J (1979) Les lesions coronaires des valvulopathies aortiques operees. Arch Mal Coeur 72: 1114

15. Laks H, Geha AS, Lundell DC, Hammond GL (1980) Combined aortic valve replacement and Myocardial revascularization. Connecticut Medicine 44: 353

16. Reed GE, Sanoudos GM, Pooley RW, Moggio RA, McClung A, Somberg ED, Praeger PI (1983) Results of combined valvular and myocardial revascularization operations. J Thorac Cardiovasc Surg 85: 422

17. Parravicini R, Modena MG, Sandiford FM (1981) Bypass aortocoronarico associato a terapia chirurgica della valvola mitrale. Min Cardioang 29: 477

18. Karp RB (1982) Mitral valve replacement and coronary artery bypass grafting. Ann Thorac Surg 34: 480

19. Pinson WC, Cobanoglu A, Metzdorff MT, Grunkemeier GL, Kay PH, Starr A (1984) Late surgical results for ischemic mitral regurgitation: Role of wall motion score and severity of regurgitation. J Thorac Cardiovasc Surg 88: 663–672

20. Berger TJ, Karp RB, Kouchoukos NT (1975) Valve replacement and myocardial revascularization. Results of combined operation in 59 patients. Circulation (Suppl. I) 51, 52: 126–131

21. Richardson JW, Kouchoukos NT, Wright JO (1979) Combined aortic valve replacement and myocardial revascularization: results on 220 patients. Circulation 59: 75

22. Nunley DL, Grunkemeier GL, Starr A (1983) Aortic valve replacement with coronary bypass grafting. Significant determinants of ten-year survival. J Thorac Cardivasc Surg 85: 705

23. Kirsch U, Rodevald G, Kalmar P (1972) Induced ischemic arrest. Clinical experience with cardioplegia in open heart surgery. J Thorac Cardiovasc Surg 63: 121

24. Minale C, Bardos P, Bourg NP, Messmer BJ (1982) Early and late results of porcine bioprostheses versus mechanical prostheses in aortic and mitral position. In: Cohn LH, Gallucci V (eds) Cardiac Bioprostheses, New York, Yorke Medical Books Publisher, pp 154–168

25. Minale C, Bourg NP, Bardos P, Messmer BJ (1984) Flow characteristics in single and sequential aorto-coronary bypass grafts. J Cardiovasc Surg 25: 12

26. Flemma RJ, Johnson WD, Lepley D Jr (1971) Simultaneous valve replacement and aorta-to-coronary saphenous vein bypass. Ann Thorac Surg 12: 163

27. Merin G, Danielson GM, Wallace RB (1973) Combined one-satage artery and valvular surgery: a clinical evaluation. Circulation (Suppl III) 47, 48: 173
28. Berndt T, Hancock EW, Harrison DC (1973) Combined aortic valve replacement and coronary bypass surgery (abstract). Circulation (Suppl IV) 47, 48: 74
29. Hultgren HN, Miyagawa M, Buch W (1973) Ischemic myocardial injury during cardiopulmonary bypass surgery. Am Heart J 85: 167
30. Assad-Morrel JL, Connolly DC, Brandenbury RO (1975) Aortocoronary artery saphenous vein bypass grafts – isolated and combined with other procedures. J Thorac Cardiovasc Surg 69: 841
31. Anderson RP, Bonchek LI, Wood J (1973) Safety of combined aortic valve replacement and coronary bypass grafting. Ann Thorac Surg 15: 249
32. Kennedy JW, Kaiser GC, Fisher LD (1981) Clinical and angiographic predictors of operative mortality. In the Collaborative Study in Coronary Artery Surgery (CASS). Circulation 63: 793
33. Baudet M, Gandjbakhch I, Rigaud M, Rocha P, Baehrel B, Bardet J, Bourdarias JP, Cabrol C (1978) Traitement chirurgical par replacement valvulaire et pontage aorto-coronaire de l'insuffiance mitrale par dysfonctionnement chronique du pilier posterieur. Arch Mal Coeur 71: 1023
34. Fox AC, Glassman I, Isom OW (1979) Surgically remediable complications of myocardial infarction. Prog Cardiovasc Dis 21: 461
35. Nunley DL, Starr A (1983) Papillary muscle rupture complicating acute myocardial infarction. Am J Surg 145: 574
36. Wisoff BG, Fogle R, Weisz D, Garvey J, Hamby R (1980) Combined valve and coronary artery surgery. Ann Thorac Surg 29: 440

Cardiac valve replacement and simultaneous myocardial revascularisation

A. FRILLING, W. BIRCKS, R. KÖRFER, K. MINAMI and H.D. SCHULTE

The routine use of coronary angiography in the evaluation of patients with valvular heart disease has demonstrated that a significant number of patients suffer from co-existing occlusive coronary artery disease. The incidence of coronary artery disease and concomitant cardiac valve disease that requires surgical therapy ranges from 8 to 56 per cent [3, 4] and increases with age, particulary after the age of 40.

In our institution the first combined procedure was performed in December 1974. At that time routine use of coronary angiography was not practicable and as in most centers only patients with angina had this invasive investigation preoperatively. Up to the end of 1983 155 patients (pts.) (105 males, 50 females; mean age: 62 years, range: 43–77 years) underwent cardiac valve replacement and simultaneous myocardial revascularisation [5].

According to the nature of the predominant disease, the patients were divided in two groups. Group I consisted of 138 pts. with predominant rheumatic valve disease and group II consisted of 17 pts. with predominant coronary artery disease.

In group I single valve replacement was performed in 124 pts. (aortic valve replacement (AVR): n = 75; mitral valve replacement (MVR): n = 49). 13 pts. underwent double valve replacement (AVR + MVR: n = 12; MVR + tricuspid valve replacement (TVR): n = 1), and 1 patient underwent triple valve replacement (AVR + MVR + TVR). The mean number of coronary artery bypass grafts was 1.6 per patient (range: 1–6 grafts per patient).

In group II mitral valve incompetence following myocardial infarction required MVR in 15 pts. In another 2 pts. AVR was performed due to hemodynamic reasons during ECC. Mean number of coronary artery bypass grafts was 2,3 per patient (range: 1–3 grafts per patient).

According to the NYHA-criteria 87 pts. were in clinical class III and 68 in clinical class IV.

Early mortality was 8,4 per cent in the whole series (155/13) – 7,9 per cent in group I (138/11) and 11,8 per cent (17/2) in group II. Regarding the period since 1979 early mortality dropped down to 6.5 per cent (137/9). Surprisingly there was no difference between the two groups. Postoperative follow-up ranged from 3

342

Table 1. Preoperative clinical status, symptoms and hemodynamic findings in patients with predominant rheumatic valve disease with coexisting coronary artery disease (group I) and in patients with predominant coronary artery disease and coexisting valve disease (group II).

| | Group I valve disease with coexisting coronary artery disease | | | Group II coronary artery disease with coexisting valve disease | | |
	aortic valve	mitral valve	multi-valvular	aortic valve	mitral valve	Total
Number of patients	75	49	14		17	155
Diagnosis predominant stenosis	58	40				
Diagnosis predominant insufficiency	10	7		2	15	
Stenosis = insufficiency	7	2	14			
Stenosis = insufficiency III	30	36	10		11	87
Clinical class (NYHA) IV	45	13	4		6	68
Angina pectoris	70	38	13		9	30
Myocardial infarction	9	2	1		15	27
Dyspnoe	55	44	12		15	126
Syncopes	16	–	2		–	18
LVEDP (mmHg)*	20,7	13,4	14,1		20,17	
Cardiac index $(1 \cdot min^{-1} \cdot m^{-2})$*	2,7	2,71	2,83		2,2	
PPA (mmHg)*	22,1	36,1	37,8		27,3	

* Mean value. Düsseldorf 1974–1983.

Table 2. Operative mortality after cardiac valve replacement, after aortocoronary bypass and after cardiac valve replacement combined with simultaneous myocardial revascularisation.

	Patients (n)	Letality (per cent)
Cardiac valve replacement (single and multiple)	1626 (84)	5,2
Aortocoronary bypass	1614 (34)	2,1
Cardiac valve replacement and simultaneous aortocoronary bypass	137 (9)	6,5

( ) died during the early postoperative period. Düsseldorf 1978–1983.

months to 8 years with an average of 2 years; there were 4 late deaths.

Our results show, that valve replacement and simultaneous revascularisation can be performed with acceptable risk. Comparing the operative mortality of combined operation (6,5 per cent) and the mortality of isolated valve replacement or bypass surgery, there is no significant difference between each type of operation [2, 6].

Furthermore there is no difference in operative mortality concerning patients operated for rheumatic valvular disease with concomitant coronary artery disease or predominant coronary artery disease and concomitant valvular disease (mostly mitral insufficiency). Against it Assad-Morell [1] found out, that mitral valve insufficiency following myocardial infarction entails much higher operative mortality.

The type of valve disease and the number of bypasses performed have no significant influence on the early postoperative mortality.

On the other hand the operative mortality depends on the preoperative clinical class.

Our results implicate, that simultaneous myocardial revascularisation shows significant better clinical results when performed in patients suffering from acquired valve disease and concomitant coronary artery disease.

References

1. Assad.Morell JL, Connolly DC, Brandenburg RO, Giuliani ER, Schattenberg TT, Pluth JR, Barnhorst DA, Wallace RB, Danielson GK (1975) Aorto-coronary artery saphenous vein bypass grafts. J Thorac Cardiovasc Surg 69: 841
2. Ciaravella JM, Ochsner JL, Mills NL (1977) Combined procedure of coronary artery bypass grafting and valve repair. Ann Thorac Surg 23: 20
3. Coleman EH, Soloff LA (1970) Incidence of significant coronary artery disease in rheumatic valvular heart disease. Amer J Cardiol 25: 401
4. Hancock EW (1977) Aortic stenosis, angina pectoris and coronary artery disease. Amer Heart J 93: 382
5. Körfer R, Bircks W, Horstkotte D, Kolb HJ, Loogen F, Schulte HD (1983) Cardiac valve replacement and simultanous myocardial revascularization. Z Kardiol 72: 18
6. Richardson JP, Westlake GW, Clarebrough JK (1980) Cardiac valve replacement and coronary bypass grafts. Med J Austr 1: 422

Bypass surgery for stenosis and occlusion of the left main coronary artery

H. OELERT, A. HAVERICH, S. IVERSEN, J. SCHULZE and R. HETZER

Introduction

The clinical state and long-term prognosis of patients with ischemic heart disease strongly support the superiority of the surgical treatment in contrast to conservative measures for stenosis or occlusion of the left main coronary artery [1, 2, 11, 18, 19]. Not only the symptoms of angina pectoris could be dramatically reduced but also was the life expectancy significantly prolonged. The danger to which these patients are exposed, however, is also expressed in the increased operative risk as compared to patients with other forms of coronary artery lesions [3, 5, 13, 14, 16, 20]. In this presentation I should like to report on our results of coronary artery revascularization in patients with stenosis or occlusion of the left main coronary artery. Specific value will be given to the comprehension of risk factors which directly will effect the perioperative course.

Patients and methods

From 1975 through 1981, 1.894 patients underwent coronary artery revascularization in our clinic. One hundred and fifty-four or 8.4% suffered from isolated or combined obstructive lesions of the left main coronary artery. One hundred and forty (91%) were male, 14 (9%) female. The mean operative age was 53.3 ± 6.9 years, ranging from 36 to 69 years. All patients included in this series had left main stem stenosis of at least 50%. Concomitant lesions not requiring surgical treatment were ischemic mitral incompetence in 2 instances, and one postinfarction ventricular aneurysm. Four patients had reoperation following failure of aortocoronary bypass grafting.

No patient with left main disease was clinically free from symptoms of angina pectoris. Twenty-three patients or 15% could be classified as grade II of the New York Heart Association (NYHA) classification, 103 or 67% as grade III, and 28 or 18% as grade IV. These latter patients had either pectangina at rest or were instable. Preoperative infarction had occurred once in 46% (n = 71) of the patients, twice in 7% (n = 11), and three times in 2% (n = 3). Fourty-five % (n = 69) had remained free from this complication until the time of surgical treatment.

The usual coronary risk factors – as described in Table 1 – could be demon-

Table 1. Incidence of risk factors in patients with left main coronary artery disease.

	N	(%)
Nicotine abuse	69	(45%)
Hyperlipidemia	67	(44%)
Arterial hypertension	62	(40%)
Excess weight	42	(27%)
Diabetes	29	(19%)

strated in the majority of patients; nicotine abuse was found in 69 cases (45%), followed by hyperlipidemia in 67 (44%), arterial hypertension in 62 (40%), excess weight in 42 (27%), and diabetes in 29 (19%) instances. At coronary arteriography, the following pattern of left main coronary artery disease was obtained.

In 103 patients (67%) this artery was stenosed 50% to 75%, in 36 patients (23%) 75% to 90%, and in 11 patients (7%) subtotal (Figure 1). In 4 patients (3%) complete occlusion of the left main coronary artery was present. In one of these patients (Figure 2), its complete retrograde filling could be demonstrated after contrast injection into the right coronary artery.

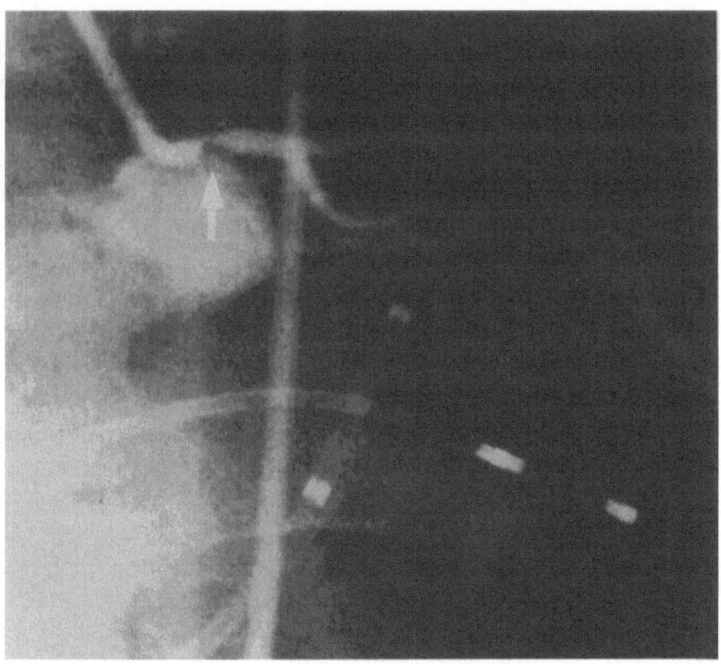

Figure 1. Left main coronary arteriogram demonstrating subtotal stenosis.

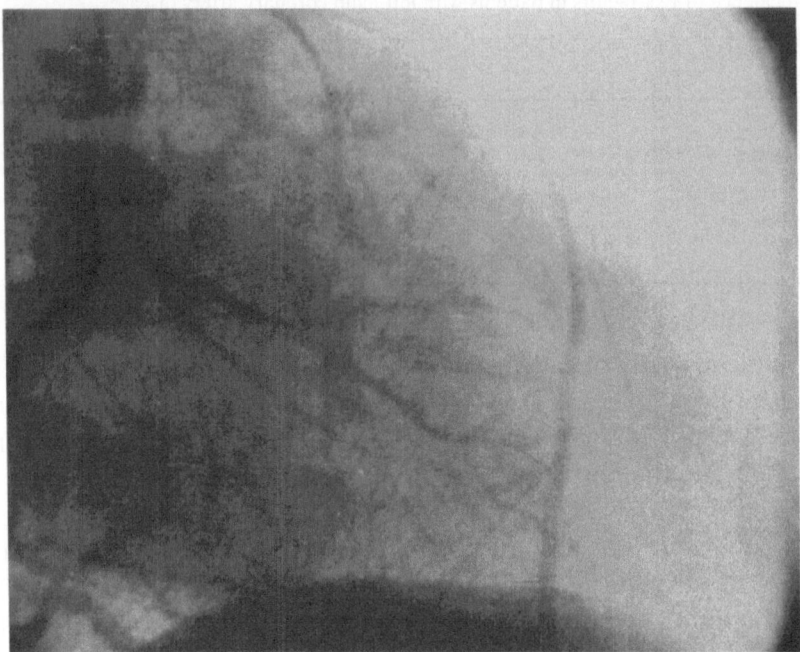

Figure 2. Retrograde filling of the complete left coronary artery system in a patient with left main coronary artery occlusion.

Localization of additional coronary artery sclerosis with more than 70% stenosis in these patients are summarized in Table 2. Only 14 patients (9%) had an isolated left main stenosis. Thirty-three times additional obstructive lesions were present in the LAD and/or circumflex artery of the left coronary artery, and 89 times in both the right and left major coronary artery branches. In a total of 60 patients, the left main stenosis was combined with a significant 3-vessel coronary artery disease.

Complete occlusion of the right coronary artery was found in 40 out of 107 patients with coronary artery disease of the right coronary artery. The import-

Table 2. Localization and incidence of additional coronary artery disease in patients with left main coronary artery stenosis.

Localization	N	(%)
Isolated LMCA	14	(9%)
LAD and/or CX	33	(21%)
RCA	18	(12%)
Right and Left CA	89	(58%)
Complete occlusion of RCA in 40 of 107 patients		(37%)

ance of the right coronary artery in the presence of stenosis or occlusion of the left main stem is documented by the fact that 103 patients or 67% had a dominant right, and only 22 (14%), and 29 (19%), resp., had a dominant left coronary artery or an equalized distribution.

The ejection fraction of the left ventricle ranged from 26% to 85% and had a mean value of $62.2 \pm 12.7\%$. A normal ejection fraction of more than 60% was found in more than $^2/_3$ of all patients (72%).

Indication for operation was the evidence of more than 50% left main stenosis in connection with the clinical and electrocardiographical signs of effort myocardial ischemia. In patients with instable angina or symptoms at rest, operative intervention was based entirely on the results of coronary arteriography.

All operations were performed on cardio-pulmonary bypass using mild perfusion hypothermia and cold potassium cardioplegic arrest. According to the multiple vessel disease in the majority of the 154 patients, a total of 353 aorto-coronary vein grafts were implanted. Using sequential bypass techniques in some patients by anastomosing 2 or more coronary arteries to one venous graft, the number of distal anastomoses/patient became higher in comparison to the number of implants, namely 2.5 versus 2.3

Results

Operative mortality within 30 days amounted to 8.4% (n = 13). Death could be attributed to cardiac causes in 5 patients each intraoperatively and early after the operation. In all these patients 2 or 3 vessel coronary artery disease had been present in addition to left main coronary artery stenosis.

Postoperatively, 50 patients or 32% required inotropic medical support. In addition the intraaortic balloon pump as circulatory assist device had to be implanted in 9 patients (6%). Four patients were resuscitated from cardiac arrest. A retrospective study of the ECG or postmortal investigation revealed the occurrence of perioperative infarction in 17 patients or 11% of the total group. Thirteen (75%) of these had sustained cardiovascular complications already before onset of extracorporeal circulation. Amongst them the 3 most important insults were:
1. arterial hypertension of systolic more than 200 mmHg,
2. arterial hypotension of less than 80 mmHg systolic,
3. atrial and/or ventricular dysrhythmias including ventricular fibrillation, occasionally induced by manual irritation of the heart.

In 10 of the 17 patients perioperative infarction was without postoperative hemodynamic consequences. However, amongst all cardiac deaths, 6 were directly related to the myocardial injury. In contrast, only 11% of all patients without perioperative myocardial infarction had experienced similar complications.

In a separate study [7], comprising 130 patients with left main stem stenosis, the early results of revascularization were analysed according to the occlusion pattern of the left and right coronary artery branches. Amongst the various groups a specifically high operative risk was found only for patients with more than 90% left main stenosis and coexistent occlusion of the right coronary artery. The hospital mortality in this group was 15% (n = 6), as was the rate of perioperative infarctions.

Although mortality and morbidity in these patients were found to be 2–3-fold higher than in the total series or other subgroups, this difference was not significant because of the small number of patients. For the same reason, it can also only be stated that early mortality was nearly twice as high in patients with lower than normal ejection fractions.

None of the 4 patients with complete occlusion of the left main coronary artery sustained a perioperative myocardial infarction or died early after the operation. Preoperatively, they all suffered from pectangina grade III and IV, whereby 2 patients had significant stenosis of the right coronary artery in addition, and another 2 patients had undergone an anterior wall infarction preoperatively.

One hundred an twenty-two or 86.5% of 141 surviving patients could be followed up over a mean observation-period of 26.4 ± 18.5 months postoperatively, ranging from 5 to 73 months. Thirteen patients (9.2%) suffered late postoperative myocardial infarction, 7 of which were lethal. None of these patients had had an isolated left main stem stenosis. Another 6 late deaths could be attributed to non-cardiac causes. Based on these results, the cumulative survival rate amounted to 71% after 5 years. This outcome is significantly different from the fate of patients with coronary artery disease but no left main stem stenosis who were operated in our institution during the same period and in whom a 5-year actuarial survival rate of 96.5% was attained. The degree of anginal symptoms could be significantly improved postoperatively. While before the operation 85% of the patients had complained severe angina during exertion or even at rest, postoperatively 88% of the survivors were found to have pectangina grade I or II according to the NYHA classification. Only 6% of each could either be classified as grade III or showed no improval of pectangina at rest. All patients with persistent clinical symptoms had apart from left main stem stenosis either an additional multiple vessel disease or complete occlusion of the right coronary artery.

Discussion

Similarly to others [1, 5, 11, 12], we have found a wide spectrum of coronary artery disease associated with left main stem stenosis. This is not only related to the history of the patients with variable symptoms of angina pectoris but also to the number and localization of previous infarctions as well as additional peripheral coronary artery disease. Of special interest in this connection is the high incidence

(40%) of the associated complete occlusion of the right coronary artery. The fact, that only 9% of all patients had an isolated left main stenosis demonstrates that this is only part of the disease in the majority of patients with coronary artery obstruction.

In the group with isolated main stenosis, no patient died, and the presumption can be made that left main disease per se does not present an increased operative risk. Similarly, complete occlusion of the left main stem does not carry significant risk factors as long as good collateral artery blood supply has developed [4, 6, 8]. At least did neither of our 4 patients die nor could a perioperative infarction be demonstrated. The increased operative mortality in our patients with left main stenosis as compared to other patients undergoing coronary artery revascularization during the same period, should primarily be related to the increased operative risk in the presence of multifocal obstructive lesions. This at least may explain the high mortality and morbidity of 15% each in patients with a combination of more than 90% left main stem stenosis and complete occlusion of the right coronary artery.

There are reports in the literature that demonstrate the occurrence of in part irreversible myocardial damage during the pre-extracorporeal circulation period in patients with instable angina pectoris [9, 10, 11, 13, 15, 17]. Accordingly, we found that episodes of hyper- or hypotension as well as atrial and ventricular arrhythmias were accompanied by a significantly increased number of perioperative infarctions. In 6 out of 10 patients who died, such cardiovascular incidences had occurred and must be made responsible for the ensuing myocardial failure. By prevention of these complications significant less perioperative infarcts and deaths have been encountered in patients with left main stenosis aggravated by multifocal coronary artery disease since the end of this study. In summary it can be stated that the operative risk in patients with left main stenosis or occlusion is only increased in the presence of additional multifocal coronary artery obstructive disease. The operative risk appears to be substantially higher when subtotal left main coronary artery stenosis is combined with complete occlusion of the right coronary artery. Similarly, in patients with left main stenosis the incidence of perioperative infractions is slightly increased as compared to patients with isolated 1- to 3-vessel disease. Following successful revascularization the actuarial 5-year survival rate amounts to 71%. Eighty-eight % of the patients are postoperatively free of symptoms and can be classified as grade I or II according to the NYHA.

Summary

The prefered treatment of left main coronary artery (LMCA) stenosis is surgical revascularization. This procedure, however, still carries an increased operative risk. This paper aims at analysing some of the risk factors which may be of

350

significant influence on the perioperative course.

From 1975 through 1981 a total of 154 patients (pts.) underwent coronary revascularization for stenosis (n = 4) or occlusion (n = 4) of the LMCA. Preoperatively, 85% of the pts. had pectangina grade III and IV (NYHA), 55% had suffered one or more myocardial infarctions. In 14 pts., LMCA disease occurred as an isolated lesion. In 33 cases additional isolated lesions were found in the LAD and/or circumflex system, 18 times in the right coronary artery (RCA), and 89 times in RCA and left coronary arteries. Complete occlusion of RCA was found in 40 pts. A total of 60 pts. had 3 vessel disease in addition to LMCA stenosis.

A mean of 2.5 distal anastomoses /pt. were constructed under cardio-pulmonary bypass and cardioplegic arrest.

Operative mortality (OM) was 8.4% (n = 13), 6.5% were related to cardiac causes. The incidence of perioperative infarcts (POI) was 11% (n = 17), in $^3/_4$ of these pts. cardiovascular complications (hypertension, hypotension, arrhythmias) had occurred before onset of extracorporeal circulation. Pts. with a more than 90% LMCA stenosis and complete occlusion of the RCA appear to be at higher risk for both OM and POI (15% each). No Om and POI occurred in pts. with either occlusion or isolated stenosis of LMCA.

Follow-up investigations (mean = 26.4 ± 18.5 months) revealed late infarcts in 13 pts. (9.2%), 7 of which were lethal. Including 6 late deaths from non-cardiac causes, cumulative mortality at 5 years was 29%. Nearly 90% of the surviving pts. had become entirely asymptomatic or had very little angina (classes I and II NYHA).

References

1. Campeau L, Corbara F, Crochet D, Petitclerc R (1978) Left Main Coronary Artery Stenosis. The Influence of Aortocoronary Bypass Surgery on Survival. Circulation 57: 1111
2. Chaitman BR, Fisher LD, Bourassa MG, Davis K, Rogers WJ, Mynard C, Tyras DH, Berger RL, Judkins MP, Ringqvist I, Mock MB, Kilip Th (1981) Effect of Coronary Bypass Surgery on Survival Patterns in Subsets of Patients with Left Main Coronary Artery Disease. Report of the Collaborative Study in Coronary Artery Surgery (CASS). Am J Cardiol 48: 765
3. Cohen MV, Gorlin R (1975) Main Left Coronary Disease (Clinical Experience from 1964–1974). Circulation 52: 272
4. Crospy IK, Wellons HA, Burwell L (1979) Total Occlusion of Left Coronary Artery. Incidence and Management. J Thorac Cardiovasc Surg 77: 389
5. DeMots H, Bonchek LE, Rosch J, Anderson RP, Starr A, Rahimtoola SH (1975) Left Main Coronary Artery Disease. Risks of Angiography, Importance of Coexisting Disease of Other Coronary Arteries and Effects of Revascularization. Am J Cardiol 36: 136
6. Goldberg S, Grossman W, Markis JE, Cohen WV, Baltaxe HA, Levin DC (1978) Total Occlusion of the Left Main Coronary Artery. A Clinical Hemodynamic and Angiographic Profile. Am J Med 64: 3
7. Haverich A, Hetzer R, Rafflenbeul W, Oelert H, Borst HG (1982) Surgical Revascularization for Stenosis and Occlusion of the Left Main Coronary Artery. Z Kardiol 71: 719

8. Hetzer R, Warnecke H, Wittrock H, Engel HJ, Borst HG (1980) Extracoronary Collateral Myocardial Blood Flow during Cardioplegic Arrest. Thorac Cardiovasc Surgeon 28: 191

9. Hetzer R, Haverich A, Rafflenbeul W, Reichelt W, Oelert H, Borst HG (1980) Surgery for Preinfarction and Early Postinfarction Angina – the Hannover Experience. In: Rafflenbeul W, Lichtlen PR, Bacon R (eds) Unstable Angina Pectoris. Stuttgart, Thieme, p 189

10. Isom W, Spencer FC, Feigenbaum H (1975) Prebypass Myocardial Damage in Patients Undergoing Coronary Revascularization: an Unrecognized Vulnerable Period. Circulation 52, Supp II: 119

11. Jones EL, King SB, Craver JM, Douglas JS, Kaplan JA, Morgan EA, Brown CM, Bradford JM, Hatcher CR (1980) The Spectrum of Left Main Coronary Disease. Variables Affecting Patient Selection, Management, and Death. J Thorac Cardiovasc Surg 79: 109

12. Lavine P, Kimbiris D, Segal BL, Linhart JS (1972) Left Main Coronary Artery Disease (Clinical Arteriographic and Hemodynamic Appraisal. Am J Cardiol 30: 791

13. Loop FD, Lytle BW, Cosgrove DM, Sheldon WC, Irarrazaval M, Taylor PC, Groves LK, Pichard AD (1979) Atherosclerosis of the Left Main Coronary Artery: 5 Year Results of Surgical Treatment. Am J Cardiol 44: 195

14. McCallister BD, Killen DA, Reed WR, Arnold M, Crockett JE, McConahay DR, Bell HH (1975) Results Following Coronary Artery Bypass in Patients with Left Main Coronary Artery Disease. Am J Cardiol 35: 153 (Abstract)

15. Moore CH, Lombardo TR, Allums JA, Gordon FT (1978) Left Main Coronary Artery Stenosis: Hemodynamic Monitoring to Reduce Mortality. Ann Thorac Surg 26: 443

16. Obermann A, Harrell RR, Russell RO, Kouchoukos NT, Holt JH, Rackley CE (1976) Surgical Versus Medical Treatment in Disease of the Left Main Coronary Artery. Lancet II: 591

17. Smullens SN, Wiener L, Kasparian H, Brest AN, Bacharach P, Noble PH, Templeton JY (1972) Evaluation and Surgical Management of Acute Evolving Myocardial Infarction. J Thorac Cardiovasc Surg 64: 495

18. Sung RJ, Mallon SM, Richter SE, Ghahramini AE, Sommer LS, Kaiser GA, Myerburg RJ (1975) Left Main Coronary Artery Obstruction – Follow-up of Thirty Patients with and without Surgery. Circulation 51: 112

19. Talano JV, Scanlon PJ, Khan M, Meadows WR, Loeb HS, Pifarré R, Gunnar RM (1974) Influence of Surgery on Survival in 145 Patients with Left Main Coronary Disease. Circulation 50: 110

20. Zeft HJ, Manley JC, Huston JH, Tector AJ, Auer JE, Johnson WD (1974) Left Main Coronary Artery Stenosis: Results of Coronary Bypass Surgery. Circulation 49: 68

Bypass surgery adjacent to streptolysis therapy

B.J. MESSMER, R. VON ESSEN, R. DÖRR, W. MERX, J. MEYER,
P. BARDOS, C. MINALE and S. EFFERT

Introduction

Immediate surgical revascularization for myocardial infarct has been the dream of every progressive cardiac surgeon ever since aorto-coronary bypass surgery became realistic in 1967. As early as 1971 Favaloro [1] reported 11 patients treated surgically for acute myocardial infarct with only one death. Bolooki [2] demonstrated in 1975 that time was the most important factor influencing the early result of such operations. The excellent results achieved by Berg [3] and Philips [4] prove that acute myocardial infarct may be treated surgically.

Introduction of thrombolysis was another step forward in treatment of acute myocardial infarct [5]. Especially selective intracoronary thrombolysis with streptokinase has proved to be an effective and potent procedure for medical revascularization during the early phase when fresh thrombotic occlusion of a major coronary artery is responsible for ischemia [6]. It has, however, been our experience that reocclusion due to the underlying and untreated arteriosclerotic lesion is high when no additional measurements were undertaken. This potential risk prompted us already in 1980 to perform early bypass surgery, and in 1981 to use additional percutaneous transluminal coronary angioplasty (PTCA) in order to prevent rethrombosis [7, 8].

Material and methods

During the four years period between March 1980 and February 1984 a total of 400 patients with acute myocardial infarct have been treated with intracoronary streptokinase using the protocol described earlier [8]. At emergency catheterization 312 patients (78%) showed complete occlusion of the relevant coronary artery while the remaining 88 patients (22%) presented a high grade stenosis but no occlusion.

Further management after successful thrombolysis consisted either in medical treatment, in PTCA, and/or in early bypass surgery.

The surgical group was comprised of 61 patients (54 males and 7 females) with an average age of 55 years (range 38–76 years). The ischemic time interval which represents the time between acute onset of clinical symptoms and successful reperfusion was 181 +/− 66 minutes in this group.

Acute ischemia was due to occlusion of the LAD in 28 patients (46%), the RCA in 27 patients (44%), and the circumflex artery in 6 patients (10%), respectively. The majority of patients had multiple vessel disease which made insertion of an average of 2,9 vein grafts per patient necessary.

Operation was performed whenever possible two to four days after thrombolysis but timing was greatly dependent upon the availability of space within the operative schedule.

Surgery was done under routine conditions in all patients using moderate hypothermia of 28 C. and cardioplegic arrest. No specific precautions were undertaken.

At surgery but prior to cardiopulmonary bypass transmural needle biopsies were taken in most patients from the formerly ischemic area in order to define the amount of hypoxic damage.

Results

Thrombolysis was successful in 86% (268 patients) of the 312 patients who presented complete occlusion at the time of initial catheterization. Early complications are listed in Table 1. Of 61 patients submitted to early surgical revascularization one patient (1,6%) with massive hemorrhagic infarct died from intractable left heart failure immediately after the procedure.

Bleeding urging for reoperation was seen in four patients (6,5%) and significant postoperative congestive heart failure in five (8,2%) two of whome were in need of the intraaortic balloon pump. Two patients suffered from an early cerebrovascular insult without sequels.

Until now one late death (1,7%) due to reinfarction occured at two months after surgery in a patient who made a complicated recovery with bleeding and severe congestive heart failure. Nonfatal reinfarction became clinically apparent in one patient (1,7%) two months after the operation.

The actuarial survival amounts to 96% at five years (Figure 1). Fifty-seven of the surviving patients are in CHA-class I and II. Only three patients are signifi-

Table 1. Relation between time of surgery and early complication.

Time of surgery (days after lysis)	No. pts.	Early death	CHF	Bleeding	CVA
0–1	10	–	3 (30%)	2 (20%)	1
2	51	1 (2%)	2 (4%)	2 (4%)	1
Total	61	1 (1,6%)	5 (8,2%)	4 (6,5%)	2

354

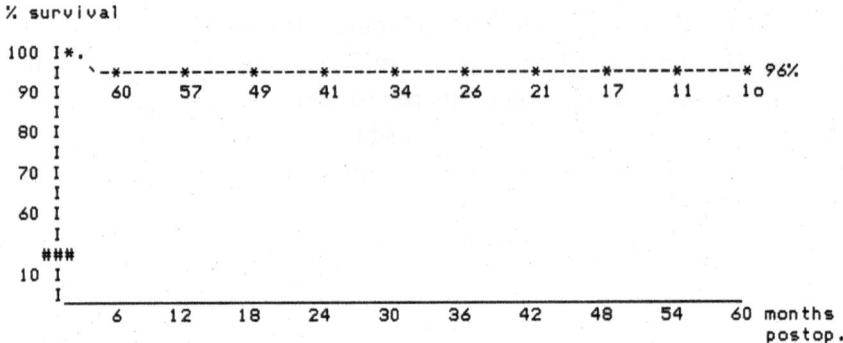

ACTUARIAL SURVIVAL OF 61 PTS.

Figure 1. Actuarial survival of 61 pts.

cantly restricted due to an LV-aneurysm in one case and rapid progression of coronary artery disease in two.

Until now 27 nonselected patients underwent recatheterization study within one year after the operation (Table 2). Of a total of 72 vein grafts inserted in these patients 7 (10%) were occluded. Out of 27 grafts to the infarct vessel 4 (14,8%) were occluded and of 45 grafts to other coronaries only 3 (6,6%) were closed. This difference is, however, statistically not significant.

No correlation could be found in the present series between the length of the initial ischemic time interval and late graft occlusion to the infarct vessel. Two graft occlusions, one each fatal and nonfatal occured in patients with an ischemia of less than two hours. Another two were recorded at recatheterization in patients with an ischemia between two and three hours but only one occured among patients with an ischemic time interval of more than three hours in spite of the fact that this group encomprises the highest proportion of recatheterization studies (Table 3).

Light and electron microscopic studies of the transmural needle biopsies demonstrate various degree of hypoxic damage as seen in Figure 2.

Table 2. Late complications: Vein graft occlusion (27 pts with recath. data).

	No. of grafts	No. (%) grafts occluded
Infarct vessels	25	4 (14,8%) n.s.
Other vessels	45	3 (6,6%)
Total	72	7 (10,0%)

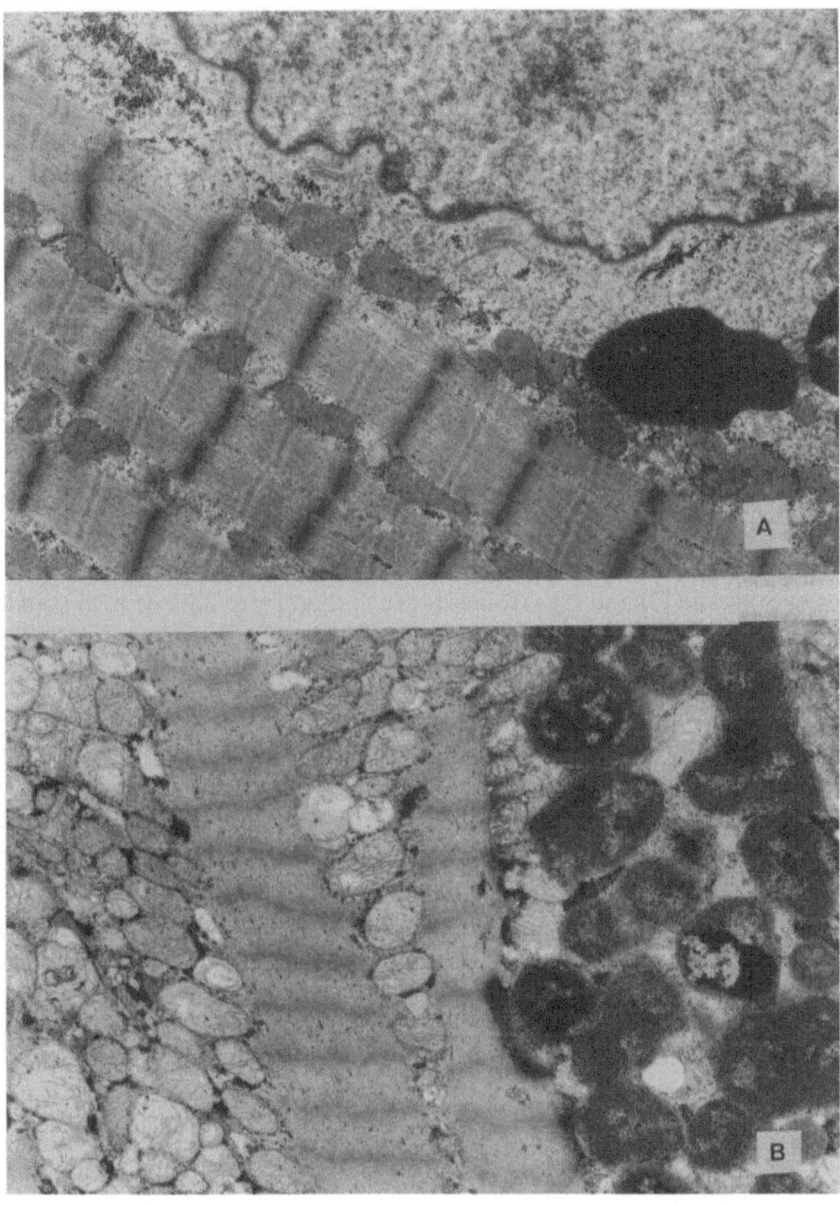

Figure 2. Transmural biopsy from formerly ischemic area. Ischemic time interval 119 min, operation three days after successful thrombolysis (Pt.H.J., 55y, male). Intact myocardium (A) but swelling of mitochondriae (B) as a result of hypoxic damage.

Table 3. Ischemic time interval and late graft occlusion to infarct vessel.

Ischemic interval (min)	No. pts. (%)	No. pts. (%) recath.	Occl. inf. graft
< 60	1 (2%)	1 (100%)	–
60–119	10 (17%)	4 (40%)	2*
120–179	18 (31%)	6 (33%)	2
180–240	21 (36%)	13 (62%)	1
>240	8 (14%)	4 (50%)	–

* One recorded at autopsy.

Discussion

Selective intracoronary thrombolysis has proved to be successful in a high percentage of patients submitted to this therapy during the very early phase of acute myocardial infarct. Similar to direct surgical revascularization as proposed by the groups of Spokane [3] and DesMoines [4] such therapy requires a high standard organization with a team of cardiologists willing to perform catheterization round the clock whenever necessary. In the vaste majority of communities and hospitals such logistics including immediate and perfect diagnosis before the patients arrival in the hospital, emergency transportation without delay to the closest center offering the possibilities for invasive study and organization of the catheterization laboratory while the patient is under his way are not available nor will they ever be. Systemic thrombolysis with either thrombokinase or a plasminogen activator has therefore been prefered by some groups with the additional argument that i.v. application can be performed even earlier [9]. Time is indeed the main factor influencing directly the extent of the ischemic damage. Microscopic studies of the biopsies taken until now from the formerly ischemic area demonstrate ischemic damage even in patients with an ischemic interval of less than two hours [10].

While early in the series patients were often submitted to surgery independently upon the ischemic time interval indication for early operation is nowadays based on an ischemia of less than four hours in patients otherwise suitable for surgery. This time limit may be exceeded in patients who demonstrate good wall function in the formerly ischemic area or in patients with persistent severe angina. A loss of R-waves in the corresponding EKG-leads and initially increased enzyme levels do not necessarily prevent from surgical intervention but in such patients we are rather restrictive with the indication. Age, however, is not a limiting factor for surgery, and the oldest patient of this series, a man of 76 years, enjoys still an excellent result at three years after the operation.

A major problem consists in the timing of operation. Surgery within 24 hours after acute ischemia and successful thrombolysis does not seem to be advantageous because of too short a recovery time taking into consideration that surgical trauma to the heart even under best cardioplegic protection does not necessarily improve the condition of the myocardium.

The significantly higher incidence of postoperative congestive heart failure in patients operated upon too early (Table 1) prompted us to postpone surgery at least to the second day after surgery. Ideal seems to be the third or fourth day while a longer term increases the risk of reocclusion which has been shown to be high as 37% in patients without further invasive treatment [11]. This high reocclusion rate is not amazing if one considers the generally high grade residual stenosis which acts as a constant threat for rethrombosis.

Late results of the combined medico-surgical therapy in this group are excellent. Compared to patients with thrombolysis alone or in combination with PTCA but no surgery the surgical group shows the best long-term results when analyzed for late mortality and reinfarction rate. In our own experience total mortality after one year was 21,2% in 204 patients who had successful thrombolysis but no additional invasive treatment. When PTCA was successful (129 pts.) mortality decreassed to 9,3% [11]. This is, however, still higher than the total mortality of the present group which amounts to 3,3% due one early and one late death.

Of major concern is the fact that the absolute number and the proportion of patients submitted to early surgery after successful thrombolysis has decreased over the past two years. This is certainly due to the fact that more and more community hospitals treat their own patients by means of systemic thrombolysis.

At first glance the immediate effect of such treatment may be advantageous for the patient but in the long range thrombolysis alone remains unsatisfactory in the majority of patients when no additional measurements such as bypass surgery or at least PTCA are performed.

References

1. Favaloro RG, Effler DB, Cheanvechai C, Quint RA, Sones FM (1971) Acute coronary insufficiency (Impending myocardial infarction and myocardial infarction) Surgical treatment by the saphenons vein graft technique. Am J Cardiol 28: 598
2. Bolooki H, Kotler MD, Lottenberg L, Dresnick S, Andrews RC, Kipnis S, Ellis RM (1975) Myocardial revascularisation after acute infarction. Am J Cardiol 36: 395
3. Berg R Jr, Selinger SL, Leonhard JJ (1981) Immediate coronary artery bypass for acute evolving myocardial infarct. J Thorac Cardiovasc Surg 81: 493
4. Phillips SJ, Kongthahworn C, Skinner JR, Zeff RH (1983) Emergency coronary artery reperfusion: A choice therapy for evolving myocardial infarktion. J Thorac Cardiovasc Surg 86: 679
5. Rentrop P, Blanke H, Köstering K, Karsch KR (1979) Acute myocardial infarction: intracoronary application of nitoglycerin and streptokinase in combination with transluminal recanalization. Clin Cardiol 5: 354
6. Merx W, Dörr R, Rentrop P, Blanke H, Karsch KR, Mathey DG, Kremer P, Rutsch W, Schmutzler H (1981) Evaluation of the effectiveness of intracoronary streptokinase infusion in

acute myocardial infarction: postprocedure management and hospital course in 204 patients. Am Heart J 102: 1181

7. Meyer J, Merx W, Schmitz H, Erbel R, Kiesslich T, Dörr R, Lambertz H, Bethge C, Krebs W, Bardos P, Minale C, Messmer BJ, Effert S (1982) Percutaneous transluminal coronary angioplasty immediately after intracoronary streptolysis of transmural myocardial infarction. Circulation 66: 905

8. Messmer BJ, Merx W, Meyer J, Bardos P, Minale C, Effert S (1983) New developments in medical – surgical treatment of acute myocardial infarction. Ann Thorac Surg 35: 70

9. Schröder R, Biamino G, Leitner ER v, Linderer T, Brüggemann T, Heitz J, Vöhringer HF, Wegschneider K (1983) Intravenous Short-term Infusion of Streptokinase in Acute Myocardial Infarktion. Circulation 67: 536

10. Schapper J, Messmer BJ, Döring V, Scheld H, Walter P, Hehrlein F (1984) Ultrastruktur des menschlichen Myokards nach AV – Bypassoperation und/oder Thrombolyse. Zeitschrift f Kardiologie 73 (Suppl. 1): 54

11. Essen R v, Uebis R, Schmidt W, Dörr R, Merx J, Effert S, Schweizer P, Erbel R, Bardos P, Minale C, Messmer BJ. Intrakoronare Streptokinase beim akuten Herzinfarkt. Dtsch Med Wschr (in press)

Emergency bypass operation after PTCA

E. KRAUSE and D. SCHERER

To prevent myocardial infarction, to save myocardium and relief the patient of angina are the purposes of Em-ACBG-procedures after PTCA-failure. The number of Em-ACBG-operations differs in several centers. A mean of approximately 7% seems realistic and may be a question of indication, Table 1, Table 2. Differences result from more or less ample indication for occlusion, dissection and spasm of the coronary vessel. Table 3 shows the characteristics of our patients population. In 39 out of 762 PTCA-patients*, emergent or urgent surgery was

Table 1. Number of Em-ACBG operations in several centers.

Reul,	Houston	35% (1979–1983)
		25,8% (Feb.–Dez. 83)
Creighton,	CINC.	11%
PTCA Registry		6,8%
Kabbani,	San Francisco	6,3%
Univ.-Cl.,	Frankfurt/M.	5,1%
Walsh,	New York	3,7%
Craver,	Atlanta	3%

Table 2. Indication for Em-ACBG operations.

Coronary occlusion	Angina
Coronary dissection	Electrographic signs
Coronary spasm	of acute injury
Myocardial Infarction	Cardiac tamponade
Low output	

Table 3. Characteristics of patient population, Frankfurt/M.

Nr. of patients	39 (5,1%)	Out of 762 PTCA procedures
Males	33	Age range 36–68
Females	6	Age range 46–61

* PTCA was performed at the Department of Cardiology University Clinics, Frankfurt/M.

necessary. Mostly 1 vessel disease was attempted, Table 4. Signs of myocardial infarction appeared in the catheterlaboratory and sometimes caused cardiogenic shock, intermittent ischemia was present in 8 cases, Table 5.

More ACBGs were done than vessels attempted, the reason is that correction of lesions caused on others then stenosed coronaryarteries and sometimes stenoses of 50% to 60% were included. 22 SVD, 14 DVD, 2 TVD, 1 QVD, Table 6.

The time from coronary occlusion during PTCA to revascularization by ACBG supply was 40 min. to 240 min. in 35 patients, and more than 240 min. in 4 patients. In the first group the patients were placed on cardiopulmonary bypass as soon as possible. The fate of the patients is shown on table 7.

Of 39 patients in whom PTCA failed 31 suffered from myocardialinfarction in the catheterlaboratory and 8 showed intermittent ischemia. After Em-ACBG-procedure 10 patients were free of MI, 27 had signs of MI in the ECG and 2 died perioperatively. In conclusion: Inspite of surgery after PTCA-attempts MI rate is high and also letality, only with signs of intermittent Ischemia after PTCA failure the results are good.

The extension of myocardial infarction seems to have direct relation for the outcome of patients, the consequency should be to dilate only such vessels which supply relatively small areas of myocardium that will not cause big MI if PTCA fails.

Table 4. Failed PTCA Vessels.

Diseased vessels: 1 vessel	33	*Vessels attempted:* LAD	24
2 vessels	4	RCA	10
3 vessels	2	RCX	3
		RD	1
		L.Main	1

Table 5. Condition of patients after PTCA.

Cardiogenic shock	4
Myocardial Infarction	31
Intermittent ischemia	8

Table 6. Em-ACBG after PTCA.

ACVB done	
Single	22
Double	14
Triple	2
Quadruple	1

Table 7. Results of EM-ACBG-Procedures after PTCA.

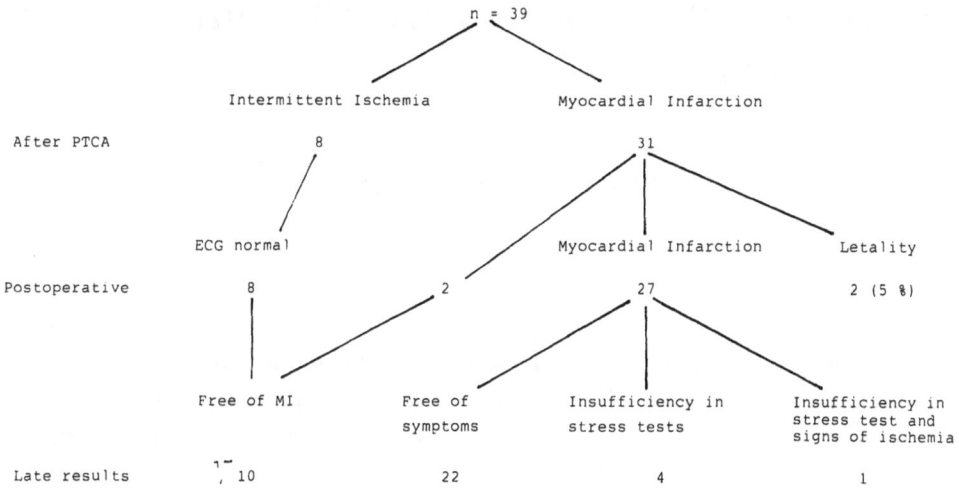

References

1. Dorros G, Cowley MJ, Simpson J, Bentivoglio LG (1983) Percutaneous Transluminal Coronary Angioplasty; Report of Complications from the National Heart, Lung and Blood Institute PTCA Registry. Circulation 67 (4)
2. Kabbani SS, Bashour TT (1984) Surgical experience following percutaneous transluminal coronary angioplasty. Texas Heart Institute Journal, Vol. 11 (2)
3. Surgery for failed PTCA (1984) Cardio 1 (No. 6)

Massive coronary artery spasm with resultant myocardial infarction after ACVB – surgery. A case report

H.-E. SCHERER, H.-J. ENGEL, E. HÖRMANN, H. OSTER and K. LEITZ

A 53 years old male patient with an isolated LAD-stenosis and mild anterior hypokinesis underwent two initially successful PTCA-procedures which were both followed by significant restenoses. Because of persistent typical effort angina, a venous bypass to the LAD was performed. Three hours after the patient returned to the intensive care unit, the ECG showed extensive ST-segment elevations in leads II, III and aVF suggesting transmural inferior wall ischemia.

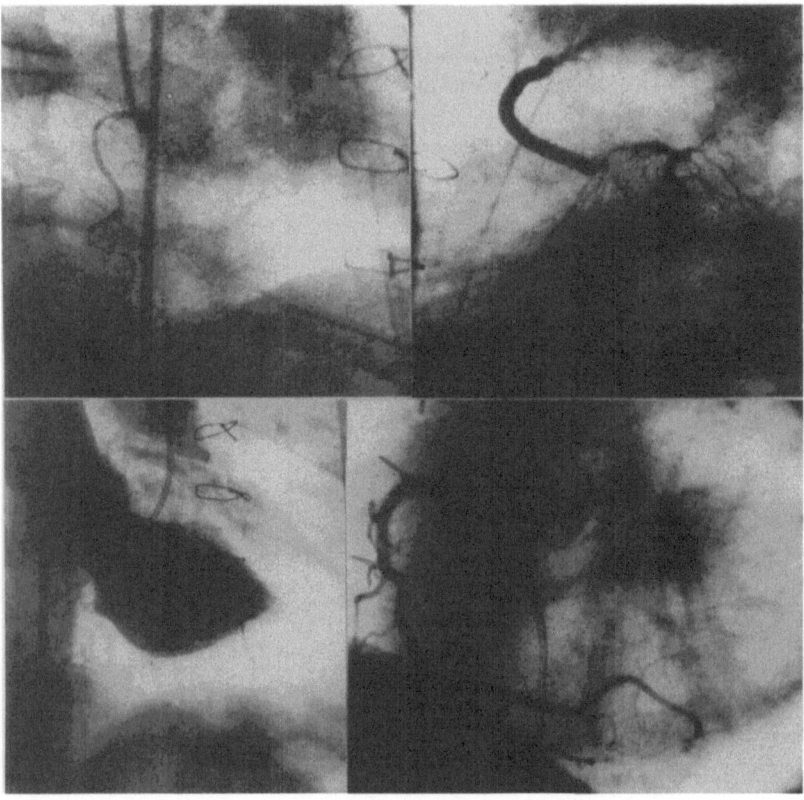

Figure 1.

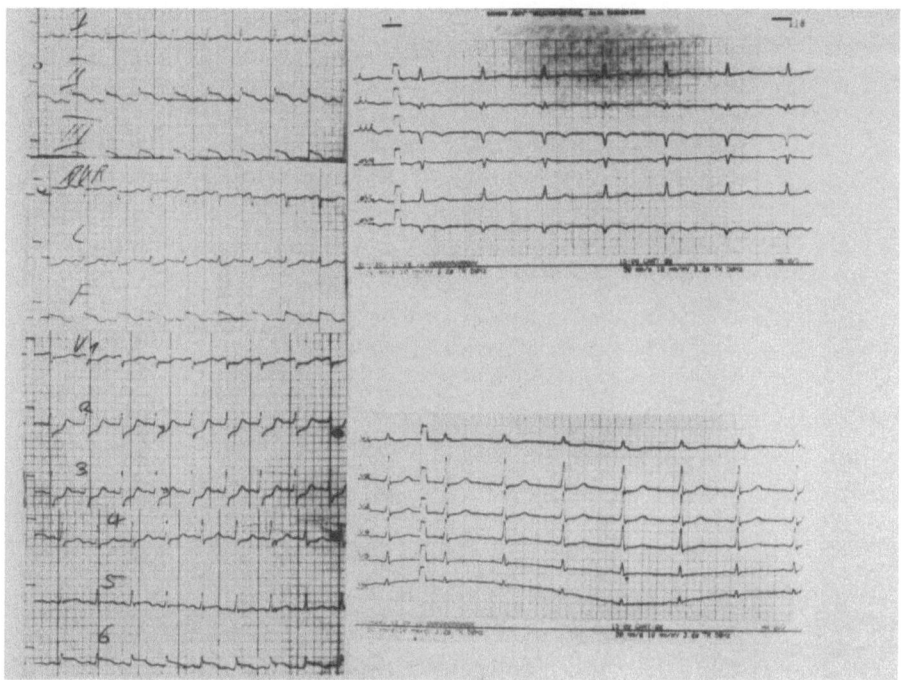

Figure 2.

Immediate control-angiography showed a massive spasm of the entire coronary system, especially of the dominant RCA. The LAD-bypass was open. Left ventriculography demonstrated inferior akinesis. Injection of 5 mg verapamil i.v. resulted in partial relief of the spasm. Continuous i.v. application of calcium-antagonists did not, however, prevent transmural inferior myocardial infarction with pathologic permanent Q-waves in the inferior leads and abnormal enzyme rise (CK, CK-MB etc.). After uneventful recovery, control-angiography was performed on the 20th postoperative day demonstrating a patent bypass to the LAD and normal left circumflex and right coronary arteries. The inferior akinesis was unchanged.

The reason of this massive coronary artery spasm remains unclear. Except the usual medical regimen the patient had obtained only urapidil i.v. to manage the preexisting hypertension, soon replaced by sodiumnitroprussid infusions. A possible interaction between these two substances may be considered.

Index of subjects